Psychiatric-Mental Health Nurse (PMH-BC™) Certification Review

Raymond Zakhari, DNP, EdM, ANP-BC, FNP-BC, PMHNP-BC, has a diverse clinical background ranging from intensive care (CCRN) to medical house calls. He began his career at Duke University Medical Center in the cardiothoracic ICU. In 2009, he founded Metro Medical Direct, the first concierge, nurse practitioner-owned house call and telehealth practice in New York City. Dr. Zakhari trained in sex therapy at the New York University School of Medicine/Langone Medical Center by Dr. Virginia Shaddock, who is the coauthor of *The Synopsis of Psychiatry*. New York-Presbyterian Hospital Department of Internal Medicine appointed Dr. Zakhari to the medical staff in Psychiatry at the Payne Whitney Clinic. His experience has included consultative services as a Sexual Assault Forensic Examiner, an officer of the New Jersey Air National Guard deployed in support of Operation Iraqi Freedom, and has held adjunct faculty appointments at the Hunter Bellevue School of Nursing, New York University, Liberty University, and Adelphi University. Dr. Zakhari hosts a podcast called "The Psychology of It All," and over the years, he has published in peer-reviewed journals and presented at both regional and national conferences, and is the author of the The Psychiatric-Mental Health Nurse Practitioner Certification Review Manual.

Psychiatric-Mental Health Nurse (PMH-BC™) Certification Review

Raymond Zakhari, DNP, EdM, ANP-BC, FNP-BC, PMHNP-BC

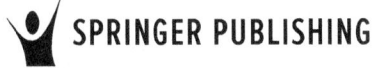

Copyright © 2022 Springer Publishing Company, LLC
All rights reserved.

No part of this publication may be reproduced, stored in a retrieval system, or transmitted in any form or by any means, electronic, mechanical, photocopying, recording, or otherwise, without the prior permission of Springer Publishing Company, LLC, or authorization through payment of the appropriate fees to the Copyright Clearance Center, Inc., 222 Rosewood Drive, Danvers, MA 01923, 978-750-8400, fax 978-646-8600, info@copyright.com or on the Web at www.copyright.com.

Springer Publishing Company, LLC
11 West 42nd Street
New York, NY 10036
www.springerpub.com
http://connect.springerpub.com/home

Acquisitions Editor: Jaclyn Koshofer
Compositor: Integra

ISBN: 978-0-8261-4535-2
ebook ISBN: 978-0-8261-4536-9
DOI: 10.1891/9780826145369

21 22 23 / 5 4 3 2 1

The author and the publisher of this Work have made every effort to use sources believed to be reliable to provide information that is accurate and compatible with the standards generally accepted at the time of publication. The author and publisher shall not be liable for any special, consequential, or exemplary damages resulting, in whole or in part, from the readers' use of, or reliance on, the information contained in this book. The publisher has no responsibility for the persistence or accuracy of URLs for external or third-party Internet websites referred to in this publication and does not guarantee that any content on such websites is, or will remain, accurate or appropriate.

Library of Congress Control Number: 2021915625

Contact us to receive discount rates on bulk purchases.
We can also customize our books to meet your needs.
For more information please contact: sales@springerpub.com

Publisher's Note: New and used products purchased from third-party sellers are not guaranteed for quality, authenticity, or access to any included digital components.

Printed in the United States of America.

To the patients who have allowed me the privilege of caring for them, and to the nurses and nursing students from whom I have learned so much and have had the privilege to teach.

Contents

Preface   *ix*
Pass Guarantee   *xi*
Acknowledgments   *xii*

PART I: FOUNDATIONAL KNOWLEDGE   *01*

1: Psychiatric-Mental Health Nursing Certification   *03*

2: Scope and Standards of the Psychiatric-Mental Health Nurse   *15*

3: Fundamental Theories of Mental Illness and Nonpharmacological Interventions   *37*

4: Neuroanatomy, Physiology, and Psychopharmacology   *71*

PART II: DISORDERS   *105*

5: Substance Use Disorders and Addiction   *107*

6: Delirium and Dementia   *129*

7: Psychotic Disorders   *151*

8: Sleep Disorders   *169*

9: Mood Disorders   *193*

10: Anxiety and Related Disorders   *211*

11: Child/Adolescent and Developmental Disorders   *241*

12: Personality Disorders   *265*

PART III: PRACTICE TEST   *291*

13: Practice Test Questions   *293*

14: Practice Test Answers   *327*

Index   *353*

Preface

The primary job of the psychiatric-mental health nurse is to work alongside the individual or family in a mostly coaching/teaching role, but increasingly in a more traditional hands-on direct care role as the population with comorbid medical conditions accesses mental health services. The board-certified psychiatric-mental health nurse is in a unique position to meet the needs of the most vulnerable patients.

The caveat for all mental health professionals is that we should be cautious that our strong desire to relieve human suffering does not pull the veil over our eyes, causing all human suffering and evil to be labeled a disorder. Treating mental illness is often very complicated. Essentially, the field of psychiatric-mental health is a secular belief system codified in the *Diagnostic and Statistical Manual of Mental Disorders*, Fifth Edition (*DSM-5*). The *DSM-5*, "the bible of psychiatry," requires the user to have confidence in what we hope for, while resting in the assurance of what we do not see. Research in the field is significantly limited due to ethical constraints and often offers correlation and association in place of cause and effect, equating statistical significance with clinically meaningful outcomes. Unlike traditional medicine, we do not have cause and effect scans and biomarkers to definitively call a disorder or illness a disease. The mind is more than just a synonym for brain; it encompasses the individual's life experience and the environment in which the person lives (their family, their role, their connection to people, and their spirituality). The various committees of the American Psychiatric Association categorize abnormal behaviors of the human condition by classifying signs and symptoms with varying degrees of duration and intensity in the hope of clearly distinguishing between mental illness and normal functioning. The things labeled disorders are social constructs articulated using biological metaphors. Each new version of the DSM represents the general morality and values of the current Western society, primarily the industrialized world. As the values of society change, morality also changes. Etiology theories range from the sociological to the physiological and are subject to the will of current sociopolitical values of an elite group of academics during a particular time in history.

Regardless of the state of the science, we can offer our patients a sense of belonging and hope. We can help them develop a skill set that allows them to navigate the complexities of this world in which suffering and uncertainty seem to be the only constants. Helping patients discover a sense of purpose and connection to something greater than themselves restores their dignity as a human being. Both patients and therapists are often very eager to bring order to chaos by labeling a group of symptoms a disorder. The clinician's eagerness to alleviate their personal feeling of powerlessness and reduce the patient's turmoil can lead to premature conclusions. The act of diagnosing and treating communicates to the patient that they are not alone in their condition, but the diagnosis must be accurate because patients will often adopt an identity congruent with the disorder.

This book helps the experienced psychiatric-mental health nurse summarize their years of clinical experience and prepares them to sit for the board certification exam in psychiatry. By doing the work of psychiatry, you have accepted a calling to enter into people's lives when they are most vulnerable. Any experienced clinician knows the work of psychiatry seeks to maintain and restore social order by mitigating maladaptive coping mechanisms that adversely affect the individual, family, and society.

Pass Guarantee

If you use this resource to prepare for your exam and you do not pass, you may return it for a refund of your full purchase price. To receive a refund, you must return your product along with a copy of your original receipt and exam score report. Product must be returned and received within 180 days of the original purchase date. Excludes tax, shipping, and handling. One offer per person and address. Refunds will be issued within eight weeks from acceptance and approval. This offer is valid for US residents only. Void where prohibited. To begin the process, please contact customer service at CS@springerpub.com.

Acknowledgments

I would like to thank Lisa Zakhari, my wife, who has stood by my side encouraging me to complete this challenge, and Zachary and Elizabeth, my children, who provided much-needed diversion and joy along the way, and who often remind me of my own words, "No one asked how you feel, just do it."

Part I

Foundational Knowledge

Psychiatric-Mental Health Nursing Certification

> ### ▸ OBJECTIVES
> - Review of self-care strategies and establishing a studying timeline
> - Evidence-based study strategies
> - Review of the ANCC test map and major content areas

INTRODUCTION

Congratulations! If you are reading this book, you have thought about getting board certified as a psychiatric-mental health nurse (PMHN). Obtaining and maintaining this credential (PMH-BC™) communicates to your colleagues and patients that you are up-to-date in your knowledge and skills of psychiatric-mental health nursing. Registered nurses who have achieved this professional designation report a sense of professional pride and achievement. Achieving the credential of a board-certified psychiatric mental health nurse conveys to your patients and colleagues that you have the expertise based on didactic knowledge and experience to call yourself an expert in the field of psychiatric-mental health nursing. Some nurses have used this credential as a foundation for professional development and growth by combining it with other certifications (Sexual Assault Nurse Examiner, Certified Legal Nurse Consultant, Certified Addiction Registered Nurse, Certified Case Manager, etc.) to carve out their unusual and fulfilling career path in which they enjoy a greater sense of autonomy. Additionally, a board-certified registered nurse (RN-BC) can take other certificate training in specific therapeutic modalities, such as cognitive behavioral therapy (CBT), dialectical behavior therapy (DBT), family systems, somatic therapy, coaching, in order to refine their skills and better help their clients. PMHN is one of the few nursing specialties that is most conducive to telehealth (tele-psych) platforms. The PMH-BC™ credential enhances a candidate's appeal for competitive psychiatric-mental health nurse practitioner programs as well.

PMH-BC™ EXAM ELIGIBILITY REQUIREMENTS

In order to obtain this certification (PMH-BC™), it is not merely sufficient to pass a test. An RN must also meet the following criteria:

- Practiced the equivalent 2 years full time as an RN with a minimum of 2,000 clinical hours in psychiatry within the 3 years before sitting for the exam.
- Additionally, the experienced psychiatric nurse must complete 30 continuing education hours in psychiatric-mental health nursing within the preceding 3 years of the board certification exam.
  - Some examples of the continuing education hours include topics related to neuroanatomy and physiology, psychopharmacology, cognitive behavioral therapy, dialectical behavioral therapy, family therapy, motivational interviewing, interpersonal therapy, psychiatric assessment, case management, and crisis intervention.

It is common to experience many feelings while embarking on this journey to validate your knowledge and achieve board certification. The decision to pursue this is often personal. Board certification as an RN is not mandatory for practice. You can still work as a psychiatric-mental health nurse without subjecting yourself to the stress and expense of this exam. Professional RNs want to communicate to the world that they are intellectually curious, self-motivated, disciplined, organized, and committed to best practices. When you are ready to rise to this challenge, this book will help you prepare for the Psychiatric-Mental Health Nurse exam. This comprehensive print and digital resource provides an overview of the exam, scope and standards of practice, and fundamental theories. It will cover topics such as therapeutic treatment and management, patient education, cultural competence, therapeutic communication, health promotion, and crisis intervention. Here are some fast facts to help allay your fears and to help you focus your efforts as you prepare for the exam:

- You have been honing your skills over the past 2 years
  - Health promotion and maintenance
  - Intake screening, evaluation, and triage
  - Case management and care coordination
  - Patient and family education and advocacy
  - Crisis intervention
  - Administering psychopharmacology and monitoring for therapeutic and adverse effects
  - Psychiatric rehabilitation and group facilitation
- Reviewing the material in this book will refresh your memory or raise your awareness of the information needed to pass the test.

STUDYING AND CARING FOR YOURSELF

Preparing to study for the exam is an important step in the process of board certification. The subject matter can appear so voluminous that it seems impossible to recall and apply everything necessary to pass the test. The following is a list of evidence-based studying techniques that can significantly increase your chance of success. The study tips draw from the field of educational psychology, adult learning theory, and cognitive behavioral theory (CBT). Review and implement these techniques before you begin preparing for the PMH-BC™ ANCC exam. **If you read and apply these strategies, you will greatly enhance your probability of success:**

- **Make time:** Studying for an important exam requires a special dedication of time. Studying for the exam will be far less effective if it is added on to existing obligations rather than having made room for it in your life. In order to effectively study for this test using the evidence-based strategies set forth, you will need to create the necessary time to cover all the essential material on a consistent and scheduled basis.
  - **Timeline:** Creating a timeline will help you prioritize your professional development. Study times should be done in blocks of 2 to 4 hours, free of all distractions. This may require you to drive to a library. The timeline will need to include travel time. When building your study plan, figure out if you are a morning or night person, and try to schedule your block time accordingly. Before you create a time budget, you will need to:
    - Create a list of all of your obligations, including as many things as possible that you do on a weekly basis (household cleaning, cooking, childcare, transporter, church, laundry, exercise, holiday gatherings, birthdays, phone calls, upcoming major life events), and then plot these on a grid with approximate time requirements.
    - Decide how soon you will be taking the test (ideally within 6 months of meeting the test eligibility criteria).
    - Review the table of contents of this book and the latest ANCC test map.
    - Identify your block of study time(s) each week.
      - What will you have to cut out or do less of?
      - Plot your study times on a calendar.
  - **Distractions:** Your studying should be free from any distractions. Ideally, you want to simulate the testing environment as much as possible. On the day of the test, you will check all of your electronic devices into a locker and pass through a metal detector. You will not be able to bring anything into the test room with you. Practice being out of touch when you are studying. Give your studies your undivided attention and avoid the following:
    - Chatting
    - Eating and drinking
    - Social media
    - Phone, smartwatch, etc.
    - Try not to be responsible for watching children when studying or wait until they are asleep

- Cognitive behavioral strategies to enhance your studying efforts (these are very similar to strategies you may have used with your patients to achieve other worthwhile goals):
  - **Visualization:** The first step in this process is to imagine in detail passing your exam. Think deeply about where you are when you find out. How would you feel? How proud would your friends and family feel? Next, visualize yourself doing the necessary work to pass. See yourself following your study timeline, blocking time to study, delaying gratification, blocking distractions, and putting off social obligations. Visualize yourself covering the various topics to be covered on the exam. Visualize yourself pressing through something difficult and the sense of accomplishment you will have.
  - **Rereading:** Reading does not mean stopping to take notes along the way. Read for the sake of understanding and to refresh. Read twice the content outlines and any associated materials you may not know well. Rereading more than twice does not increase retention and becomes a procrastination tactic that deceives the student into believing they are making progress.
  - **Note-taking:** Note-taking (particularly by hand) while going through material significantly increases retention of information. Reviewing notes and checking them against a source enhances your ability to recall. This is most helpful to do with formal classes in school or after a continuing education presentation.
  - **Rehearsing:** This technique involves explaining the concept aloud to a pretend patient, family member, or nursing student. This is best accomplished by removing all distractions from the study environment and giving undivided attention to the task at hand. It also helps to recite the material out loud, chunking it along the way.
  - **Synthesizing:** Piecing together information helps you understand the relationship between ideas and concepts. Synthesis is better than simple memorization because this will help you apply your information to various scenarios. One way to synthesize is to draw graphs or charts reflecting the core concepts. Organizing a chart will help you organize the information for easy recall. Mapping is particularly helpful when trying to remember specific steps in a procedure.
  - **Practicing:** Doing many practice questions is very useful in helping overcome test anxiety. As you practice answering questions, you will develop a habit of carefully reading the stem of the question and each of the answer choices to help you select the best answer.
  - **Self-verbalizing:** This procedure involves you verbalizing the steps that you need to follow in order to complete the task. In this process, you should whisper to yourself aloud; this strategy can work particularly well while you are actually taking the test.
  - **Justifying:** This procedure involves explaining an important concept that helps to determine if the premise and a question are true. How do you know a brief psychotic episode from schizophrenia? How do you distinguish dysthymia from major depressive disorder? Do you distinguish normal use from a substance use disorder? Explaining the distinctions between these types of questions will help you solidify in your mind the rationales for the answer to a question.

SELF-CARE

The study tips are predicated on the assumption of consistent and adequate attention to basic physiological, psychological, and sociological needs. Human beings require consistent care for optimal performance.

- **Sleep:** Impaired or inadequate sleep hinders your ability to learn and retain information. It is imperative that you get adequate and consistent sleep, particularly when preparing for an exam or enduring something particularly stressful (Feldman & Kubota, 2015). On average, 6 to 8 hours is recommended per night. As a PMHN, one of the most common areas you will counsel your patients about is the importance of sleep hygiene. Some common recommendations include:
  - Avoiding screens 2 hours before going to bed
  - Setting a cool enough room temperature
  - Going to bed at the same time each night
  - Ensuring the room is as dark as possible
  - Implementing a white noise
  - Turning on a fan to keep the air circulating
  - Sleeping naked or with minimal clothing
  - Taking any medications for sleep as prescribed
  - Avoiding alcohol and caffeine
- **Radical acceptance:** Forgiving yourself for all of the time you have previously wasted and all the obligations you have failed to meet is essential (Feldman & Kubota, 2015). You must forgive yourself in order to release this burden from your mind as you prepare for the exam.
- **Avoid extremes:** Engaging in marathon study sessions has been shown to reduce retention by as much as 30% (Rohrer & Pashler, 2007). It is better to study for shorter periods over more time so that your hippocampus can consolidate your memory, make it easier to retrieve through your limbic pathway during times of stress (like the ANCC exam).
- **Enhance self-efficacy:** As a PMHN many theoretical models and treatment plans rely heavily on the concept of the belief in oneself or the therapist's expressed belief in the patient's likelihood of success. Build your confidence in your study effort and test-taking ability to significantly increase your chance of success (Feldman & Kubota, 2015). If you are sitting for board certification, you have likely passed many exams containing much more detailed content than the ANCC exam. Also, convince yourself how much you love studying and taking tests. This may require some effort. You might want to build yourself a reward system. Eventually, you may truly enjoy studying.
- **Eating:** It is important to eat consistent meals and avoid concentrated sweets that can surge and plunge your blood sugar (Hasegawa et al., 2017). It is also best to avoid very heavy meals before a study or test session. Caffeine is helpful if this is something you usually drink. Trying coffee for the first time just before the exam is not a good idea. Gum chewing has also been found to be minimally helpful while studying or taking a test (Hasegawa et al., 2017). It can also be a great distraction if you are blowing bubbles or making any noise with them. If you do chew gum, do it very quietly.

- **Exercise:** Engaging in consistent physical activity for at least 20 minutes can significantly increase your mental acuity and ability to retain information. Exercise can also help you build the necessary structure into your day as you prepare for the exam (van Dongen et al., 2016). While exercising, you should not be trying to study by listening to lectures or reading. Fast classical music has been shown to enhance retention by stimulating various neurons. This controversial theory is called the Mozart effect (Hetland, 2000; Nantais & Schellenberg, 1999).
- **Relationships:** It will be vital that you pay attention to close relationships. These people have been and will be your support system. Social interactions can also significantly reduce stress and remind you of your higher purpose in life. Avoid announcing your test date to anyone beyond your immediate family because it creates unnecessary pressure.
- **Personal hygiene:** Attending to hygiene helps make your study efforts more deliberate. You should prepare for your study sessions as if you are going to work. The ritual of preparation for the task helps organize the mind and prepares it for the task at hand. While showering, shaving, brushing your teeth, and putting on your deodorant, visualize what your study session will be like. Visualize the topics that might be covered, the practices you will do, and how long the study session will take. Some people who work from home even dress up as if they are going into the office because it makes them more productive. Studying in your boxers or bathrobe does not prepare the mind and body for serious work.

▶ COGNITIVE DISTORTIONS

Cognitive distortions can be your biggest downfall in preparing for this exam. It can be very helpful to be mindful of the ones that you are using to self-sabotage your success. A cognitive distortion is a habit of mind used to interpret circumstances without regard for supporting evidence in order to substantiate how we think or feel. Often people assume incorrectly that their thoughts and feelings are facts. Thoughts and feelings are not facts; they are merely data. By understanding that our thoughts and feelings are not necessarily facts, we can allow our minds to deal with reality rather than substituting our own fantasies be they hostile or otherwise. This is a list of the most commonly used cognitive distortions:

- **All or nothing thinking:** Seeing things in categories of all good or all bad. Performance that is less than perfect is interpreted as a complete failure.
- **Overgeneralizing:** Inflating a single negative event into a larger never-ending pattern of defeat, for example, creating a self-fulfilling prophecy.
- **Negative mental filter:** Dwelling on negative details to the exclusion of positive aspects, even when the positive aspects are more objectively prominent.
- **Disqualifying the positive:** Rejecting positive experiences by insisting that they don't count. For instance, handling an interpersonal challenge effectively and maturely then concluding that it was just luck.
- **Jumping to conclusions:** Interpreting events without evidence to support the assessment.

- **Mind-reading:** Believing that others hold a view of you without confirming the belief or entertaining an alternate explanation. For example, thinking your boss is angry with you because he did not greet you. His behavior, in fact, may have been unrelated to you, perhaps related to a preoccupation with some other problem.
- **The fortune-teller error:** Predicting the future in a negative way as if it were preordained to turn out badly, conversely interpreting the future in a positive way as if it were preordained to turn out well.
- **Catastrophize:** Exaggerating the importance of negative events until they are seen as overwhelming. This increases a person's sense of helplessness and hopelessness.
- **Emotional reasoning:** Believing that your emotions reflect the state of the world. For instance, when depressed, believing that the world is going to hell in a handbasket or when happy, things are looking up, and you are going to hit it big.
- **Essentializing:** Seeing a situation as a reflection of your core self, for example, rather than thinking you made a mistake, you think you're a loser. Or conversely, coming up with a solution immediately makes you an expert. This distortion can also be applied to other people; for example, if someone forgets your name, you may conclude that that person is very self-centered and shallow or that you are of such low stature your name is not worth being remembered.
- **Personalizing:** Believing yourself to be the cause of external events even though it is unlikely that you are responsible for them. For example, when a child season argument between the parents, the child concludes it is their fault. This distortion is particularly common in people with a history of abusive parents or spouses or being in close relationships with people with substance use disorders.

▶ EXAM PREP EXERCISE

The time has come to put your CBT skills to good use and help yourself achieve your goals:
- Write an example for each cognitive distortion a client (or you) may believe as you prepare for your test. Next, write what evidence you have that supports or refutes this distortion. This exercise should have reduced your anxiety and raised your confidence in preparing to take this test. When you find your mind wandering, refer back to the evidence.

ABOUT THE AMERICAN NURSES CREDENTIALING CENTER (ANCC) PSYCHIATRIC-MENTAL HEALTH NURSE BOARD CERTIFICATION EXAM

- ANCC is a subsidiary of the American Nurses Association (ANA), serving as the independent professional credentialing body for professional nursing practice. The organization accredits healthcare organizations that provide and approve continuing nursing education. The ANCC offers both APRN and RN board certification exams for a variety of specialties, including PMH-BC™ and PMHNP-BC qualifications.

- Passing the exam allows the RN to use the board-certified (BC) designation post-nominally: for example, *Raymond Zakhari, BSN, RN, PMH-BC*. The ANCC is the only credentialing body to offer a board certification (BC) exam for psychiatric-mental health nursing.
- The test is administered at various Prometric Testing Centers (prometric.com) around the world. You can only schedule your exam once you have received the Authorization to Test (ATT) from ANCC. Your ATT is only sent *after* your online application has been completed and your transcripts have been validated by ANCC.
- **New exam release:** A new exam is released every 2 to 3 years on average. **Content on the PMH-BC™ exam is based on the *DSM 5*.** It is always best to check the website for the latest test content map.
  - Each ANCC exam has several versions.
  - Each version of the exam is randomly assigned.
  - The exam is not computer adaptive.
  - Most of the exam questions will be multiple choice.
    - There are alternate format questions including drag and drop, extended multiple-choice questions where you are asked to pick more than one correct answer, hot-spot questions in which you will be asked to identify a structure in response to a test question, that is, which lobe of the brain is responsible for executive functioning? You would have to click on the lobe of the brain represented in a diagram.
  - The test will have 150 questions. Twenty-five of the questions are not graded; rather they are only used for statistical validation purposes. Only 125 questions are scored.
  - The time limit is 3 hours to complete the test. Once the clock starts, there is no way to pause the time, even if you go to the bathroom. Once the allotted time expires, the test will automatically shut down.
  - **Unanswered questions are marked as incorrect.**
  - You can mark and return to questions within the allotted time.
  - There will be separate time allocated for a computer tutorial before the exam begins.
  - Sample ANCC exams are available on the website to try before you sit for the exam. The sample test can be taken as many times as you wish.
- ANCC *can* take 4 to 6 weeks to process a completed application. During slower times of the year, it may take as little as three weeks. Peak application season is from April to July and from November to January.
  - **Scheduling your exam:** Waiting to schedule your exam may limit your time selection options. Schedule your exam as soon as you receive your ATT.
    - **Make sure you have created your studying timeline before you apply to the test, and that you have started studying.**
      - If you must test on a certain day, you can broaden your search to another testing center; you may have to look in another state.
    - **Missed appointment or expired ATT:** You will be considered a no show; your testing window automatically expires. Call the testing center Prometric as soon as possible and then contact ANCC. ANCC will allow for one reschedule, but you will be charged a rescheduling fee.

- **Pass/fail:** You will find out immediately whether you passed or failed the exam. Once you complete your exam and leave the room, the proctor will have a printout containing your unofficial result. An official result will be mailed to you. The unofficial result cannot be used as proof of passing for any official purpose.
  - **If you fail:** The ANCC allows you to retake the exam up to 3 times in 12 months, but there must be at least 60 days between attempts. You must wait five days (after taking your exam) to reapply to test.
  - **Reapplying:** You must resubmit all materials as if you were applying for the first time and pay all the associated fees again.

▶ PMH-BC™ TEST CONTENT MAP

- The test is focused on your ability to critically think and choose the best answer given the circumstance with the limitations imposed.
- The test will include 150 questions, of which 125 will be scored. The test is divided according to the nursing process (assessment, planning, implementation, and evaluation), with the majority of questions (39%) coming from the implementation section. The assessment and planning are equally dense, comprising 44% of the total questions (22% each). The evaluation section refers to the outcomes as a result of the implementation and comprises 18% of the questions. These categories are represented and distributed as follows:

- Assessment and diagnosis (33 questions of which 27 are scored questions)
  - Psychosocial developmental stages
  - Physiological causes of psychiatric symptoms
  - Psychiatric disorders
  - Coping skills and defense mechanisms
  - Mental status exam and assessment tools
- Planning (33 questions of which 27 are scored questions)
  - Client-centered care
  - Patient education concepts
  - Cultural competence including gender identity/sexual orientation, religious beliefs, and ethnicity
  - Therapeutic communication barrier management
  - Treatment planning and resource utilization
- Implementation (57 questions of which 49 are scored questions)
  - Treatment modalities and frameworks
  - Complimentary alternative modalities and interventions
  - Case management and coordination of care
  - Medication management, including therapeutic and adverse effect monitoring
  - Psychoeducational group facilitation (motivational interviewing and relapse prevention)
  - Health promotion (tobacco cessation, substance use prevention, and self-care)
  - Crisis intervention and emergent situations

- Evaluation (27 questions of which 22 scored questions)
  - Effectiveness of intervention
  - Legal and ethical considerations
  - Quality improvement/process improvement
  - Outcome measurement

DISSECTING QUESTIONS

In order to choose the best possible answer, you must know exactly what you are being asked. The majority of questions will be multiple choice. Multiple-choice questions consist of three parts. They are the entire question, the stem (the essential information of the question), and the answer choices (one correct and three distractors). **ALWAYS READ THE ENTIRE QUESTION AND ALL THE ANSWERS BEFORE SELECTING ANYTHING!**

- Do not read into the question.
- Do not assume information that is not presented (i.e., do not overanalyze).
  - If the information is not given, assume it is not needed and has no effect on the answer.
- **Step 1:** Is the question asking you to recall a fact or apply information? Moreover, is the question asking you to do something or find out something?
  - Are there any keywords in the question such as: avoid, best, except, not, initial, first, most, least, of the following (are you looking for correct answers or wrong answers)?
- **Step 2:** Can you apply Maslow's Hierarchy of Needs? Just because this is a psychiatric exam, you cannot forget that physiological needs always take priority over psychosocial needs. Remember to choose the safest answer and consider what would happen if each answer is chosen. (Does the answer actually answer the question?)
- **Step 3:** Is the answer choice an assessment or implementation. For the exam assessment type answers, include when you are gathering more information either by physical exam (including vital signs, weights, finger sticks, screening test, etc.), requesting a provider order a diagnostic test, or by interviewing the patient or collateral sources. Implementation answer types include when you administer medication, provide psychoeducation, initiate restraints or seclusion, or hold a medication. Also, consider if the assessment or implementation matches the stem of the question.
  - The lab calls the PMHN on the acute psychiatric unit to report a client has an absolute neutrophil count of 700 has been taking his clozapine 500 mg daily. What should the PMHN do first?
    a) Hold the next dose and notify the psychiatric-mental health nurse practitioner.
    b) Move the patient to a private room.
    c) Instruct the patient on the importance of taking his medication exactly as prescribed.
    d) Remind the patient of the importance of proper hand hygiene.

The stem of this question deals with agranulocytosis in someone taking clozapine. The question asks for an implementation. The stem is asking about a physiological condition. The answer should be a physiological intervention that addresses the stem and should not make the problem worse. Based on this information, the correct answer is A.

Moving the patient to a private room may also be appropriate, it does not address the potential of making the situation worse. Instructing on the importance of medication adherence would worsen the problem in this case, reminding of good hand hygiene while helpful and related to the agranulocytosis would not take priority over holding the medication.

- **Step 4:** Select the correct answer: Remember to eliminate answer choices after you have read the entire question and all the choices to increase your odds of selecting the correct answer. Do not second guess your answer choice unless you have a compelling reason (e.g., you recall an essential concept that directly relates to the stem, or you have a clearer understanding of the question that you did not initially have).
  - Most people change the correct answer to the wrong answer rather than a wrong answer to the correct answer.
  - If you are unsure about an answer choice, you can mark the question to come back to it for later review.
- Final tips about choosing the correct answer:
  - If you have two answers that seem equally good, choose the least expensive, least invasive option that allows you to answer the question. For example, if your choice is between a CT scan of the head or a focused neurological exam, the latter will likely be the best option. **(There are no scans or biomarkers in psychiatry that can diagnose a psychiatric condition. Once something appears on a scan, it becomes a neurological condition.)**
  - See if the answer choices have something in common or are very similar. If two answers are very similar, they are likely incorrect. If all three are related, they too can usually be excluded.
  - Be mindful of results that are wide-ranging. Middle-of-the-road values are usually correct.
  - Make sure the answer fits the question. It is common to have excellent distractors that do not address the stem or task in the question.
  - When answering "all of the following are true except" type of question, remember that you are looking for a wrong answer.
  - Finally, err on the side of caution without assuming very remote risk. Answers should be evidence-based, and not based on anecdotal or unusual or atypical situations.

WHAT TO DO AFTER YOU HAVE PASSED YOUR BOARDS

Let me be the first to congratulate you on a job well done. Savor the moment of accomplishment and treat yourself to a reward. Then:

- Digitize your transcripts and save them in a cloud platform such as Dropbox or Google Docs.

- Scan a copy of your degree or certificate (create a digital record-keeping system of continuing education earned to maintain your certification, and track expiration dates and recertification requirements).
- Scan copies of all your certifications.
- Update your resume to reflect your new credentials (First Name Last Name PMH-BC).
  - Consider creating a professional social media profile on LinkedIn or other professional networking sites.
- Start looking for conferences and make your plans to attend. This certification is just the beginning of the learning that will continue for the rest of your life.
  - Start daydreaming and investigating how you can use your credential for entrepreneurial endeavors to create a fulfilling career.

REFERENCES

Feldman, D. B., & Kubota, M. (2015). Hope, self-efficacy, optimism, and academic achievement: Distinguishing constructs and levels of specificity in predicting college grade-point average. *Learning and Individual Differences*, 37, 210–216. https://doi.org/10.1016/J.LINDIF.2014.11.022

Hasegawa, Y., Tachibana, Y., Ono, T., & Kishimoto, H. (2017). Flavour-enhanced cortisol release during gum chewing. *PLOS ONE*, 12(4), e0173475. https://doi.org/10.1371/journal.pone.0173475

Hetland, L. (2000). Listening to music enhances spatial-temporal reasoning: Evidence for the "Mozart Effect" *Journal of Aesthetic Education*, 34 (3/4), 105. https://doi.org/10.2307/3333640

Nantais, K. M., & Schellenberg, E. G. (1999). The Mozart Effect: An Artifact of Preference. *Psychological Science*, 10(4), 370–373. https://doi.org/10.1111/1467-9280.00170

Politte, L. C., Huffman, J. C., & Stern, T. A. (2008). Neuropsychiatric manifestations of multiple sclerosis. *Primary Care Companion to the Journal of Clinical Psychiatry*, 10(4), 318–324. https://doi.org/10.4088/PCC.v10n0408

Rohrer, D., & Pashler, H. (2007). Increasing retention without increasing study time. *Current Directions in Psychological Science*, 16(4), 183–186. https://doi.org/10.1111/j.1467-8721.2007.00500.x

van Dongen, E. V., Kersten, I. H. P., Wagner, I. C., Morris, R. G. M., & Fernández, G. (2016). Physical exercise performed four hours after learning improves memory retention and increases hippocampal pattern similarity during retrieval. *Current Biology*, 26(13), 1722–1727. https://doi.org/10.1016/J.CUB.2016.04.071

Scope and Standards of the Psychiatric-Mental Health Nurse

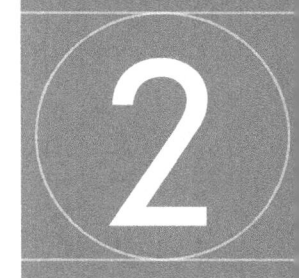

> **OBJECTIVES**
> - Identify types of leadership styles
> - Identify quality improvement process
> - Practice laws and ethical principles
> - Key position statements from professional organizations
> - Cultural awareness related to special populations

INTRODUCTION

The primary objective of the psychiatric-mental health nurse (PMHN) is to establish a therapeutic alliance with the patients in their care. Therapeutic alliance is the best predictor of a successful treatment outcome regardless of the therapeutic technique or psychopharmacological choice. In order for the PMHN to retain and maintain professional viability, they must remain vigilant, ensuring patient safety, applying evidence-based practice, and promoting efficient resource utilization.

The American Nurses Credentialing Center board certification exam map identifies common domains of specialty nursing unique to the PMHN certification. These specific domains of the professional role PMHN remain the most overlooked material by test-takers. This overlooked content relates to specific leadership styles, quality improvement and safety, practice inquiry, technology and information literacy, health delivery systems, ethics, law, and scope and standards specific to the work of behavioral health nursing.

HEALTH PROMOTION ACCORDING TO U.S. GOVERNMENTAL ENTITIES

- U.S. Centers for Disease Control and Prevention (CDC), Department of Health and Human Services (DHHS) tracks public health trends, aggregates data, and publishes mandates for public health and safety:

- **Health Insurance Portability and Accountability Act of 1996 (HIPAA):** Legislated privacy and security laws to protect personal health identifiers from disclosure without express consent from the patient or responsible party. HIPAA guarantees patients four fundamental rights:
  - Patients have a right to be made aware of HIPAA protection of confidentiality.
  - Patients may have access to their medical records.
    - The DHHS regards psychotherapy notes as not part of the medical record, and therefore not subject to patient access.
    - Prescription medications, session start and stop times, frequency of treatment, test results, summaries and prognosis, consultation reports are considered part of the general medical records.
  - To request an amendment to their record.
  - To require permission for disclosure of personal health information.
- **Nurse Practice Act:** Delineated by each state board of nursing to expressly define the work of professional nurses. The Nurse Practice Act defines the state's duty to protect the public from unsafe nursing practice, delineates practice privileges, licensure process, explicit restrictions, and educational requirements for licensure by defining basic competencies.
  - **Licensure:** A process by which an agency of state government grants permission to individuals accountable for the practice of a profession. This allows the professional nurse to practice in the state.
  - Provides title protection (i.e., identifies who may be called a "Professional Registered Nurse")
  - Grants legal authority and establishes mandates for RN practice
  - Subject to public hearing review before enactment
  - Disciplinary actions
    - Practicing without a license or proper collaboration or supervision
    - Fraud
    - Falsification of records, inaccurate records, incomplete records
    - Deviation from standards of care
    - Failure to apply nursing judgment

SCOPE OF PRACTICE

- Scope of practice delineates who may do what, when, where, how, and why as governed by the terms of the state's professional license and as described in the Nurse Practice Act.
- **Certification:** A credential that allows for specialty title protection (e.g., PMH-BC™), granted by a professional organization certifying that an individual meets the minimum requirements of professional practice specified by the profession, communicates mastery of specialty knowledge. The American Nurses Credentialing Center, a subsidiary of the American Nurses Association (ANA), is the only certifying body for psychiatric nursing. Certification is subordinate to licensure. The state licensure may expressly forbid a particular

function regardless of the mastery demonstrated by achieving certification. (Note: Certification is not required for practice unless the Nurse Practice Act requires it for licensure.)
- **State exceptions to confidentiality:** Usually enacted as a result of case law as decided by the state judicial system.
    - Intent to harm self or others
        - Duty to warn potential victims in imminent danger (Tarasoff principle, 1976)
    - Attorney involved in litigation
    - Records released to insurance companies
    - Answering court orders, subpoenas, or summons
    - Mandatory reporting of diseases
    - Child or elder abuse
- **Informed consent:** Governed by state laws, a communication process (respecting the patient's right to autonomy) between patient and provider that clearly explains the risks and benefits of a particular treatment, the condition (diagnosis and prognosis) being treated, the risks and benefits of refusing the proposed treatment, and alternatives to the proposed treatment.
    - Emancipated minors are persons under the age of 18 and must be married, a parent, or legally emancipated through court proceedings and/or self-sufficient and living away from the family home (depending on individual state laws).
- **Capacity:** A clinical decision (not a legal designation) based on an evaluation by a state qualified evaluator (often a mental health professional) to determine the patient's ability to understand new information, circumstances, and meaningfully interact with the information and express rational thoughts related to the situation (Tunzi, 2001). A capacity determination can be made by a nonmental healthcare provider directly caring for the patient. For example, a surgeon planning to operate on a patient can make the determination as to whether the patient has the capacity to consent to the surgery. The process of obtaining an informed consent requires that the clinician document the explanation provided and that the patient understands the situation and the risks and benefits of having or not having the procedure. The determination of capacity is a situational determination (i.e., capacity to consent or assent [allowing for or failing to object] to treatment for or to accept or refuse treatment).
- **Competency:** A legal designation (not a clinical impression) regarding a person's ability to make reasonable decisions regarding their well-being (person or property). All persons of legal age are presumed competent until a court declares the individual incompetent (Black, 1999). If deemed incompetent, a guardian must be appointed.
- **Involuntary Commitment Criteria:** A process (which differs from state to state) of forcing an individual to receive a psychiatric evaluation. The patient retains all civil liberties except the ability to come and go as they please. General criteria include:
    - Person must have a diagnosed psychiatric disorder.
    - Person poses harm to self or others as a result of the psychiatric disorder.
    - Person is unaware or unwilling to accept the nature and severity of the disorder.
    - Treatment is likely to improve functioning.

PROFESSIONAL ORGANIZATIONS

- **American Nurses Association (ANA), American Psychiatric Nurses Association (APNA).**
  - Most specialties have their own national organizations.
  - **Standards of practice:** An official reference explicitly stating the rights and privileges regarding the type of practice. It further defines the PMHN roles and actions, identifies competencies assumed among members of the profession, guides the manner in which professional practice is judged, reflects expectations of care, can be used to legally describe the work of the profession, and when a deviation has occurred and may contain specific practice protocols and specify actions.

- **American Nurses Association (ANA)/American Nurses Credentialing Center (ANCC)**
  - ANA believes that patients' interests are best served by a healthcare system in which many different types of qualified professionals are available, accessible, and working together collaboratively; the patient retains the right to choose their healthcare provider (Houser & Oman, 2011).
  - Scope of practice should reflect a professional's true expertise.
  - **Protecting and advancing scope of practice**
    - Protecting and advancing scope of practice for nurses is a major initiative of ANA.
    - The PMH-BC™ should demonstrate mastery of the following skills unique to their specialty:
      - Monitor quality indicators
        - Incorporate evidence-based practice principles into daily practice
        - Review quality outcomes of care
      - Provide culturally sensitive care
        - Increase personal cultural sensitivity and awareness when assessing patient's perception of illness and health
        - Consider cultural interpretations of the various roles in healthcare delivery
    - Professional role
      - Advocacy
        - Stand up for patients' rights and empower them to self-advocacy
        - Reduce the stigma of mental illness
        - Help patients receive available services
        - Participation in professional organizations (American Nurses Association (ANA), International Society of Psychiatric Nurses (ISPN)
      - Utilization of information technology
      - Work collaboratively within and across organizations

LEADERSHIP STYLES

Nurses should be leaders and engage with health professions to transform and redesign healthcare (Brinkert, 2010; Institute of Medicine, 2001; Schmitt, Blue, Aschenbrener, & Viggiano, 2011).

- **Transformational leadership:** A style marked by a charismatic ability to communicate vision and secure buy-in from stakeholders.
- **Situational leadership:** A style marked by flexibility and adaptability to the context of the situation, able to engage at various levels with key stakeholders and address their concerns.
- **Autocracy (authoritarian leadership):** A style marked by motivated, independent, self-directed individual who prefers to give specific directions and exert control over a situation with little to no input from those in their charge.
- **Democratic leadership:** A style marked by emphasizing team process, valuing input from stakeholders, decisions are made by consensus.
- **Laissez-faire leadership:** A style marked by indecision and ambiguity, suited to figure head individuals who have very experienced, autonomous, and self-directed subordinates.
- **Servant leadership:** A style marked by "follow me" rather than "forward march." In this approach, the leader works alongside their subordinates, adapting to fill in gaps, and may inadvertently enable poor performers.
  - NPs are educated to lead interdisciplinary teams as full partners in care
  - Design, implement, evaluate, and advocate to redesign healthcare systems
  - Engage in evidence-based clinical practice
- Utilize ethical principles
- Pursue professional development
  - Publishing
  - Presenting
  - Clinically supervise/precept
    - Mutual respect and interactive learning with Mentees
  - Continuing education conferences
  - Critical thinking through deliberate inquiry
  - Enhance self-awareness with respect to interpersonal and intrapsychic exchanges
- Participate in policy making at local, state, and national levels
  - Testifying at hearings
  - Attend lobbying events
  - Engage the media
  - Phases of policy making include an inclusive and collaborative process of formulating, implementing, and evaluating (Rich, 2018)
- Teaching and coaching
  - Teach to reduce risk and promote health
  - Coach for health behavior changes

- Maintenance of nurse–patient relationship
  - Cultivate an environment of trust and mutual respect
  - Establish and maintain healthy professional boundaries
  - Use principles of therapeutic communication
- Management of health status
  - Health assessments
  - Take health histories

HEALTH PROMOTION AND MAINTENANCE

- Assessment
  - Mental status exam
  - Distinguishing variations of normal from abnormal
  - Family system evaluation and collateral evidence gathering
  - Disease prevention education
- Planning
  - Helping identify feelings and behaviors
  - Treatment planning and coordination of care
  - Case management providing oversight and authorizing services and benefits
- Intervention
  - Therapeutic interventions—help patients identify community resources for mental health
  - Psychoeducation and psychopharmacology education of patients
  - Mental health promotion and education
  - Teaching coping strategies
  - Outreach services designed to connect the individual or family to support networks and access entitlements.
- Evaluation with respect to outcome of the intervention
  - Monitoring for therapeutic and adverse effects of psychopharmacology
  - Reduced harm and risk-taking behaviors
  - Examples include keeping appointments, taking medication, attending to basic needs, developing social networks, finding purpose and meaning in work, recreation, and manifesting mature defense mechanisms

ETHICS

A branch of philosophy (epistemology) that describes moral principles that govern how a person carries out an obligation, responsibility, or duty to self and fellow man
- Ethical principles that govern decision-making

- **Autonomy:** The right to self-govern free from external control or influence
  - Patient must be involved in decision-making to the full extent of their capacity (mutual decision-making)
  - Patients have a right to refuse treatment (unless ruled incompetent by a civil authority who can mandate retention and treatment over objection)
  - Patients have a right to be treated in the least restrictive manner/setting
- **Beneficence:** Doing good, promoting well-being
- **Nonmaleficence:** Doing no harm
- **Veracity:** Conformity to facts, truthfulness, accuracy
- **Justice:** The quality of being equitable and reasonable
- **Respect:** Regard for the feelings, wishes, rights, and traditions of others

- Ethical decision-making in dilemmas
  - **Dilemma:** Situations in which there are two or more justifiable alternatives, both are of similar risk and benefit. Providers have an ethical duty to disclose errors, accidents, injuries, and positive test results to patients. The following are crucial issues to consider that illustrate the implications of an ethical dilemma:
    - As a result of disclosure, the patient may have legal recourse for financial restitution.
    - Individuals may suffer harassment or discrimination.
    - Individuals may request reasonable accommodations.
    - Opportunity for personal support from peers.
  - **Deontological theory:** An action is judged as good or bad on its merits regardless of consequence. This is the most common approach to ethical decision-making in most instances that affords the greatest deference to the individual's autonomy.
    - Patients have a right to know what is happening during their treatment.
  - **Teleological theory:** The goodness and badness of an action is based on the foreseeable consequences (the end justifies the means). This approach is less often used as it often trumps the individual's right to self-determination.
  - **Virtue ethics:** Actions are based on moral (ethical) principles.

CULTURAL COMPETENCE

Implies people should be treated as unique individuals by considering their social context when providing care. More accurately, the term "cultural awareness" dictates using the knowledge of the individual's cultural experience to inform the clinician's interpretation of the signs, symptoms, and perceptions while applying the ethical principle of respect (cultural sensitivity).
- **Culture:** Beliefs, values, behaviors, and characteristics common among members of a group.

- **Culture-bound syndromes:** Transient nonpathological behaviors associated with a culture. It is essential for clinicians to be mindful of these phenomena as not to inaccurately label a psychiatric disorder (e.g., a patient indicates she must consult with her deceased ancestors to guide her care).
- **Cultural health determinants:** Families pass along norms, beliefs, and values related to essential functions of daily living (food, shelter, safety, belonging, and education).
  - **Ethnicity:** A self-identified descriptor of race, tribe, nation, or community in which the individual shares common beliefs and values.
  - **Environmental determinants of health:** Safety of the immediate surroundings, climate, air and water quality, stability of financial resources, socialization, crime, transportation, cleanliness, and climate control.

SPECIAL POPULATIONS

People in this population are often in circumstances they would have never chosen but may find themselves in as it may still be better than what the alternative seemingly normal situation may have been. Often these individuals, if assessed, would score high on the Adverse Childhood Events scale. Using a trauma-informed approach will enhance the therapeutic alliance:
- Homeless
  - Risk factors include:
    - Families usually headed by single female parent
    - Limited education
    - Underemployment
    - Teen mothers
    - Mental illness, substance use disorder, domestic violence, undocumented immigration status, child abuse survivors
    - Emergency shelter
    - Transitional housing
    - No or pending loss of primary night-time residence within 14 days without social safety net
    - Families with children or unaccompanied youth who are unstably housed and likely to continue in that state
    - "People who are fleeing or attempting to flee domestic violence, have no other residence, and lack the resources or support networks to obtain other permanent housing" (Housing for Urban Development, 2012)
- **Sexual minorities and classification:** In order to best serve this population, one should attempt to understand a situation with an empathic attitude towards the patient's point of view and experience. Currently, clinicians should inquire about the patient's preferred personal pronouns (PPP) and address them accordingly.
  - **Sexual orientation:** The object of attraction (physical, emotional, or romantic) stratified on the Kinsey scale from 0 to 6. Zero is exclusively heterosexual, and six is exclusively homosexual.

- **Asexual:** Not attracted to either sex
- **Bisexual:** Attracted to people of both sexes
- **Heterosexual:** Attracted to people of the opposite sex
- **Homosexual:** Attracted to people of the same sex
- **LGBTQ:** Lesbian, gay, bisexual, transgender, and queer or questioning
- **Newer mnemonic:** LGBTQIA—lesbian, gay, bisexual, transgender, queer OR questioning, intersex, and asexual or allied
- **Sexual identity:** The manner in which a person identifies psychologically along continuum from female to male, including the object of attraction.
  - A male, who represents himself as a man, who is attracted to men exclusively, may define himself as a gay man
  - A female, who represents herself as a woman, and is attracted to men, may define herself as a straight woman
- **Sex:** The biological manifestation based on external genitalia and chromosomal composition female (XX), male (XY).
- **Gender identity:** An individual's deep perception along the continuum of normative (*cis*) constructs ranging from masculinity to femininity named by the individual.
  - **Hypothetical example:** A man who traumatically loses his genitalia in an accident can still identify as a man; however, if the person (XY) elects to have gender affirmation surgery (removing/ reconstructing or altering parts of the body to align with the gender identity), the individual may identify as a trans-woman. The individual does not have to be transitioning either surgically or hormonally in order to identify as trans.
- **Gender identity disorder:** A diagnostic term that describes a person's experience of significant gender dysphoria (discontent with their biological sex). It is no longer considered a mental disorder in *DSM 5* (because one's gender should not be considered a pathology but rather the distress caused is the condition for which therapy is provided).
  - Some healthcare experts, institutions, and regulatory agencies recommend a best practice strategy of asking patients how they identify (male, female, trans-male, trans-female, agender, binary, gender-nonconforming, etc.), and their preferred personal pronouns (she/her, he/him, them/they, proper nouns, etc.)
  - Gender is an excluded criterion from Delusional Disorders in *DSM 5* by consensus of expert opinion based on the psychiatric literature, however, debates persist among leading experts.
  - **Cisgender:** Has a gender identity consistent with their sex regardless of the orientation.
  - **Transgender:** A person has a gender identity that is inconsistent with their sex.
    - **FtM:** A person who was biologically female (XX) at birth, who identifies as male.
    - **MtF:** A person who was biologically male (XY) at birth, who identifies as female.

- **Gender fluid:** A person who expresses personal gender changes based on their experience and perception.
- **Nonbinary:** A person who does not strictly identify as male or female.
- **Agender:** A person who does not identify with any gender.
- **Transsexual:** An older, sometimes preferred term by some who have permanently changed or seek to change their body through medical interventions including but not limited to hormones and surgery.

FORENSICS AND CORRECTIONAL INSTITUTIONS

- **Forensic nursing:** The practice of nursing intersecting the legal system with healthcare may provide direct services to patients, consultative services to agencies, and expert testimony in healthcare-related investigations such as sexual assault, wrongful death, and standards of care. The nurse–patient relationship is based on the crime committed and the investigation necessary.
  - **Forensic:** The application of scientific knowledge to a legal problem
  - **Forensic science:** Application of science methodologies to answer legal questions, for example, vital signs measures, standard assessment or practice procedures, health assessment techniques, etc.
  - **The nurse in this role is adversarial with the patient and aligned with the justice system.** The PMHN involvement is:
    - Requested by a court
      - Material or fact witness
      - Expert opinion
      - Amicus brief (friend of the court, the nurse cannot have a personal interest in the outcome of the case in order)
    - Requested by an attorney
      - Asked to review case law and litigation
      - Asked to explain thinking disorders and patterns, impaired cognition, and mental health disorders as they may relate to a crime
  - **Forensic risk assessment:** A psychiatric evaluation performed in emergency department after arrest but before confinement to a correctional facility, intended to protect the public from persons with a known mental disorder having had violent or antisocial behaviors leading to legal trouble.
- **Correctional nursing:** The relationship with the patient is based on the offender's health, unlike a forensic encounter, and the nurse is aligned with the patient.
- **Self-disclosure:** Takes the attention away from the patient and their problems and may trigger countertransference issues which may lead to a violation of professional boundaries (this should be avoided, especially in forensic and correctional settings).
  - The clinician should remain calm, objective, neutral, and self-reflective in dealing with a population (rapists, pedophiles, murders, and other criminals) that may trigger an emotional response. The PMHN should compartmentalize their emotions and debrief after the fact.

QUALITY IMPROVEMENT

- Monitoring, identifying problems, and measuring outcomes that establish new parameters for improved performance with the aim of improving quality of care, reducing complications, and enhancing patient satisfaction.
- **Risk management:** A process used to identify potentially litigious practices due to adverse patient outcomes, focusing primarily on system errors and passive safety measures.
- **Sentinel event reporting:** Triggers a root cause analysis (RCA) for unexpected adverse outcomes that are reportable to health officials and regulating bodies charged with public protection. RCA aims to identify all the contributing factors that resulted in the sentinel event.
  - Inpatient suicide
  - Unanticipated death
  - Sexual assault of a staff member, visitor, or vendor
  - Improper procedure on the wrong patient, wrong procedure
  - Unintentional retained objects
  - Fire or unanticipated environmental hazard in a patient care area

PREVENTION

- Reducing morbidity and mortality due to disease or condition
- **Primary prevention:** Healthy people provided general advice (balanced diet, seat belts, exercise, and helmets)
  - Regulations against drunk driving
  - Workplace safety measures
  - Environmental protections
  - General measures for mental health (hobbies, friendships, purpose, etc.)
- **Secondary prevention:** Looking for disease in a group at risk (sensitivity is key)
  - Blood pressure screening
  - **Mental health screenings:** PHQ-9, MOCA, Mental Status Exam
  - Sexually transmitted infections
  - Long-acting injectable to prevent recurrence of psychosis symptoms
  - Taking medications: naltrexone, buprenorphine, methadone
- **Tertiary prevention:** Reducing disease progression in one who is diagnosed, often after acute treatment and stabilization
  - Drug alcohol rehabilitation
  - Support groups
  - Therapy
  - Psychoeducation

HEALTH BEHAVIOR GUIDELINES

- Healthy behaviors that benefit the majority of the population regardless of comorbidity
- **Exercise**: Provides both physical and mental benefits, reduces comorbidity, enhances quality of life, most effective treatment for depression and anxiety
  - Check with a healthcare provider before starting an exercise program
  - Begin gradually; set expectations and do not expect overnight results
  - Strive for sustainability and enjoyment
  - Exercise should be sufficiently taxing to generate sweat and increased heart rate but not so much that the individual cannot carry on a conversation
  - Encourage 4–5 days per week to include both aerobic and anaerobic
    - **Encourage self-awareness:** To reflect on one's beliefs, thoughts, emotions, motives, biases, and limitations, and how these may influence behavior

ADVANCED DIRECTIVES

- **Living will:** A document detailing the patient's instructions and preferences for end-of-life care in the event that they are not able to make their wishes known. This is not legally binding and some states.
- **Healthcare power of attorney**: A legal document indicating an individual (healthcare proxy, durable medical power of attorney, surrogate) to make medical decisions on behalf of the incapacitated patient. This document is effective once the patient has been determined to be incapacitated and/or mentally unable to communicate in a deliberate manner. The document must be signed by the patient and witnessed by two adults.
- **Power of attorney:** A legal document in which a patient appoints an individual to make all (person and property) decisions on their behalf should they become incapacitated. This document must be notarized.

ANTICIPATORY GUIDANCE

- A tailored prevention framework to reduce morbidity and mortality.
- Assumes information provided in a timely manner will reduce morbidity and mortality along the life span. The need for information is determined and a systematic manner.
- Bright futures web-based aggregated guidelines for anticipatory guidance based on the premise that every child deserves a healthy and optimal relationship with a healthcare provider.
- Eliciting information from key individuals regarding the unique needs of the patient based on age, disease, or developmental milestone: Medication adherence, car seat safety, water safety, seat belts, helmets, immunization schedule, and red flags.

- **Health-specific:** Assisting individuals to meet the healthcare challenges across the life span.
  - Anticipated decline and death and grieving
  - Anticipated disease progressions such as Alzheimer's or psychotic disorders
  - Coping with catastrophic injuries
  - Exploring risk of domestic violence
  - Survivor coping after divorce or death
  - End-of-life planning

KNOWLEDGE CHECK: CHAPTER 2

1. Which of the following is characteristic of the leadership competency for the psychiatric-mental health nurse?

   A. Participating in a community-focused program that promotes mental health and reduces the risk of mental health problems
   B. Evaluating the appropriate use of seclusion and restraints in caring for a mentally ill patient
   C. Developing an age-appropriate treatment plan
   D. Modifying the treatment plan based on the patient's needs

2. A state's Nurse Practice Act specifies which of the following?

   A. Who may use the title registered nurse and what they can do
   B. Restricts the practice of psychologists and other mental health professionals
   C. Regulates the ability of family members caring for loved ones
   D. Provide oversight for service and benefits provided to patients

3. Which of the following may govern the practice of the psychiatric-mental health nurse?

   A. Statutory law
   B. The U.S. Constitution
   C. Certification
   D. City ordinances

4. Which of the following allows the psychiatric-mental health nurse to practice in a state?

   A. Certification
   B. Licensure
   C. Credentialing
   D. Graduation

5. Which statement is true regarding the scope of practice?

   A. The scope of practice defines the registered nurse's role, actions, and competencies, varying from state to state
   B. Guarantees patient's rights to receive care from a registered nurse
   C. The scope of practice provides a way to judge the nature of the care provided
   D. Delineates practice protocols for mental institutions

(See answers next page.)

1. A) Participating in a community-focused program that promotes mental health and reduces the risk of mental health problems
Participating in a community-focused program that promotes mental health exemplifies a leadership competency. Evaluating the appropriate use of seclusion and restraints, developing an age-appropriate treatment plan, and modifying the treatment plan based on clients' needs are clinical competencies rather than a leadership core competency.

2. A) Who may use the title registered nurse and what they can do
The state Nurse Practice Act does not provide for oversight of services and benefits provided to patients, nor does it regulate the practice of non-nurses, including family members caring for loved ones.

3. A) Statutory law
Statutory laws made by state governmental entities govern the practice of a profession within a state. The U.S. Constitution, certifications, and city ordinances do not govern professional practice within states.

4. B) Licensure
Licensure allows a professional to practice their profession in a state. Certification designates the successful completion of a course of study. Credentialing is a process that verifies minimum levels of professional competence to ensure public safety. Graduation is a ceremony offered by an educational institution in accordance with established criteria of completion.

5. A) The scope of practice defines the registered nurse role and actions, identifies minimal competencies held by all registered nurses, and varies from state to state
Patient's rights are not governed by the nurse's scope of practice. It does not provide a way to judge the nature of care provided rather this is the function of standards of care. Practice protocols are delimited by local institution's governing board and must meet the minimum standards of care.

6. Which of the following statement is true regarding standards of care?
   A. Standards of care delineate the minimum levels of acceptable performance and a way to judge the nature of care provided by a professional
   B. Standards of care dictate the qualifications of the registered nurses
   C. Standards of care identify competencies assumed to be held by all registered nurses
   D. Standards of care denote specialty training of a professional

7. Amid the COVID-19 pandemic, the psychiatric-mental health nurse is providing follow-up psychoeducation regarding medication therapeutic and adverse effects. The patient wants to have a video visit through their non-HIPAA (Health Information Portability and Accountability Act) secure video chat. Which of the following can be discussed during the visit?
   A. Patient's name
   B. Patient's diagnosis
   C. Address
   D. Phone number

8. According to the Health Information Portability and Accountability Act (HIPAA), which of the following entities can receive personal health identifiers without express consent from the patient?
   A. The patient's next of kin
   B. The patient's health insurance company
   C. The patient's clergy
   D. The patient's attorney

9. The following situation requires patient consent to release medical information:
   A. If the client reveals intent to harm self or others
   B. Records to the insurance company
   C. Responding to court orders, subpoenas, or summons
   D. Next of kin wanting to help the patient make decisions

10. The psychiatric-mental health nurse is witnessing consent for a patient who will have electroconvulsive therapy (ECT). Which of the following requires the patient's capacity to consent to treatment?
    A. The procedure is covered by the patient's insurance
    B. The patient understands the purpose, risks, benefits, and alternatives of the proposed treatment
    C. The next of kin agree with the proposed treatment
    D. The patient has a therapeutic alliance with the person performing the procedure

(See answers next page.)

6. A) Standards of care delineate the minimum levels of acceptable performance and a way to judge the nature of care provided by a professional

Qualifications and competencies of the registered nurse are reflective of the scope of practice. Specialty training is denoted by the process of achieving certification.

7. B) Patient's diagnosis

Personal health identifiers include name, address, and phone number. Patient diagnosis is not considered a personal health identifier.

8. B) The patient's health insurance company

The patient must consent to release personal health identifiers to the next of kin, clergy, and an attorney. Patient consent is not required to release personal health identifiers to a patient's health insurance company.

9. D) Next of kin wanting to help the patient make decisions

Medical information may be released to parties needing to know to prevent harm to self and others, arranging for payment from the health insurance company, and in response to court subpoenas or summonses. The patient must consent to release medical information to the next of kin, helping to make healthcare decisions.

10. B) The patient understands the purpose, risks, benefits, and alternatives of the proposed treatment

The insurance coverage, agreement by the next of kin, and therapeutic alliance are not considered in the patient's assessment of decision-making capacity to consent to treatment.

11. Which of the following ethical principles deals with promoting the well-being of a patient?

    A. Justice
    B. Beneficence
    C. Nonmaleficence
    D. Autonomy

12. Which of the following ethical principles would conflict if the treatment team wanted to implement a therapeutic deception for the good of the patient?

    A. Beneficence
    B. Nonmaleficence
    C. Justice
    D. Veracity

13. A patient who is refusing psychiatric treatment has their case adjudicated. The judge orders treatment over objection for the good of the patient. Which ethical principle is trumped?

    A. Beneficence
    B. Nonmaleficence
    C. Justice
    D. Autonomy

14. Actions judged based on their inherent value regardless of their consequence is based on which ethical decision-making approach?

    A. Teleological theory
    B. Deontological theory
    C. Virtue ethics
    D. Justice principle

15. An action that is judged good or bad based on the consequence demonstrates which ethical decision-making approach?

    A. Teleological theory
    B. Deontological theory
    C. Virtue ethics
    D. Justice principle

(See answers next page.)

11. B) Beneficence
The principle of beneficence is that of doing good for the patient. Justice is the principle of equity. Nonmaleficence is the principle of first doing no harm. Autonomy is the principle of respecting the individual's right to self-determination.

12. D) Veracity
Veracity is the ethical principle of truthfulness and non-deception, either by omission or by commission. Beneficence is the principle of doing good. Nonmaleficence is the principle of first doing no harm. Justice is the principle of equity.

13. D) Autonomy
Autonomy is the principle of respecting the individual's right to self-determination. Beneficence is the principle of doing good. Nonmaleficence is the principle of first doing no harm. Justice is the principle of equity.

14. B) Deontological theory
Deontological theory considers the inherent value regardless of consequences. The teleological approach allows the ends to justify the means. Virtue ethics is an approach to ethical decision-making that considers the moral character of the individual rather than the action. Justice is the principle of equity.

15. A) Teleological theory
The teleological approach allows the ends to justify the means. Deontological theory considers the inherent value regardless of consequences. Virtue ethics is an approach to ethical decision-making that considers the moral character of the individual rather than the action. Justice is the principle of equity.

REFERENCES

American Nurses Association. (2015). *Code of ethics for nurses*. Retrieved from http://www.nursingworld.org/codeofethics

American Nurses Association. (2018). *Scope of practice, American Nurses Association*. Retrieved from https://www.nursingworld.org/practice-policy/scope-of-practice/

American Nurses Credentialing Center. (n.d.). *Psychiatric-mental health nurse practitioner (Across the Lifespan) certification (PMHNP-BC) | ANCC*. Retrieved from https://www.nursingworld.org/our-certifications/psychiatric-mental-health-nurse-practitioner/

Black, H. C. (1999). *Black's law dictionary*. New York, NY: West Publishing. doi:10.2307/1066423

Brinkert, R. (2010). A literature review of conflict communication causes, costs, benefits and interventions in nursing. *Journal of Nursing Management, 18*(2), 145–156. doi:10.1111/j.1365-2834.2010.01061.x

Centers for Disease Control and Prevention. (2017a). Deaths and mortality-U.S. Retrieved from https://www.cdc.gov/nchs/fastats/deaths.htm

Centers for Disease Control and Prevention. (2017b). *Immunization schedules*. Retrieved from https://www.cdc.gov/vaccines/schedules/index.html

Department of Housing and Urban Development. (2012). *Changes in the HUD definition of "Homeless" National Alliance to End Homelessness*. Retrieved from https://endhomelessness.org/resource/changes-in-the-hud-definition-of-homeless/

Houser, J., & Oman, K. S. (2011). An implementation guide for evidence-based practice. Sudbury, MA: Jones and Bartlett Learning LLC.

Institute of Medicine. (2001, March). Crossing the quality chasm: A new health system for the 21th century. *IOM, 14*, 1–8.

Institute of Medicine. (1999). *To err is human*. Retrieved from http://www.nap.edu/openbook.php?record_id=9728

Patient Protection and Affordable Care Act, 42 U.S.C. § 18001 et seq. (2010).

Rich, R. F. (2018). Social science information and public policy making. Washington, DC: Routledge. doi:10.4324/9781351306324

Schmitt, M., Blue, A., Aschenbrener, C. A., & Viggiano, T. R. (2011). Core competencies for interprofessional collaborative practice: Reforming health care by transforming health professionals' education. *Journal of the Association of American Medical Colleges, 86*(11), 1351. doi:10.1097/ACM.0b013e3182308e39

Tarasoff v. Regents of University of California, 17 Cal. 3d 425 (Cal. 1976)

Tunzi, M. (2001, July15). Can the patient decide? Evaluating patient capacity in practice. Retrieved from https://www.aafp.org/afp/2001/0715/p299.html

Fundamental Theories of Mental Illness and Nonpharmacological Interventions

3

> ### ▶ OBJECTIVES
> - Review the Health Belief Model (HBM)
> - Transtheoretical model and the process of change
> - Motivational interviewing paired with stages of change
> - Maslow's hierarchy of needs
> - Relapse prevention model
> - Stages of development
> - Nursing theorists
> - Therapeutic alliance
> - Nonpharmacological modalities, including psychotherapy and complementary and alternative interventions

INTRODUCTION

The focus of this chapter is on the psychosocial theories that guide psychotherapy and explain potential motivations for human behavior. Biological factors and psychopharmacology are addressed explicitly in separate chapters and will incorporate physiological theories of neuroanatomy and physiology as they relate to mental illness.

The principles of physiology and pathophysiology are the foundation for much of the work that is done in nursing and medicine. The field of psychiatric-mental health is more accurately labeled behavioral health. The scientific evidence demonstrating a cause-and-effect relationship remains limited. The entire diagnostic process in psychiatry is by exclusion. The aim of psychopharmacology treatment is to mitigate the physical signs and symptoms which are thought to cause a maladaptive coping behavior pattern. The approach to medication selection remains trial and error despite advances in pharmacogenomic testing.

In order for the work of therapy to unfold and healing to occur, the psychiatric-mental health nurse (PMHN) must develop a therapeutic relationship with the client and family system in order to build a therapeutic alliance. Working knowledge of psychosocial theories will help the nurse elicit and organize essential information and develop a care plan. The theoretical models and conceptual frameworks help the PMHN make sense of the client and family system's behavior, which at times can seem at odds with wellness.

Psychotherapy is a nonspecific shorthand term used to refer to nonpharmacological interventions such as individual talk therapy, group therapy, and family therapy intended to help clients heal or recover. The theoretical frameworks presented in this chapter serve as the foundation for most of the work of psychotherapy. Therapists will often draw from a varied pool of theories and interventions with the intent of personalizing care. This approach is known as eclectic psychotherapy. As a board-certified PMH-BC™, you have a professional obligation to lifelong learning in order to enhance your competency in various psychotherapeutic interventions. Each type of therapy presented requires specialized training combined with supervised clinical practice in order to achieve mastery.

HEALTH BELIEF MODEL (HBM)

- A conceptual framework to explain health behaviors and guide behavioral interventions to promote health (Maiman & Becker, 1974)
- Key concepts:
  - **Perceived susceptibility:** One's belief regarding the chance of getting a condition
  - **Perceived severity:** One's belief of how dangerous a condition and its sequelae would be if it happened
  - **Perceived benefits:** One's belief in the efficacy of the advice to reduce disease impact
  - **Perceived barriers:** One's belief about the cost of the advised action, that is, "what do I need to give up?" (time, money, image, status) to implement the recommendation
  - **Cues to action:** Something that activates or enhances readiness to change or implement the new behavior or stop an existing behavior
  - **Self-efficacy:** One's confidence in one's ability to successfully perform the health behavior change

▶ CLINICAL VIGNETTE

What questions might the PMHN ask of the family regarding the following vignette in trying to answer key concepts of the Health Belief Model?

A 16-year-old boy has started smoking cigarettes, socializing with freshman college kids, and hooking up with various classmates. His parents are worried that he will become addicted to smoking, perhaps try other substances, contract a sexually transmitted infection, or get a girl pregnant. The boy rationalizes his behavior by saying everyone else is doing it, and he fits in better with the older people.

TRANSTHEORETICAL MODEL (TTM)

- A stage-based model for behavior change over time is drawn from major theoretical frameworks and conceptual models (Prochaska & Diclemente, 1986; Prochaska & Velicer, 1997).

- Key concepts:
  - **Stages of change:**
    - **Precontemplation:** No intention to take action within the next six months; denial that a problem exists
    - **Contemplation:** Acknowledges that a problem exists and intends to take action in the next six months
    - **Preparation:** Intends to take actions within the next 30 days and has taken some behavioral steps to plan
    - **Action:** Engaging in behavior change for less than six months
    - **Maintenance:** Sustained behavior change more than six months
  - **Decisional balance:** Acknowledge ambivalence is normal in the process of change
    - **Pros:** Considers the benefits of making the desired change
    - **Cons:** Considers the cost of making the desired change
  - **Self-efficacy:**
    - **Confidence:** Ability that one can engage in the behavior change in various situations
    - **Temptation:** Likelihood of engaging in unhealthy behavior in various situations
    - **Importance ruler:** On a scale of 1 to 10, "How important is it for you to make this change?" (1 being least important and 10 most important)
      - Ask this question first to gain insight into underlying factors and reasoning for why it is at the current level of importance.
    - **Confidence ruler:** On a scale of 1 to 10, "How confident are you that you will be able to make this change?" (1 not confident at all and 10 extremely confident
      - If the client gives an answer of <7, inquire why their confidence is not lower. This will enhance self-efficacy as they give you examples and reasons of how they arrived at seven and may move higher on the confidence ruler as they hear themselves explain all the hard things in life they have overcome.
  - **Process of change**
    - **Consciousness raising:** Discovering and accepting facts in support of the health behavior change (e.g., *"I recognize that my drinking is causing me health problems."*)
    - **Dramatic relief:** Experiencing negative emotions such as fear, anxiety, worry that goes along with the unhealthy behavioral risks (e.g., *"I am afraid if I don't drink to calm my nerves, I won't be able to socialize."*)
    - **Self-reevaluation:** Incorporating behavior change as an essential feature of one's identity as a person (e.g., *"I am a responsible mother, and that means I do not use alcohol to cope with life."*)
    - **Environmental reevaluation:** Recognizing the positive impact of healthy behavior on the social and physical environment and or recognizing the negative impact of the unhealthy behavior (e.g., *"As a result of not getting drunk after a stressful day I did not spend the next day recovering and was able to meet my deadline at work."*)
    - **Self-liberation:** Making a firm commitment to change (e.g., *"Today is the day where I say enough is enough and I stop using."*)
    - **Helping relationships:** Developing social support for healthy behavior change (e.g., *"I am going to attend Alcoholics Anonymous meeting and join Big Vision so I can make friends and socialize without alcohol."*)

- **Counter conditioning:** Liberally substituting a healthy alternative behavior or cognition for an unhealthy behavior or automatic negative thought (e.g., *"Instead of drinking when I feel happy or sad, I will call a friend and get dessert, or get a spa treatment, or do the longer workout I have been putting off."*)
- **Reinforcement management:** Implementing a rewards structure for positive behavior change and reducing rewards or aversive reinforcement for unhealthy behaviors or transient lapses (e.g., *"I earned my chip at Alcoholics Anonymous; I got my weight loss pendant from Weight Watchers; I will plan a mental health day off of work if I don't call out sick for 3 months"*)
- **Stimulus control:** Reducing environmental cues to engage in unhealthy behavior and adding cues to remind to engage in healthy behavior (*e.g., "I am going to cancel my wine club membership and give away all my bottles."*)
- **Social liberation:** Recognizes social norms have changed in a direction that supports the desired healthy behavior (e.g., *"It is getting impossible to smoke anywhere anymore, perhaps I should just quit."*)

MOTIVATIONAL INTERVIEWING (MI)

- A therapeutic technique to get people unstuck and encourage a health behavior change that uses elements of cognitive behavioral therapy (CBT) and the HBM and is often paired with the transtheoretical model. MI attempts to elicit the client's internal motivation for change and to frame the benefit of the change in a manner congruent with the client's values (Table 3.1; Miller & Rollnick, 2012).
- Listen for **change talk** as the client articulates the
  - **Desire for change:** The client expresses a preference for change "I would like to. ., I want to ..., I wish ..."
  - **Ability to change:** The client makes statements about capability "I could ..., I can ..., I might be able to ..."
  - **Reasons to change:** The client is making specific arguments for change "I would probably feel better if I ..."

Table 3.1 Motivational Interviewing versus Traditional Counseling

Motivational Interviewing (Patient is the Expert on Themselves)	Traditional Counseling (Sage on the Stage)
Partnership: Forms a partnership with the client, honoring their expertise and perspective, noncoercive	**Confrontation**: Involves override of the client's impaired perspective, imposes awareness of "reality" which the client cannot see or is unwilling to admit
Elicitation: Assumes the resources and motivation to change are intrinsic to the client. Elicit motivation by drawing on the client's perceptions, goals, and values	**Instruction**: Assumes the client lacks knowledge, insight, skill necessary for change; the therapist provides enlightenment
Autonomy: Affirms the client's capacity and rights to self-direction, facilitating informed choice	**Expert**: The provider tells a patient what ought to be done

- **Need to change:** The client makes statements expressing an obligation to change "I ought to..., I have to..., I really should ...."
- **Other expressions:** Clients may also express commitment to or tell of an action they have taken in the direction of the desired change.

APPLYING THE FOUR PRINCIPLES OF MI

- **Express empathy:** Radical acceptance, reflective listening, ambivalence is normal; use client's own words (e.g., *"What you are going through sounds difficult, and it has served well enough to get to this point, it is normal to feel conflicted, you may have some very intense feelings."*)
- **Develop discrepancy:** Amplifying from the client's perspective, the discrepancy between present behavior and their desired goal, create cognitive dissonance; client rather than therapist should present the arguments for change (e.g., *"If I am understanding you correctly, you are sick and tired of feeling sick and tired but know that you cannot continue doing these things, and you want to make a better future?"*)
- **Roll with resistance:** Avoid arguing for change, resistance not directly opposed, invite a new perspective; the client is the primary resource for solutions and signals therapist to respond differently (e.g., *"I understand change can be very difficult, and you may not be ready now; is there something that would need to change before you are ready; what made you want to come for help?"*)
- **Support self-efficacy:** Therapist expresses their belief in the client's ability to make the necessary change when ready (e.g., *"You have told me all the hard things in your life that you have overcome, and I believe when you are ready you will be able to make the necessary changes."*)

MASLOW'S HIERARCHY OF NEEDS

- A psychological theory that prioritizes human physiological needs over psychological needs before the client can reach their full potential while ensuring the survival of the species (Figure 3.1; Maslow, 1969)
  - **Physiological:** Food, water, air, sex, sleep
  - **Safety:** Protection from physical harm, nature, psychological harm
  - **Love and belonging:** Companionship, friendship, intimacy
  - **Self-esteem:** A sense of accomplishment, self-worth
  - **Self-actualization:** Achieving full potential, creative activities, the pursuit of improvement, contributing to social well-being
- When a patient cannot meet their physiological and safety needs, they usually meet the criteria for hospital admission
  - Hospitalization provides for basic physiological and physical safety needs
  - The sense of belonging can develop in a milieu

```
                    /\
                   /  \
                  / Self\
                 /-actualization\
                /(future-oriented)\
               / hope, societal improvement\
              /─────────────────────────────\
             /        Self-esteem            \
            /(positive regard for self and well-being)\
           /───────────────────────────────────────────\
          /           Love and belonging                \
         /       (socialization and assimilation)        \
        /─────────────────────────────────────────────────\
       /                 Safety needs                      \
      /         (environmental exposure and harm)           \
     /───────────────────────────────────────────────────────\
    /                Physiological needs                      \
   /           (essential nutrients and procreation)           \
  /─────────────────────────────────────────────────────────────\
```

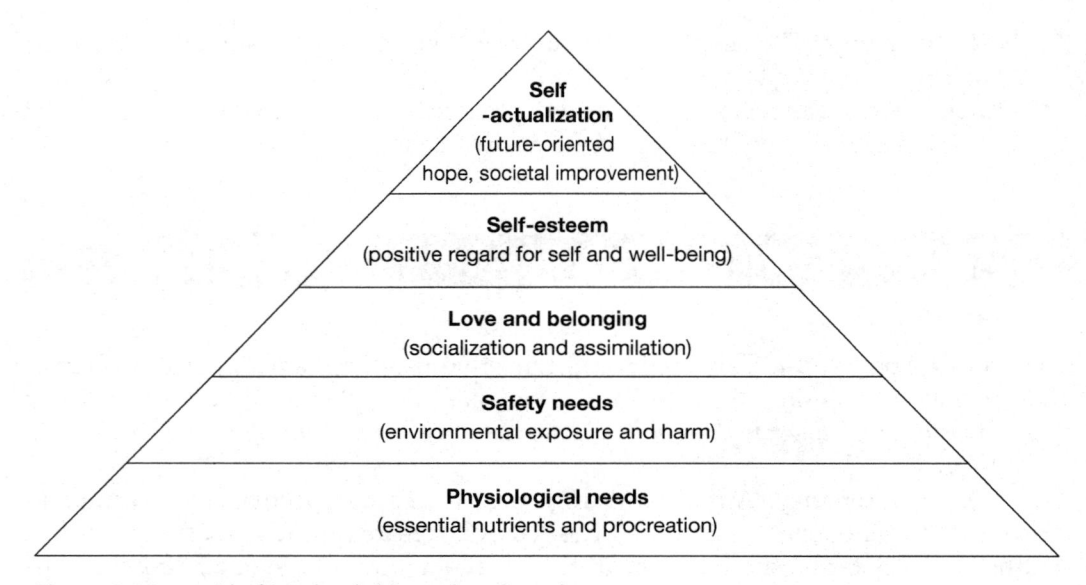

Figure 3.1 Pyramid of Maslow's hierarchy of needs.
Source: Adapted from Maslow, A. H. (1969). Psychology of science: A reconnaissance. Anna Maria, FL: Maurice Bassett Publishing.

- **Partial hospital programs, continuous day treatment programs, and intensive outpatient programs** focus on the needs of belonging, and as patients gain function, they gain self-esteem
- **Vocational rehabilitation, psychodynamic therapy, psychoanalysis** focus on patients' work through self-actualization

▶ CLINICAL VIGNETTE

A 60-year-old female who has increasingly been isolating herself, neglecting her basic needs, unable to get food, and maintain her shelter, presents to the emergency department when an ambulance was called for an odd smell coming from her apartment. The patient is soiled, dehydrated, with impoverished speech, and tearful. The neighbor reports she has been progressively reclusive since the death of her husband a year ago.

According to Maslow's hierarchy of needs, what elements must be addressed in the plan of care for this individual? What questions should the nurse ask? What services will need to be put into place to assure this patient's safety and well-being? Does this patient meet involuntary hospitalization criteria?

● RELAPSE PREVENTION

- A social-cognitive model describing determinants of relapse (Larimer, Palmer, & Marlatt, 1999)
- **High-risk situations:** The immediate precipitant to relapse
  - **Negative emotional states:** Anger, anxiety, depression, frustration, loneliness, and boredom

- **Interpersonal conflict:** With significant others, family members, superior, romantic interest, loss
- **Social pressure:** Direct and indirect environmental cues, being around the vice
- **Positive emotional states:** Associated with the vice as a solution or enhancer of well-being (e.g., a reward for a day's work, seductive advertising)
- **Coping strategy:** A person's response to a high-risk situation
  - **Effective:** Leaving a high-risk situation, positive self-talk, calling a friend, planning another activity, contingency planning, avoidance of high-risk situations
  - **Ineffective:** Using the vice as the coping strategy, lingering in a high-risk environment, minimizing potential harms
- **Self-efficacy:** Belief in one's ability to effectively cope and the expectation about the outcome
- **Abstinence violation effect (AVE):** Cognitive restructuring in which the lapse is distinguished from a relapse and seen as an isolated mistake, one of the two sequences can follow:
  - The client resumes abstinence behavior despite negative feelings of failure (e.g., "*I was doing so well on this diet, I ate a cookie, it tasted good, but I can get back on track and start from right where I am and move forward.*")
  - The client decides to negate sobriety and attempts to quell negative emotional state by further lapses (e.g., "*I was doing so well on this diet, and then I ate a cookie, then I feel bad and I want to feel better, so I eat the rest of the cookies.*")

THE PROBABILITY OF RELAPSE IS CONTINGENT ON THE COPING STRATEGY

- **High probability:** High-risk situation→ <u>ineffective coping strategy</u>→ poor self-efficacy → lapse → AVE → relapse
- **Low probability:** High-risk situation ←<u>effective coping strategy</u> ←increased self-efficacy ←decreased probability of relapse

SOCIAL LEARNING THEORY

- Learned behaviors occur in a social context; expectations and outcomes reinforce the behavior and increase sustainability (Bandura, 1989).
- Key concepts:
  - Cognition and environmental factors can reinforce learning. The patient acts in a certain way and receives positive feedback increases the likelihood that the behavior continues.
  - **Direct experience:** The patient learns a healthy behavior and likes the result, increased likelihood of continuing the behavior.
  - **Vicarious learning:** The patient observes a negative consequence to a behavior, reduces the likelihood that the behavior will be adopted. Patient has learned not to do the potentially harmful behavior.

PSYCHOLOGICAL STAGES OF HUMAN DEVELOPMENT

- Stage-based theory of personality development (Table 3.2; Erikson, 1956)
  - Does not need to master the prior stage to move to the next stage. However, subsequent stages will reflect the failed stage (Sadock, B., Sadock, V., & Ruiz, 2015)
  - Tasks can be mastered at any time if previously failed
- Each stage comes with a developmental crisis. The crisis arises as the individual's needs conflict with society's needs
- Mastery of the stage results in the acquisition of fundamental virtues
- Ages are an approximation and can overlap slightly

▶ COGNITIVE THEORY (JEAN PIAGET 1896–1980)

- Human development progresses from cognition to learning and then moves to comprehending.

KEY CONCEPTS

- **Schemas:** Building blocks of knowledge. The child develops a mental representation of the world (units of information relating to aspects of the physical world)
- **Adaptation:** A process that enables the transition from one stage to another
  - **Equilibrium:** A force that moves the development along; happens when a child's schema can deal with the new information by assimilation.
  - **Assimilation:** Uses an existing schema to deal with a new object or situation (e.g., an 18-month-old child sees a bald-headed man with a bowtie and immediately starts crying, saying "no doctor, no doctor").
  - **Accommodation:** When the child is unable to assimilate the new information into an existing schema, they form a new one (e.g., the 18-month-old child's mother explains that even though the man is wearing a bowtie and is bald, he is not a doctor because he is not giving the child a shot. The child then learns not every bald-headed man with a bowtie is going to give him an injection.)
- **Stages of cognitive development**
  - **Sensorimotor (birth to 2 years):** The child learns that an object still exists even if he cannot see it.
  - **Preoperational (2 to 7 years):** The child learns a symbolic representation of either pictures or words. A child cries if when he says cookie and receives a picture of the cookie rather than the cookie.
    - Egocentricity with difficulty taking the viewpoint of another.

Table 3.2 Erikson's Stages of Development

Age and Developmental Stage	Developmental Task	Mastery	Virtue Existential Questions	Failure	Potential Mental Disorders
0–1 year Infancy	Trust vs. mistrust	Trusting and optimistic	Hope Can I trust the world?	Mistrusting, paranoid, suspicious	Dysthymia Schizotypal Personality Addictive predisposition
2–3 years Toddlerhood	Autonomy vs. shame and doubt	Good self-control and will power asserts independence	Will Am I OK the way I am?	Inadequacy, dependent on others, shame in their lack of ability	Obsessive compulsive personality disorder Paranoid Personality
4–6 years Childhood	Initiative vs. guilt	Goal-directed, motivated, a sense of purpose, leadership skills	Purpose What am I here for?	Feels like they are a bother to others, remain followers, lack self-initiative	Inhibition Fear, timidity Somatization
7–12 years Middle childhood/ school-aged	Industry vs. inferiority	Competent, confident in one's abilities to achieve goals	Competency Can I do things?	Society is too demanding, inferiority complex, may not reach full potential	Dependent personality
13–20 years Adolescence	Identity vs. role confusion	Able to commit self to others despite differences,	Fidelity Who am I, and what do I hope to be?	I do not know what I want to be when I grow up. Where do I belong?	Antisocial Personality Borderline Personality
21–35 years Early adulthood	Intimacy vs. isolation	Happy, committed relationships, feeling safe in a relationship	Love Am I able to love? What is love?	Avoiding commitment, isolating, loneliness, fear of partner commitment.	Schizoid Personality Disorder Avoidant personality
36–65 years Adulthood	Generativity vs. stagnation	The desire to be part of the broader community, leave a legacy, feeling useful	Care Can I make my life mean something for the greater good?	Low interest in work, going through the motions, lack of interest in the broader community, disconnected, nothing to contribute	Narcissistic Injury Dependency Avoidance
>66 Late adulthood	Ego integrity vs. despair	Positive life review, satisfied with accomplishments, sense of closure, and death without fear	Wisdom Was it OK for me to be whom I have been?	Negative life review, dissatisfied with life that was led, hopelessness and depression	Isolation and desperation

Source: Reproduced with permission from Erikson, E. (1956). The problem of ego identity. *Journal of the American Psychoanalytic Association, 4,* 56–121.

- **Concrete operations (7 to 11 years):** Children start to work things out in their head, develop number conservation (four quarters is the same as $1.00, is the same as 100 pennies.)
- **Formal operations (11 years and older):** Abstract thinking and hypothesis testing. Algebra is possible If $X + 8 = 10$, $x = 2$

▶ SULLIVAN'S STAGES OF INTERPERSONAL DEVELOPMENT

- Herbert "Harry" Stack Sullivan (1892–1949) (Table 3.3; Sullivan, 1955).
- Personality is within an energy system
  - Tension is the potential for action (e.g., anxiety, premonitions, drowsiness, hunger, sexual excitement)
    - The tension created by a biological imbalance between the person in the environment
      - Not always on the conscious level
      - Partial distortions of reality

Table 3.3 Sullivan's Stages of Interpersonal Development

Stage	Age	Developmental Task	Means of Accomplishing	Psychopathology Failing to Accomplish
Infancy	Birth–18 months	Oral gratification	Sucking, chewing, crying, feeding	Psychosis, addiction, paranoia
Childhood	18 months–6 year	Delayed gratification	Toilet training	Dysthymia, depression
Juvenile	6–9 years	Social skills/peer relationships	Interactive play/pretend play	Schizoid/schizotypal personality
Preadolescence	9–12 years	Same-sex relationships	Gender-specific play: Boys rough and tumble, shooting games; Girls play school and house	Gender identity dysphoria
Early adolescence	12–14 years	Opposite sex relations	Sexual development, the curiosity of the opposite sex	Gender identity disorder, anxiety, paraphilia, fetishes
Late adolescence	14–21 years	Developed self-identity	Vocationally focused, defines self through accomplishment	Narcissistic personality disorder

Source: From Sullivan, H. (1955). *The interpersonal theory of psychiatry.* New York, NY: W.W. Norton & Company. Retrieved from https://content.taylorfrancis.com/books/download?dac=C2004-0-01296-0&isbn=9781136439292&format=googlePreviewPdf.

- Energy transformations are the actions themselves (in response to tension)
  - Personality develops within a social context
  - Personality depends on the presence of other people
  - Development depends on the individual's ability to establish intimacy with another person
  - Anxiety can interfere with satisfying interpersonal relationships
  - Healthy development entailed experiencing intimacy and loss toward another person
- Interpersonal relationships and experiences constitute the self-system that influences personality development
- To understand behavior, one must understand the relationship and the person's life
- **Primary drivers of behavior** (why do we do the things we do?)
  - **Physical needs** *(Maslow's level one):* Food, air, sex, sleep
  - **Safety needs** *(Maslow's level two):* Safety broadened to mean conforming to social norms of the individual's reference group
    - Mental illness occurs when self-satisfaction interferes with the self-system
    - Relieving anxiety is the driver behind actions and creates a sense of interpersonal security

▶ SIGMUND FREUD

- Father of psychoanalysis; emphasis on the intrapsychic conflict between structures of the mind (Id, Ego, and Superego). Fantasy, instincts, urges, and urges (sexual and aggressive) drive people's thoughts and behaviors (Table 3.4)
  - **Id:** Primitive pleasure-seeking mind, food, sex, survival; seeking immediate satisfaction
  - **Ego:** Conscious mind, rational mind, reality-based, employs defense mechanisms.
    - Thinking process
    - Reality tests
    - Employs defense mechanisms as a means of protecting the integrity of the mind
      - Without defense mechanisms, the mind becomes psychotic

Table 3.4 Psychosexual Stages of Development (Sigmund Freud)

Stage	Age	Developmental Task	Means of Accomplishing	Psychopathology Failing to Accomplish
Oral	0–18 mo	Oral gratification	Sucking, chewing, crying, feeding	Psychosis, addiction, paranoia
Anal	18 mo to 3 y	Delayed gratification	Toilet training	Dysthymia, depression
Phallic	3–6 y	Sexual exhibitionism	Interactive play/pretend play	Sexual identity disorders
Latency	6–16 y	Socialization and identity development	Mastery of psychosocial and motor skills	Narcissistic personality disorder, borderline personality disorder

Source: Adapted from Freud, S. (1905). *Three essays on the theory of sexuality* (7 Standard ed., pp. 123–246). New York, NY: Basic Books.

- Superego:
    - The Ego's ideal state
    - Morality
        - Right versus wrong
        - Guilt versus shame
        - Moral obligations versus fantasies
        - *The therapist attempts to function in the role of an external Super ego*
- Conflicts are resolved through defense mechanisms (Table 3.5)

Table 3.5 Defense Mechanisms

Defense Mechanism	Unconscious Process Used to Reduce Anxiety	Example
Denial	Refusing to believe a painful reality	A partner denies the evidence of a love affair
Displacement	Shifting an impulse toward a more acceptable object	Kicking the dog in response to being disciplined
Rationalization	Self-justifying explanation instead of reality which is perceived as threatening	An alcoholic who says she only drinks socially
Projection	Disguising one's impulse by attributing to others	"All guys do this"
Reaction formation	Switching unacceptable impulses into the opposite impulse	Displacing angry feelings with extreme friendliness
Regression	Retreating to a previously mastered developmental stage	A child reverts to thumb-sucking or bedwetting in response to a new stressor (new baby, new school)
Conversion	Psychological angst is manifest as a physical symptom	Abdominal pain with no organic etiology
Dissociation	Outer body experience, disconnected from the physical world	Becoming inattentive or daydreaming or freezing during an acute stress
Humor	Seeking a funny aspect in a stressful situation to reduce associated anxiety	Daughter-in-law overhears mother-in-law complaining about her housekeeping, and daughter-in-law blurts out "she cannot cook either"
Intellectualization	Considering an emotional issue in intellectual terms	A terminated employee acknowledges the business sense and identifies the benefits of the termination in order for the business to succeed
Undoing	Behavior in an attempt to correct a past unacceptable behavior	The physically abusive spouse comes home with flowers
Sublimation	Substituting a socially acceptable constructive activity for a robust contrasting impulse	One with anger management issues may take up intense exercising

NURSING THEORISTS

- **Jean Watson:** Clinical Caritas guides the practice of nursing and is essential in creating a therapeutic relationship and alliance for healing
  - Results in satisfying basic human needs
  - Promotes individual and family growth
  - Radical acceptance for the patient
  - Creating an environment that allows for achieving full potential
- **Madeleine Leininger:** Cultural care
  - Patients have the same basic needs regardless of culture
  - Culture provides the context for care and the meaning of suffering
    - Values
    - Beliefs
    - Generational experiences
    - Gender roles
    - Religion
- **Hildegard Peplau**: Theory of interpersonal relationships
  - A personal relationship is emphasizing the nurse–client dyad as the foundation to practice. The emphasis was on the give and take of the nurse–client relationship, creating a shared experience between the nurse and client; the work of the nurse therapist includes facilitating through observation, description, formulation, interpretation, validation, and intervention (Peplau, 1992).
  - Similar principles as in motivational interviewing: Asking open-ended questions, reflective listening, developing a menu of options, consider the pros and cons of the status quo and proposed change, affirming and validating.

BIOPSYCHOSOCIAL MODEL

The practice of nursing emphasizes a holistic approach when providing care. The biological premise of mental illness is based on the theory when neurons malfunction symptoms are manifest (Stahl, 2013). Behaviors can alter brain chemistry which in turn can also permanently alter the neuronal response. For example, risk-taking behavior may provide the feeling of an adrenaline rush. When the rush is over, the body will return to the baseline state of rest, but when this behavior is repeated over time consistently, cravings and withdrawal symptoms may develop. Alternatively, genetic mutations, neuronal dysfunction, receptor insensitivity may also produce many of the symptoms associated with psychiatric disorders leading to maladaptive behaviors. For these reasons, the etiology of a psychiatric disorder is insufficiently accounted for by one theory. In order to capture the broad array of underlying variables that may be causing signs and symptoms, a biopsychosocial model serves as the most common framework to address mental illness. Within the biopsychosocial model, the PMHN must consider predisposing, precipitating, perpetuating, and protective factors in each of the three domains that comprise this framework.

Table 3.6 Etiology of Mental Illness Grid

Domain	Predisposing Factors	Precipitating Factors	Perpetuating Factors	Protective Factors
Biological				
Psychological				
Sociological/ environmental				

- **Biological:** Age, race, sex, weight, comorbid conditions, toxins, infection, medications, nutrition, hydration
- **Psychological:** Resilience, history of abuse, neglect, trauma, parental attachment, self-efficacy, self-esteem, automatic thoughts, delusions, perceptions, neurodevelopmental stage, aspirations, coping mechanisms, therapeutic alliance, transference
- **Social/environmental:** Housing, safety, relationships, financial resources, educational resources, accessibility, support systems, legal status, cultural assimilation

A biopsychosocial approach to mental illness requires a thorough assessment across the domains of life to develop an accurate understanding of the client (Table 3.6).

NONPHARMACOLOGICAL TREATMENTS

Nonpharmacological treatments are sometimes referred to as talk therapy. Talk therapy is commonly referred to as psychotherapy and can include group therapy, family therapy, and complementary alternative therapies. As the nurse provides care in a holistic and integrative fashion, it is essential to become well versed in nonpharmacological treatments. A purely psychopharmacological approach to mental illness does not take into account environmental and interpersonal stressors and the coping mechanisms used to mitigate adverse effects. An integrated approach is the most beneficial in treating psychiatric disorders.

Many patients are resistant to the use of psychopharmacology initially and are more receptive to nonpharmacological interventions, particularly in dealing with children, pregnancy, and the geriatric population. Psychopharmacology in some cultures bears a stigma that serves as a psychological barrier to care. People may seek therapy for a variety of reasons beyond self-discovery and individual betterment. Some common reasons people seek therapy include loss, interpersonal conflicts, symptom management such as panic and phobia, and unfulfilled life expectations, particularly around significant transitions. Another common reason for nonpharmacological therapy is to help patients with personality disorders, particularly narcissistic and borderline personality disorders. Often nonpharmacological therapy is court ordered by the legal system or as a contingency of continued employment. The primary goal in therapy is to establish and maintain a therapeutic alliance (Table 3.7).

- **Therapeutic alliance:** A psychodynamic phenomenon characterizing the perceived bond between the patient and therapist. Most predictive factor in a successful outcome.

Table 3.7 Three Phases of Therapy

Phase/Purpose	Therapist Behavior	Client Behavior
Orientation ■ The nurse listens to the client and develops a general impression of the situation then validates the findings by checking with the client for accuracy	■ Identify goals ■ Establish boundaries ■ Set expectations ■ Outline treatment options ■ Expected timeline ■ Build trust	■ Reluctance to disclose ■ Avoidant ■ Guarded ■ Ambivalence ■ Elation ■ Resistance ■ Flight into health
Working/treatment ■ The nurse may help the client through experiential learning, developing coping strategies	■ Prioritizing goals ■ Health monitoring ■ Symptom management/distress tolerance ■ Facilitate coping ■ Reevaluate ■ Counter-transference	■ Transference ■ Increased resistance ■ Increased ambivalence ■ May threaten early termination ■ May test boundaries
Termination ■ The interaction may be mutually beneficial for the nurse and the client	■ Summarize progress and care ■ Promote self-care ■ Remind of effective coping strategies ■ Strengthen self-efficacy ■ Referrals ■ Identify signs of relapse & when to seek care again	■ Signs and symptoms return remerge ■ Provocation ■ Regression ■ Resistance to termination

- Key elements include:
  - Mutual trust
  - Mutual respect
  - Attentiveness
  - Reflective listening
  - Eye contact
  - Summarizing
  - Validating
  - Affirming

▶ INDIVIDUAL THERAPY

The most common form of nonpharmacological treatments is based on a host of theoretical frameworks. Historically, the most common framework informing individual talk therapy was the psychoanalytic model popularized by Sigmund Freud ("the talking cure"). The most common form of nonpharmacological therapy currently is CBT developed by Aaron Beck. CBT has served as a foundation on which many other nonpharmacological therapies build. Other nonpharmacological therapies include dialectical behavioral therapy (DBT) originated by Marsha Linehan, existential therapy originated by Viktor Frankl, humanistic therapy originated by Carl Rogers, interpersonal therapy (IPT) originated by Gerald Klerman and Myrna Weissman, and eye movement desensitization and reprocessing (EMDR) originated by Francine Shapiro. The various elements of these therapeutic approaches are expanded and adapted into group and system (family) therapy settings.

- **Psychoanalytic therapy** (Sigmund Freud 1856–1939)
  - Based on the premise that unconscious motivations and instinctual drives cause the implementation of defense mechanisms
  - Change happens by promoting greater insight and awareness regarding defense mechanisms (see Table 3.5)
  - Based on speculation of psychodynamic developmental factors that may have occurred earlier in life, particularly within the first 5 years
  - Traditional psychoanalysis is conducted over many years and consists of hour-long sessions four times a week
- **Cognitive behavioral therapy** (Aaron Beck 1921–present and Arnold Lazarus 1932–present)
  - Focuses on present events and maladaptive responses/behaviors (Figure 3.2)
  - Uses many tools to collect data between therapeutic sessions emptied to capture the client's expectations, perceptions, and interpretations of events that are leading to distress
  - Helps the client to view reality more objectively by examining cognitive distortions and automatic thought patterns
  - The aim is to change the client's irrational beliefs, cognitive distortions, and dysfunctional thought patterns by implementing contrary behaviors
  - Typical exercises include exposure, systematic desensitization, problem-solving, role-playing, and enhancing the locus of control
  - Socratic questioning and diaries capture data that provides grist for the mill of the therapeutic session

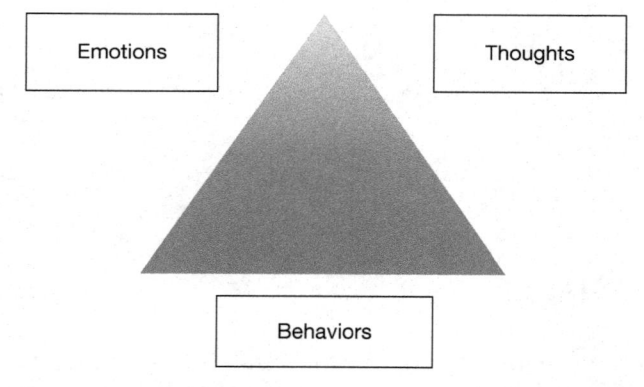

Figure 3.2 Cognitive behavioral therapy triangle. Emotions can affect behaviors and thoughts; thoughts can affect emotions and behaviors; behaviors can affect emotions and thoughts. Triggering a change in one construct will trigger a change in the other two.

- **Dialectical behavioral therapy** (Marsha Linehan 1943–present)
  - Most common and effective therapy for clients with borderline and narcissistic traits
  - Building on the CBT premise of behavioral activation

- Aims to regulate emotions, increase distress tolerance, develop self-management and interpersonal skills, and promote mindfulness
  - Reduce nonsuicidal self-injurious behavior (NSSIB), decreased passive fatigue, decreased crisis generating behavior, decrease self-invalidation, increase emotional awareness and communication.
- **Existential therapy** (Viktor Frankl 1905–1997)
  - Socratic questioning to enhance reflection and self-confrontation
  - Based on the premise of finding purpose in one's life and circumstances
  - Emphasizes accepting reality and responsible decision-making
  - Aims to have the client live an authentically consistent life focusing on the present and future aspirations based on desire and one's moral framework
    - **Socratic questioning:** A method of eliciting information and facilitating the discussion within the frame of therapy. The goal is to understand the problem from the client's perspective and to help the client discover the discrepancy between the status quo and the desired outcome. This form of questioning helps illuminate the cognitive distortions and defense mechanisms that are causing the problems that have led to the need for behavioral healthcare. Socratic questions can be used in any type of talk therapy.
      - **Clarification questions**: Helps clients identify their beliefs or examine them at a deeper level.
        - "What do you mean when you say … ?"
        - "What makes you say that?"
        - "Are you saying … or … ?"
        - "Can you say that another way?"
        - "What makes you think or act in this way?"
        - "What does this say about you?"
      - Probing assumptions for evidence; building a menu of options can help the client have more insight to build upon previously held beliefs or develop new, more adaptive beliefs.
        - "How did you come to this conclusion?"
        - "What else could we assume?"
        - "How can you verify or disprove … ?"
        - "What would happen if … ?"
        - "If this happened to a friend or family member would you have the same thoughts about them?"
        - "Are these the only explanations?"
        - "Are these reasons good enough?"
        - "Would … stand up in court of law as evidence? How might it be refuted in court?"
        - "What evidence is there to support what you are saying?"
        - "Has anyone in your life ever expressed a different opinion? Why do you think that is?"
      - Broadening the client's perspectives; inviting other possibilities can help clients see that there are other equally valid perspectives that promote locus of control and sense of safety.
        - "What alternative ways of looking at this are there?"
        - "What does it do for you to continue to think this way?"

- "Who benefits from this?"
- "What is the difference between ... (this perspective) and ... (that perspective)?"
- "What makes is this perspective better than that perspective?"
- "What are the strengths and weaknesses of ... ?"
- "How are ... and ... similar?"
- "What would ... say about it?"
- "What if you compared ... and ... ?"
- "How could you look at this another way?"
  - Analyzing and considering consequences helps a client examine potential outcomes of their beliefs and behaviors to see if they are desirable, clients may realize that their beliefs are causing their distress. Some examples include:
    - "Then what would happen?"
    - "What are the positive and negative consequences of that assumption or belief?"
    - "How does your belief affect your life (e.g., relationships, daily functioning, job, school)?"
    - "How does this belief fit with what we've learned in session before?"
    - "What makes this ... important?"
    - "What can we assume will happen if you continue to live according to this belief?"
    - "What would it mean if you gave up that belief?"
    - "How would you benefit by changing this belief?"
- **Summarizing and synthesizing:** The nurse should convey empathy and continually enhance the therapeutic alliance by being transparent about why particular questions are asked and take time to reflect what was heard. This can help ensure that the nurse and the client are of similar understanding of the problem. During this phase, the client is able to look at the new information in a holistic light. Some examples include:
  - "Let me make sure I understand. It sounds like you believe ... and that this is why ..."
  - "How does what we talked about today fit with your previous belief ... "
  - "What are your reactions to the evidence that we looked at?"
  - "What do you think you should do with this new information?"
  - "What would it look like if you were to change your belief?"
- **Humanistic therapy** (Carl Rogers 1902–1987)
  - Sometimes called "patient-centered therapy"
  - Assumes man is good
  - Builds on the CBT technique of Socratic questioning to induce positive emotions and the existential therapy emphasis on purpose and meaning
    - Specific aims include facilitating self-directed growth toward self-actualization (Maslow) and finding meaning in life and circumstances
    - Gratitude journals:
      - "What surprised me today?"
      - "What moved me today?"

- "What inspired me today?"
  - Encouraging socialization behaviors, loving kindness meditation, altruism, savoring (dwelling on positive events) rather than rumination (dwelling on negative events and consequences)
- **Interpersonal therapy** (Gerald Klerman 1928–1992 and Myrna Weissman (1940–present)
  - Socratic questioning to examine interpersonal issues that are creating current distress
  - Manualized and time limited: Focuses on the present and interpersonal distress
  - Specially developed for symptoms of depression, effective in adolescents and adults
- **Eye movement desensitization and reprocessing** (Francine Shapiro 1948–present)
  - Builds on CBT constructs of behavioral activation and exposure therapy, distraction, reflection
  - Distraction by bilateral stimulation of both cerebral hemispheres by moving eyes back and forth between two points, or alternating tapping between hands, or stereo sounds alternating between ears
  - Commonly used in post-traumatic stress disorder to achieve adaptive resolution
  - The patient must be able to tolerate and narrate their trauma
  - **Phase 1—desensitization** (while remaining attentive to present physical sensation or activity)
    - Visualize the trauma
    - Verbalize negative thoughts and maladaptive beliefs
    - Ask the client to block out negative thoughts, breathe deeply, and then verbalize what he or she is thinking, feeling, or imagining
  - **Phase 2—installation phase:** The client increases the intensity of positive replacement thoughts of the original negative thought or emotion
  - **Phase 3—body scan:** The client then visualizes the trauma alongside the positive thought and then scans their body mentally to identify any physical areas of tension

▶ GROUP THERAPY (IRVIN YALOM, 1931–PRESENT)

- Group therapy builds on CBT and psychoanalytic constructs (defense mechanisms)
  - 10 therapeutic (curative) factors of group psychotherapy
    - **Universality:** Participants discover others with similar circumstances, thoughts, feelings, behaviors. Premised on Maslow's hierarchy need for belonging
    - **Altruism:** Provides an opportunity to help participants progress in something. Premised on mature defense mechanisms
    - **Interpersonal learning:** Interactions with other people provide opportunities to learn about relationship dynamics and intimacy
    - **Imitative behaviors:** Allows participants to copy the behaviors of others. The behavior may be adaptive or maladaptive
    - **Group cohesiveness:** Participants develop an attraction to other group members, and a sense of belonging is enhanced

- **Catharsis:** The opportunity to openly express previously suppressed feelings, thoughts, and insights
- **Existential factors:** Participants learn to find meaning in loss and suffering and learn to deal with the frustrations of reality rather than reverting to a previous pattern of avoidance
- **Corrective refocusing:** Participants can visit issues related to the family of origin through the recapitulation of family dynamics as they arise within the group. The group serves as a substitute family where group members are siblings, and the facilitator is the parental figure
- **Installation of hope:** Participants can witness changes in other group members, allowing them to actualize the possibility of personal change and a better life
- **Increased development of social skills:** The group provides a natural laboratory for immediate feedback regarding the effectiveness of an individual's adaptive or maladaptive behavior

- **Five phases of group dynamics:** When forming the psychodynamic group, the leader/facilitator must identify the purpose, goals, and membership criteria and size of the group. Obtaining informed consent of each before participation to explain the risks and benefits of such a group, including breach of confidentiality, obligations of attending, and plans for aftercare. The phases of group dynamics are similar to the three phases of individual therapy in which early phases are marked by hesitancy and reluctance pending the development of a therapeutic alliance. Transference and counter transference among group members frames the working phase of the group process and is demonstrated in cohesiveness and catharsis. The termination phase differs in that reemergence of symptoms is less likely because group members can provide immediate feedback and remind of previously acquired skills.
    - **Forming:** Feeling guarded, anxious, and fearful regarding issues of self-disclosure and acceptance is common among peers. Therapeutic alliance needs to develop among group members. Identify goals, expectations, and boundaries in this phase.
    - **Storming:** Participants in this phase will demonstrate resistance and sabotaging behaviors, issues related to clique formation, and loss of control will begin to surface. The leader should allow for expression of both positive and negative feelings and help the group to examine nonproductive behaviors and underlying conflicts.
    - **Norming:** Group members have overcome initial resistance and begin to develop cohesion. Open and spontaneous communication occurs, and the group norms are solidified.
    - **Performing:** The primary objective and work of the group become more focused, members begin to engage in creative problem solving, interpersonal learning takes place in the group is unified toward goal achievement.
    - **Adjourning:** Active termination process in which leaders and members express their feelings about each other in regards to termination, review achieved goals and outcomes and identify future work remaining.

▶ FAMILY THERAPIES

- A system-based approach focusing on feedback loops that are perpetuating maladaptive behaviors and inhibiting adaptive behaviors. The process by which all family members operate is known as the family system
  - Premised on the idea that any individual member must feel understood within the context of the family system
  - Family systems operate on a set of rules (be they overt or covert). The therapist seeks to learn and discover these rules.
    - **Boundaries:** Protective mechanisms that maintain the functional integrity of the family unit, individuals, and sub-systems within the family
      - **Rigid boundaries:** Cause estrangement long-term or disengagement in the short term
      - **Diffuse boundaries:** Causes enmeshment and parentification of children
      - **Clearly defined boundaries:** Individuals maintain their unique identities while communicating love and belonging to all the members of the system
    - **Circular causality:** A feedback loop characterized by a series of actions and reactions which perpetuate a problem
    - **Homeostasis:** Familial tendency to resist change in order to maintain a steady state, even if the state is one of dysfunction
    - **Adaptability:** The family's tendency and ability to change when necessary or remain the same in the midst of change
- **Family systems therapy (Murray Bowen, 1913–1990):** Assumes an individual's behavior serves a role or function within the family unit, perpetuating or protecting against dysfunction. The goal of treatment is to increase familial awareness among individuals. The increased awareness allows individual to perceive their self-worth separate from the role they play in the family. Record family dynamics on a genogram which allows for visual representation of relationships and hierarchies.
  - **Key concepts:**
    - **Self-differentiation:** Perceiving one's intrinsic value rather than depending on external relationships and circumstances to derive self-worth
    - **Triangles:** A dyadic relationship that extends to a triad in order to reduce stress within the dyad more commonly occurs in morphostatic (less adaptable) families
    - **Nuclear family:** Characterized in families where the parental units level of differentiation is reflective of familial differentiation (e.g., if parents perceive their intrinsic self-worth, those in their care will also perceive their self-worth)
    - **Transmission process:** Passing along dysfunctional behaviors throughout generations of the family unit
    - **Projection process:** Parental differentiation is transmitted to the most susceptible child (parent derives their self-worth from the relationship with a child, creates an enmeshed dyad)
    - **Cutoffs:** The breaking of contact with the family of origin
    - **Birth order:** An influencing factor in familial interactions and individual personality characteristics

- **Structural family therapy (Salvador Minuchin, 1913–1990):** Drawing from family systems therapy in which the therapist's role is to gain an understanding of familial transactions in order to implement a change of organization in order to manage problems more effectively. Symptoms are a product of dysfunctional transaction patterns within the family. The family structure is a frame created by functional demands that articulate the transactional processes (dyadic, triangulation, transmission, projection, cutoffs, and boundary type) within the system.
- **Strategic therapy (Jay Haley, 1923–2007):** A psychoanalytically informed behavioral therapy approach in which symptoms represent metaphors reflecting problems within the hierarchical structure. Symptoms are a means of communication within the family system. This therapy aims to help family members behave in a manner that will not perpetuate problem behaviors and thereby reduce symptoms.
  - Interventions are problem-focused with less emphasis on symptomatology
  - Behavioral interventions prescribed that target the necessary sequence of interactions that maintain the problem behavior
  - Socratic questioning elicits the necessary information
  - **Directives:** Tasks and behaviors designed with the expectation of family members compliance
  - **Reframing belief systems:** Providing/eliciting an alternative vocabulary to label problem behaviors in a more positive light (e.g., meddling reframed as concerned).
  - **Paradoxical directives:** Assigning a negative task/prescribing the problem to a resistant family member with the expectation of noncompliance (e.g., wife nags husband from the minute he wakes up until the time he goes to bed because she cares about his well-being. Husband shuts down and becomes avoidant. Tell the wife she can only nag her husband a particular time of the day [6 pm–7 pm]; after that, she has to save it for tomorrow.) The idea is that the wife forgets to nag him at the assigned time, and the problem is reduced. Paradoxical exercises should be used with caution.
- **Solution-focused therapy (Steve de Shazer, 1940–2005; Bill O'Hanlon, 1952–present; and Insoo Berg, 1934–2007):** A family therapy approach premised on elements of CBT in which the therapist is capitalizing on solutions that it previously worked while enhancing individual and familial self-efficacy. This strength-based approach uses Socratic questioning to elicit necessary information and to probe for possibilities of solution.
  - **Miracle question:** "If a miracle were to happen tonight while you are asleep, and tomorrow morning you awoke to find that the problem no longer existed, what would be different?"
    - "How would you know if the miracle took place?"
    - "How would others know if the miracle took place?"
  - **Exception-finding questions:** Inquiring about a time in life when the problem did not exist helps the family move toward solutions by noting exceptions to the problem pattern of behavior.
  - **Scaling questions:** "On a 1 to 10 scale with one being the worst and ten being the best how would you rate your feelings now." (This helps people realize incremental changes over time).
    - "On a scale of 0 to 10 with 0 being unimportant and 10 being of the utmost importance, how important is it to make this change now?" This allows the

therapist to elicit what is more important and less important and uncover other perpetuating behaviors.

▶ COMPLEMENTARY AND ALTERNATIVE THERAPIES

- Increasing in popularity, patients are drawn to this type of treatment because they perceive more control over decision-making. There is also increased stigma (in certain social circles) associated with allopathic remedies, associated costs of traditional prescriptions, and unmet expectations associated with failed remedies of traditional treatment. Evidence supporting the use of complementary and alternative treatments is limited and depends on each specific modality or supplement. Safety for use during pregnancy and lactation is unknown and inadvisable according to standard medical practice in the United States.
  - **Mind–body interventions:** These therapies include guided imagery, meditation, yoga, and biofeedback.
    - Biofeedback has the most evidence to date and operates on the premise of raising awareness and learning somatic quieting as noted in CBT. Physiological effects are notable on vital signs and brain waves.
      - The person learns to control autonomic functions such as breath, heart rate, and perception.
      - Measure improvement through a reduction in signs, reports of symptoms (intensity and frequency).
      - Yoga draws on similar elements of biofeedback of raising awareness, controlling muscle tension and breath
      - Meditation drawing on elements of biofeedback raises awareness with an attempt to reduce involuntary reactivity to the environment, helping the individual gain an increased sense of control. Physiological effects are notable on vital signs and brain waves.
  - **Manipulative physical interventions:** Interventions such as acupressure and acupuncture, massage, and reflexology are increasingly accessible, seen as possibly helpful and not harmful; patients have readily embraced them.
    - Acupressure and acupuncture, based on tenets of Chinese medicine, in which the practitioner corrects vital energy (Chi) throughout the body. Studies regarding efficacy are mixed.
      - Alterations in brain chemistry may occur by the release of neurohormones and neurotransmitters triggered by tactile stimuli.
    - Massage: Enhances circulation and lymphatic drainage. It is covered by some insurance providers, qualifies for FSA and HSA card use when prescribed for specific conditions.
      - Reflexology is thought to exert similar effects. However, the theory underpinning the practice is based on Chinese medicine.
  - **Biological therapies:** Interventions in this modality include herbal products, vitamins, nutraceuticals, and aromatherapy. Evidence supporting the use of these products is limited, and risk of harm is potentially unknown, mainly when used in combination with other medications. These products are not regulated by any

authority. There is tremendous variability among products. Inform patients of potential risks related to contamination and toxicity.
- **Fish oils:** May contain a combination of omega-6 and omega-3 fatty acids. Known risk of bleeding with NSAIDs, warfarin, garlic, and ginkgo (if taken in highly potent supplement form). SSRIs also can inhibit platelet reuptake of serotonin which inhibits aggregation. It should be stopped before surgery.
- **Melatonin:** Commonly used for jetlag, adverse effects are dose-dependent, contents of the product are variable. Known interactions include: NSAIDs (increased risk of bleeding), beta-blocker (slowed heart rate), Valerian, Kava Kava, alcohol increased CNS suppression.
- **Tryptophan:** Used for pain, depression, headache, obesity. Known risks include increased risk of serotonin syndrome when used in conjunction with SSRIs, MAOIs, St. John's Wort.
- **Sam-e (*S*-adenosyl-L-methionine):** A naturally occurring compound found in all cells, used for depression and pain. Adverse effects include manic symptoms, movement disorders, and serotonin syndrome.
- **Omega-3 fatty acids:** Used for attention deficit hyperactivity disorder, inflammatory conditions, circulatory problems. Known to interact adversely with NSAIDs and anticoagulants. Bleeding risk is compounded when used with SSRIs. Should be stopped before surgery.

KNOWLEDGE CHECK: CHAPTER 3

1. A psychiatric-mental health nurse is facilitating a group for at-risk teens who have been mandated to attend meetings as part of their addiction treatment. A member of the group states that his problem is not that bad, and he can stop anytime he chooses. Using on occasion is just a way to have fun with friends. Which concepts of the Health Belief Model best describes the group member's readiness to change?

   A. Perceived severity and perceived barriers
   B. Self-efficacy and perceived benefits
   C. Cues to action and perceived susceptibility
   D. Self-efficacy and perceived susceptibility

2. A member attending a teen addiction treatment group for the first time expresses gratitude for being court ordered to attend the recovery group instead of serving prison time, and he realizes how out of control he was while using. Which Health Belief Model concept is demonstrated?

   A. Perceived severity and perceived barriers
   B. Self-efficacy and perceived benefits
   C. Cues to action and perceived severity
   D. Self-efficacy and perceived susceptibility

3. A 30-year-old man with three past psychiatric hospitalizations for schizoaffective disorder presents for follow-up in the partial hospital program. Before discharge, the patient received court-ordered Zyprexa Relprev 300 mg IM X 1. The patient tells the psychiatric-mental health nurse that he is aware that smoking can "make him need more medication." In which stage of change is the patient?

   A. Precontemplation
   B. Contemplation
   C. Preparation
   D. Action

4. The psychiatric-mental health nurse is caring for a 20-year-old man with bipolar I disorder. The patient indicates that he does not have a problem because he can accomplish so much during his manic episodes. Which stage of change is the patient in?

   A. Precontemplation
   B. Contemplation
   C. Preparation
   D. Action

(See answers next page.)

1. A) Perceived severity and perceived barriers
The member is expressing the belief regarding the seriousness of the condition as minimal and that the cost of abstaining from the addiction is reducing time with friends. Self-efficacy is an individual's belief in his or her innate ability to achieve a goal, and perceived benefits refer to the individual's perception of the effectiveness of an action to reduce a threat or illness. Perceived susceptibility is the individual's perception of acquiring disease or illness, and cues to action are stimuli necessary to trigger a health-promoting behavior.

2. C) Cues to action and perceived severity
The member describes the trigger that activated the ability to take action and the seriousness of the condition and sequelae. Perceived barriers are the belief in the tangible and psychological costs associated with the advised behavior. Perceived severity is the individual's belief of how serious a condition and its consequences are. Self-efficacy is an individual's belief in his or her innate ability to achieve a goal.

3. B) Contemplation
He is in the contemplation stage: The patient has indicated that a problem exists but has not expressed a desire to change. Precontemplation—in this stage, people do not intend to take action in the foreseeable future (defined as within the next 6 months). Preparation (determination)—in this stage, people are ready to take action within the next 30 days. Action—in this stage, people have recently changed their behavior (defined as within the last 6 months) and intend to keep moving forward with that behavior change.

4. A) Precontemplation
The patient is in the precontemplation stage; in this stage, people do not intend to take action in the foreseeable future (defined as within the next 6 months). The patient denies the problem and has no intention of making a change. Contemplation—in this stage, people intend to start healthy behavior in the foreseeable future (defined as within the next 6 months). Preparation (determination)—in this stage, people are ready to take action within the next 30 days. Action—in this stage, people have recently changed their behavior (defined as within the last 6 months) and intend to keep moving forward with that behavior change.

5. The psychiatric-mental health nurse is explaining the risks and benefits of long-acting injectable antipsychotics to a patient with a history of medication nonadherence. The patient is asking logical questions that demonstrate he can understand the facts. Which process of changing represents the patient's position?

   A. Social liberation
   B. Reinforcement management
   C. Self-liberation
   D. Consciousness raising

6. A patient was prescribed naltrexone and bupropion for binge eating disorder by her primary care provider. The patient has lost 4 pounds since her last visit 1 month ago. The patient states that sometimes she finds it very difficult not to binge eat when her emotions are intense and expresses doubt in her ability to make a lasting change. The best response is:

   A. "I can increase your dose of medication or augment you with another medication."
   B. "On a scale of 1 to 10 how important is this change for you to make?"
   C. "Give me an example of something in your life that you are most proud of achieving."
   D. "Would you like a referral to a dietician?"

7. A 35-year-old female with personality disorder not otherwise specified takes quetiapine 50 mg qhs for sleep and 12.5 mg q6h PRN for anxiety. She tells the psychiatric-mental health nurse that no one seems to understand how much stress she is under and would like to change providers. The best response is:

   A. "Do you think you need your medication adjusted?"
   B. "It sounds to me like you are frustrated and do not feel listened to."
   C. "I can give you a list of three psychiatrists whom you can choose from to give you the care you want."
   D. "It will take some time for the medication to reach full effect before you are feeling better."

8. Which of the following is a therapeutic technique to facilitate a health behavior change in a 28-year-old male with substance use disorder who is in denial regarding the severity of his habit?

   A. Solution-focused therapy
   B. Strategic therapy
   C. Psychopharmacology with naltrexone 50 mg daily
   D. Motivational interviewing

(See answers next page.)

5. D) Consciousness raising

The patient is in the consciousness raising stage (i.e., increasing awareness about healthy behavior and discovering and accepting facts in support of the health behavior change). Social liberation—environmental opportunities that exist to show society is supportive of healthy behavior. Reinforcement management—rewarding the positive behavior and reducing the rewards that come from negative behavior. Self-liberation—commitment to change behavior based on the belief that achievement of the healthy behavior is possible. Consciousness raising—increasing awareness about healthy behavior.

6. C) "Give me an example of something in your life that you are most proud of achieving"

The patient is expressing low self-efficacy; by asking about past successes, the patient's self-efficacy may be enhanced. Although augmenting the medication may be possible, the patient is experiencing the positive effects of the medication (weight loss).

7. B) "It sounds to me like you are frustrated and do not feel listened to"

Express empathy by affirming the client's feelings and demonstrating reflective listening by using her words to gain insight into her motivations. Asking if she needs her medication adjusted invalidates her feelings, as does giving her an answer about medication efficacy. Offering her a list of referrals may communicate a lack of commitment to the therapeutic relationship if done without exploring underlying motivation.

8. D) Motivational interviewing

Motivational interviewing will allow the psychiatric-mental health nurse to hear the client's reasons for maintaining the status quo as well as elicit his reasons for what it would take to trigger a desire to change. Solution-focused therapy is a goal-directed psychotherapy based on direct observation of a series of precisely constructed questions. Strategic (family) therapy does not focus on the individual but the social structure. Psychopharmacology may be appropriate, but the naltrexone is not indicated as the substance is not specified.

9. A 65-year-old female was discovered in her apartment by police, who called an ambulance for transport to the hospital after her neighbors had not seen her in several days. The patient received IV hydration, and her labs show microcytic hypochromic anemia. She is admitted to inpatient psychiatry for evaluation and treatment of what is thought to be a hoarding disorder. Which need is of primary concern to the psychiatric-mental health nurse?

   A. Adequate nutrition, hydration, and safety planning
   B. The patient feeling a sense of belonging
   C. The patient attends psychosocial rehab groups
   D. The patient requires forms for the Family Medical Leave Act

10. A 60-year-old man with alcohol use disorder in remission presents to the psychiatric emergency department and is very distraught. He tells the psychiatric-mental health nurse that he was at his daughter's wedding and called upon to make a toast. The waiter had handed him the champagne glass, and he took a sip of alcohol for the first time in 10 years. Which of the following is the best response from the psychiatric-mental health nurse?

    A. "Don't worry; it was only one drink."
    B. "How have you been able to maintain your sobriety for so long?"
    C. Tell the patient he will be admitted to inpatient rehab.
    D. Start the patient on naltrexone 50 mg daily for alcohol use disorder.

11. A 25-year-old female, admitted to an extended observation psychiatric unit, observes that another patient is placed on 1:1 observation status after expressing suicidal ideations to her psychiatrist. The patient rings the call bell to tell the psychiatric-mental health nurse that she would like to have 1:1 observation because she, too, is feeling suicidal. Which of the following is the best response from the psychiatric-mental health nurse?

    A. "What is your plan to commit suicide?"
    B. "I will place you on 1:1 status; your safety is very important to us."
    C. Call the provider on call for an order of Haldol 5 mg and Ativan 2 mg PO X 1 now.
    D. Put the patient in therapeutic seclusion to prevent self-harm.

12. A middle-school girl who is timid to take any risks, prefers solitary activities, and does not ask questions of her teachers for fear that she is bothering them likely did not master which developmental stage?

    A. Trust versus mistrust
    B. Autonomy versus shame and doubt
    C. Industry versus inferiority
    D. Initiative versus guilt

(See answers next page.)

9. A) Adequate nutrition, hydration, and safety planning

Physiological needs must take priority over psychological needs. According to Maslow's hierarchy, physiological needs include sex, food, water, warmth, and rest, followed by safety needs, then psychological needs of love and belonging, esteem needs including prestige and feelings of accomplishment, and finally, self-actualization defined as achieving one's full potential and using creative energy.

10. B) "How have you been able to maintain your sobriety for so long?"

The patient is expressing a fear of relapse. Enhancing the patient's self-efficacy by having him reflect on the effective strategies that have been previously working for him will reduce his risk of relapse. Telling a patient not to worry is invalidating. It is not appropriate to admit a patient to inpatient rehab as he has not relapsed but lapsed. Starting the patient on naltrexone for daily use may be appropriate as part of enhancing sobriety, but the Sinclair method, in this case, is a more tailored response and does not negate his adaptive coping mechanisms for the past 10 years.

11. A) "What is your plan to commit suicide?"

Patients may express suicidal ideation, but the psychiatric-mental health nurse must engage in a therapeutic conversation to assess lethality, means, coping strategies, and protective factors; the act of making time for the assessment can communicate psychosocial support and meet the underlying need of safety and belonging. Before requesting a treatment, a complete assessment is necessary.

12. D) Initiative versus guilt

Failing to master the stage of initiative versus guilt inhibits the development of purpose and virtue, and children remain followers, lack self-initiative, and can feel like they are a bother to others. Middle-school children are in the stage of development of industry versus inferiority and moving toward identity versus role confusion.

13. A 66-year-old registered nurse, who retired from psychiatry 3 years ago, spends much of her time watching television. She is easily irritated by those interrupting her shows and has no desire to engage in any activities or identify with a broader community. Which developmental stage did she fail to master?

    A. Generativity versus stagnation
    B. Ego integrity versus despair
    C. Industry versus inferiority
    D. Initiative versus guilt

14. A woman who discovers her husband has committed suicide in the middle of the night decides to tell her 4- and 6-year-old children the next morning that the reason daddy is not here today is that he went to work. What might they assume when mommy says she is going to work?

    A. Going to work means you are not coming home
    B. Mommy will come home, as has been the case in the past
    C. When someone cannot be seen, then they cease to exist
    D. Daddy will come home when mommy goes to work

15. A client has been in therapy for generalized anxiety disorder with depressive symptoms. Treatment has included both psychopharmacology and interpersonal psychotherapy. The patient abruptly reports a reemergence of the symptoms that have been in remission. In what phase of therapy is this an expected finding?

    A. Orientation
    B. Working/treatment
    C. Termination
    D. Acclimation

(See answers next page.)

13. A) Generativity versus stagnation

Mastering the developmental stage of generativity versus stagnation leads to the development of caring as a virtue and a desire to be a part of a broader community, leave a legacy, and feel useful. Failing to master this stage yields a lack of interest in the broader community and feelings of leading a disconnected existence with a nothing to contribute.

14. A) Going to work means you are not coming home

Children in this stage are considered preoperational and have an organized schema that has helped them understand that when people go to work, they come back. Thinking at this stage is egocentric and magical. Introducing this new accommodation to the children will make them think that when mommy goes to work, she will not be returning home.

15. C) Termination

During the termination phase of a therapeutic relationship, the client may experience reemergence of symptoms previously in remission as a manifestation of regression and resistance to termination. During the orientation phase, the patient may demonstrate symptoms of a reluctance to disclose, avoidance, guardedness, ambivalence, and elation. During the working treatment phase, the patient may manifest transference, increased resistance, increased ambivalence, and threaten early termination.

REFERENCES

Bandura, A. (1989). Human agency in social cognitive theory. *The American Psychologist*, *44*, 1175–84. https://doi.org/10.1037/0003-066x.44.9.1175

Erikson, E. (1956). The problem of ego identity. *Journal of the American Psychoanalytic Association*, *4*, 56–121. Retrieved from http://www.pep-web.org/document.php?id=apa.004.0056a

Larimer, M. E., Palmer, R. S., & Marlatt, G. A. (1999). *Relapse prevention: An overview of Marlatt's Cognitive-Behavioral Model*. Retrieved from https://pubs.niaaa.nih.gov/publications/arh23-2/151-160.pdf

Maiman, L. A., & Becker, M. H. (1974). The Health Belief Model: Origins and correlates in psychological theory. *Health Education Monographs*, *2*(4), 336–353. https://doi.org/10.1177/109019817400200404

Maslow, A. H. (1969). *Psychology of science: A reconnaissance*. Maurice Bassett Publishing.

Miller, W., & Rollnick, S. (2012). *Motivational interviewing: Helping people change*. Retrieved from https://books.google.com/books?hl=en&id=o1-ZpM7QqVQC&oi=fnd&pg=PP1&dq=motivational+interviewing+Miller+and+Rollnick+1991&ots=c0DheLglGW&sig=6MiIOC64-2W4Ytd-Tllo3FJ8fGw

Peplau, H. E. (1992). Interpersonal relations: A theoretical framework for application in nursing practice. *Nursing Science Quarterly*, *5*(1), 13–18. https://doi.org/10.1177/089431849200500106

Prochaska, J. O., & Diclemente, C. C. (1986). *Toward a comprehensive model of change*. In *Treating addictive behaviors* (pp. 3–27). Boston, MA: Springer US. https://doi.org/10.1007/978-1-4613-2191-0_1

Prochaska, J. O., & Velicer, W. F. (1997). The transtheoretical model of health behavior change. *American Journal of Health Promotion*, *12*(1), 38–48. https://doi.org/10.4278/0890-1171-12.1.38

Sadock, B., Sadock, V., Ruiz, P. (2015). *Synopsis of psychiatry* (11th ed.). New York: Wolters Kluwer | Lippincott Williams & Wilkins.

Stahl, S. M. (2013). *Stahl's essential psychopharmacology: Neuroscientific basis and practical applications*.

Sullivan, H. (1955). *The interpersonal theory of psychiatry*. New York. Retrieved from https://content.taylorfrancis.com/books/download?dac=C2004-0-01296-0&isbn=9781136439292&format=googlePreviewPdf

Neuroanatomy, Physiology, and Psychopharmacology

OBJECTIVES

- Nervous system anatomy and physiology overview
- Neurotransmitters and their functions
- Neuroimaging
- Genomics
- Neuropsychological testing
- Describe pharmacokinetics across the life span
- Describe the pharmacodynamics of psychotropic medication
- Explain the role of inducers and inhibitors
- Describe dose ranges and specific monitoring associated with:
  - Antipsychotics
  - Antidepressants
  - Mood stabilizing agents
  - Anxiolytics
  - Stimulants

FAST FACTS

- Brains contain approximately 150 billion neurons
- Axons transmit information from the brain, and dendrites receive information from the body
- Neurotransmission is the process of electrical information moving across synapses by chemical means
- The more caudal (inferiorly) the brain, the more primitive functions it controls. For example, the brain stem and spinal cord organize life-preserving reflexes, promote arousal or sleep, and process sensory input and motor output (hand to stove, pain, withdraw) interneuron mediated
- The hypothalamus regulates eating, drinking, sexual behavior, aggression, temperature, and the endocrine system
- The limbic system includes the amygdala, septal area, hippocampus, cingulate gyrus that control emotions
- **Frontal lobe:** Reasoning, planning, parts of speech, movement emotions, problem-solving, and personality
- **Parietal lobe:** Touch, pressure, temperature, pain, and perception

- **Temporal lobe:** Recognition, hearing, and memory
- **Occipital:** Vision
- **Cerebellum:** Movement, balance, and posture
- **Brainstem:** Respirations, heart rate, and blood pressure

INTRODUCTION

The psychiatric-mental health nurse must be familiar with neuroanatomy, physiology, and psychopharmacology because they are often in the role of preparing patients for procedures and providing psychoeducation and anticipatory guidance. The advances in brain research that have occurred over the past three decades serve as the foundation for the theories guiding behavioral health in the biopsychosocial model approach of mental healthcare. Researchers have increasingly become aware of the role of genetics and epigenetics in neuroanatomy and physiology as they relate to the development of mental illness. Despite these advances, the field of psychiatry remains in its biological infancy. Biological findings move a condition from the field of psychiatry to the specialties of neurology, immunology, rheumatology, or endocrinology.

Diagnosis by exclusion is the manner in which a psychiatric disorder is classified. The prescribing of psychopharmacology is theoretical; selection utilizes trial and error with consideration for adverse effects, acceptable side effects, and desired response. For this reason, the classifications are termed disorders, organized by clusters of symptoms rather than individual disease states. In order to classify a biological disease state, the test findings must be reproducible, empirically quantified, and discretely documented. Developing a systematic approach to assessing symptoms using validated measures will greatly increase the likelihood of consistent classification and objective measures of the efficacy of treatment. The work of the psychiatric-mental health nurse requires an integrative holistic approach in caring for the mind from a neuropsychologically informed and culturally sensitive perspective. The primary objective is to reduce distressing symptoms in the patient in order to restore or preserve maximal function.

The arena of psychopharmacology is the mainstay of contemporary psychiatric care in the United States. Now, shortsightedly, modern psychiatry is primarily concerned with answering the question of what constitutes a disorder. Psychopharmacology attempts to alter the neurochemical environment to cause a change in signs and symptoms and hopefully downstream behaviors. Medications alone do not cause an individual to become a high functioning, well-adjusted, and productive member of society.

THE NERVOUS SYSTEM

- **Brain:** Comprised of two halves known as hemispheres
  - **Cerebral cortex (gray matter):** Composed of neuronal cell bodies (soma) and dendrites, contains synapses, gyri, and sulci associated with cholinergic system, functional arousal, learning, and memory.
    - **Dysfunctions:** Alzheimer's disease, frontotemporal dementia, vascular dementia

- **White matter:** Comprised of myelinated axons, contains commissures, a bundle of nerve fibers connect the right and left side called the "corpus callosum," also involved in associations within a hemisphere
  - **Sulci:** Shallow grooves
  - **Fissures:** Deep grooves
- **Frontal lobe:** Reaches full maturity in the mid to late 20s; may begin to atrophy in the 60s; controls voluntary movement, ability to project future consequences due to current behaviors, governs according to social cues, distinguishes similarities and differences.
  - **Broca's area:** In the dominant hemisphere of the brain and is associated with speech production (fluency); a dysfunction in this area is sometimes associated with stuttering, expressive aphasia (in which the person knows what they want to say but is unable to say it).
  - **Dysfunctions:**
    - Incongruent affect
    - Decreased motivation
    - Impaired judgment and attention
    - Confabulation
- **Cerebrum:** Comprises the majority (83%) of the brain, both right and left hemispheres, separated by the central sulcus. The brain has 52 subdivisions, referred to as Broadman's areas.
  - **Left hemisphere:** Controls most of the right side of the body functions and is the dominant hemisphere in most people
  - **Right hemisphere:** Controls most of the left side of the body functions
  - **Basal ganglia (corpus striatum):** Regulates the feedback system to stabilize the information transmitted from the central nervous system (CNS) to skeletal muscles
    - **Dopaminergic pathways:**
      - **Mesocorticolimbic:** Transmits dopamine to the prefrontal cortex and the midbrain. Disorders in this pathway include attention-deficit/hyperactivity disorder (ADHD), addiction, and schizophrenia
      - Aversion-related thoughts
      - Reward-related thoughts
        - Incentive (wanting)
        - Pleasure
        - Positive reinforcement
      - Executive function
    - **Nigrostriatal:** Transmits dopamine from substantia nigra, also in the midbrain, and to the putamen and caudate nucleus. Disorders in this pathway include movement disorders such as chorea and Parkinson's disease.
      - Motor function
      - Associative learning
    - **Tuberoinfundibular:** Transmits dopamine from the hypothalamus to the pituitary gland and influences the secretion of prolactin-releasing hormone. The primary disorder in this pathway is hyperprolactinemia, in which prolactin is released, causing lactation.
    - **Putamen:** Comprised of afferent (sending) pathways exerting an inhibitory effect on the thalamus (GABA); dopamine is associated with desire and movement

- **Learning:** Rule-based tasks, observational learning, integration of information
- **Movements:** Planning, execution, and sequencing
- **Caudate nucleus:** Innervated by dopamine neurons from the substantia nigra, integrates spatial information and working memory with motor behavior: limb movements speed, accuracy, and posture. The dopamine and GABA pathways affect motivation, sleep, and emotional response.
- **Dysfunction of basal ganglia-associated structures:**
    - Tourette's syndrome
    - Parkinson's disease
    - Cognitive impairment
    - Inattention
    - Choreiform movements
    - Ruminations
    - Bradykinesia
    - Hyperkinesia
    - Dystonia
- **Temporal lobe:** Contains the diencephalon (thalamus and hypothalamus). Contains the components of the **limbic system** and Wernicke's area (associated with comprehension)
    - **Amygdala:** Processes memory and emotional responses or mood (e.g., fear, anxiety, aggression)
    - **Thalamus:** Receives sensory (touch, audio, visual) inputs, serves as the gateway to the cortex, provides a functional delay of impulses to keep from overwhelming the cortex
        - **Dysfunction:** CVA can alter the perception of inputs, unresponsiveness, alterations in sleep–wake, and receptive aphasia
    - **Hypothalamus:** Directly above the brain stem; regulates homeostasis and hormones, controls the pituitary gland by secreting releasing hormones, also creates oxytocin and vasopressin
        - **Controls:** Autonomic nervous system, emotional response, temperature, hunger, thirst, sexual behavior, sleep–wake, and memory
        - **Pituitary gland:** Master gland of the body and controlled by the hypothalamus to maintain homeostasis by the release of hormones.
            - **Anterior:** Growth hormone, FSH, LH, adrenocorticotropic hormone, TSH, prolactin
            - **Posterior:** Release oxytocin and vasopressin
- **Parietal lobe:** Sensory area integration, sense of touch, attentiveness, spatial awareness, conscious awareness of the opposite side of the body, language
    - Sensory functions extend into the temporal lobe, and for this reason, there is some overlap in sensory input processing: secondary association with auditory functions, gustatory (taste), balance, and smell
- **Occipital lobe:** Primary visual cortex, receives stimuli via optic tracts, interprets color, form, and movement of visually perceived objects
    - Sensory functions extended into the temporal lobe via the ventral tract interpreting the "what" aspect of the object in view. The dorsal stream extends toward the parietal lobe interpreting "where" aspect of the object in view

- **Cerebellum (hindbrain):** The brain behind the brain makes up 11% of the total mass; its primary function is to coordinate movement, proprioception, maintain posture and equilibrium
  - **Dysfunction:** Loss of trunk control
- **Brain stem:** Automatic programmed reflexive behaviors; all cranial nerves come from the brain stem and integrates sensory input from the head, neck, and face
  - **Ventral tegmental area:** Dopaminergic cell bodies originate from within, associate with reward circuits (cognition, motivation, and orgasm), and extend to the temporal lobe
  - **Midbrain:** CN III, IV, forms the border to the diencephalon (thalamus and hypothalamus), and the metencephalon (pons and cerebellum)
  - **Pons:** Contains the locus coeruleus and synthesizes norepinephrine; CN V (sensory input from face, mastication), CN VI: eye movement (abduction), CN VII: facial muscle movement/expressions
  - **Medulla oblongata:** CN VIII–XII, contains the cochlear, vestibular, nuclei, and reticular formation, exerts autonomic control over the body
    - Receives input from cortex, innervates the thalamus, hypothalamus
    - Regulates involuntary movement, reflexes, muscle tone, and vital signs
- **Central nervous system**
  - Spinal cord and brain
- **Peripheral nervous system**
  - Peripheral nerves that connect to the central nervous system from the periphery (muscles and glands)
  - Cranial nerves outside the brainstem
  - **Autonomic nervous system:** Regulates bodily functions to maintain homeostasis, conveys information from the central nervous system to the peripheral nervous system, and regulates involuntary movements (regulates vital signs for the situation at hand: shunting blood, altering body temperature, vascular tone, heart rate, peristalsis, muscle tone); emotions
  - **Sympathetic nervous system:** Excitatory prepares the body for fight, flight, or freeze during stress
    - Thoracolumbar origination
    - **Ganglia**: Closer to spinal cord
      - Shorter preganglionic fibers, longer postganglionic fibers
    - Stress response is all or nothing
  - **Parasympathetic nervous system:** Inhibitory allows for resting, digesting, and orgasming
    - Craniosacral origination
    - **Ganglia:** In the effector organs
      - Longer preganglionic fibers, shorter postganglionic fibers
  - **Somatic nervous system:** Comprised of spinal nerves and cranial nerves, responsible for voluntary movements, conducting impulses from the CNS to the periphery (skeletal muscles)
    - **Afferent fibers:** Relay sensations (add information to the brain) from the body to the CNS
    - **Efferent fibers:** Relay commands from (exit information from the brain) the CNS to the body

- **Neurons:** Nervous system cell comprised of a cell body (soma), nucleus, and two types of fibers (dendrites transmit information to the soma, axons transmit information from the soma)
  - Some fibers are covered with a myelin sheath (formed by Schwann cells in the peripheral nervous system)
  - **Ranvier node:** A gap between myelin sheaths (uninsulated ion channels)
    - **Sensory type (afferent):** Receptors respond to stimuli and conduct to the CNS (associations in the brain and spinal cord, interprets information (taste, touch, sight, sound), trigger motor neurons)
    - **Motor type (efferent):** Transmit from the CNS to the glands and muscles
- **Glial cells:** Non-neuronal cells in the central nervous system
  - **Microglial-phagocytes:** Clean up cellular debris
  - **Astrocytes:** Star-shaped cells, provides nutrients, maintains extracellular ionic balance, involved in growth and repair of nerve cells to maintain blood-brain barrier
  - **Oligodendrocytes:** Forming myelin sheath in the CNS to coat the axon
  - **Ependyma:** Lines the spinal cord and ventricles, creates cerebrospinal fluid (CSF) circulated by cilia, contribute to the blood-brain barriers
- **Cranial nerves:** Twelve sensory-motor nerves that emerge directly from the brain (CN I and II) and brainstem (III—XII)
  - **Dysfunction:** See Table 4.1 for cranial nerves and corresponding tests for dysfunction

TABLE 4.1 Cranial Nerves

Cranial Nerve	Name	Test (Dysfunction)
I	Olfactory	Smell (anosmia)
II	Optic	Visual Fields (hemianopsia)
III	Oculomotor	Coordinated eye movements, eyelid droop, pupil dilation (diplopia, strabismus, mydriasis, ptosis)
IV	Trochlear	Downward medially (diplopia)
V	Trigeminal	Ophthalmic, maxillary, mandibular to allow chewing (neuralgia, cluster headache, zoster)
VI	Abducens	Eye movement: downward gaze (diplopia)
VII	Facial	Facial expression, touch sensation (paresis, palsy, CVA)
VIII	Vestibulo-cochlear	Hearing and balance (nystagmus, deafness, ataxia)
IX	Glossopharyngeal	Gag reflex, taste, salivation (aspiration)
X	Vagus	Vital signs, vocal tone, swallowing (dysphagia, dysreflexia)
XI	Accessory (spinal)	Shoulder shrug, head turning (winged scapula, unable to shrug, reduced ROM turning head)
XII	Hypoglossal	Tongue movement (tongue fasciculation, deviation)

CVA, cerebrovascular accident; ROM, range of motion

- **Neurotransmitters:** Chemicals created from dietary substrates that transmit information between neurons and meet the following four criteria (Sadock, B., Sadock, V., & Ruiz, 2015):
  - **Presence of the chemical within the cell:** The chemical is either synthesized by the Neurontin or is taken up from other cells but release it
  - **Stimulus-dependent release:** It is released in appropriate quantities by the neurontin upon stimulation
  - **Action on postsynaptic cell:** Exogenous application of the substance in appropriate amounts mimics the action of the endogenously released substance on the postsynaptic cell
  - **Mechanism for removal:** A specific mechanism exists to remove the substance from the synaptic cleft either by degradation or reuptake
- **Neurotransmission:** Triggered by an electrical process, impulses are transmitted between neurons via the axon by releasing neurotransmitters (chemicals), which stimulate further neuronal activity (neurotransmission)
  - See Table 4.2 for a summary of neurotransmitters

Table 4.2 Neurotransmitters: Effect, Agonist, Antagonist, and Associated Pathology

Neurotransmitter (NT)	Effect	Agonist	Antagonist	Associated pathology
Acetylcholine (Ach)	**Increases** heart rate, secretions, sweating, salivation, memory, muscle contractions	Varenicline nicotine, donepezil memantine pilocarpine	Atropine, benztropine, scopolamine	**Decreased:** Dementia **Increased:** Parkinsonian
Norepinephrine (NE)	**Increases** heart rate, alertness, wellbeing. **Decreases** pain sensitivity, circulation	Amphetamines, cocaine, SNRIs, MAOIs, pseudo-ephedrine, albuterol, bupropion	Receptor blockers (alpha, beta, non-dihydro-pyridine calcium channel)	**Increased:** Anxiety **Decreased:** Depression
Dopamine (D)	**Increases** sense of wellbeing, satiety. **Decreases** hunger and cravings	Amphetamines, cocaine, SNRIs, MAOIs, pseudo-ephedrine, albuterol, bupropion	Antipsychotics	**Increased:** Psychosis **Decreased:** Parkinson's disease, anhedonia, addiction
Serotonin (5-HT)	**Increases** wellbeing, satiety, reduces pain perception	Amphetamines, cocaine, SNRIs, MAOIs, pseudo-ephedrine, albuterol, bupropion	Atypical antipsychotics	**Decreased:** Depression, obsessive compulsive disorder, anxiety **Increased:** Serotonin syndrome

(continued)

Table 4.2 Neurotransmitters: Effect, Agonist, Antagonist, and Associated Pathology (*continued*)

Glutamate	Most common **excitatory** NT, heightens perception (usually taste)	Domoic acid (naturally occurring in fish and shellfish)	Ketamine, dextromethorphan, memantine	**Increased:** Psychosis, mood lability, seizures **Decreased:** Impaired memory, negative symptoms
Gamma-aminobenzoic acid (GABA)	**Inhibitory, increases** sleepiness, **decreases** anxiety, alertness, memory, muscle tension	EtOH, barbiturates, benzodiazepines, baclofen, sedative hypnotics, sodium oxybate (GHB)	flumazenil	**Decreased:** Anxiety
Opioids (neuropeptides)	**Increases** sedation, **decreases** anxiety, and pain perception	Narcotics	Naloxone, naltrexone	**Decreased:** Lower pain tolerance
Cannabinoids*	**Increases** hunger, **decreases** satiety, motivation, sex drive	Dronabinol, tetrahydrocannabinol	N/A	**Increased:** Insatiability, apathy
Histamine	**Increases** alertness, stomach acid, skin sensitivity	N/A	Antihistamines (diphenhydramine), H2 Blockers (famotidine), antipsychotics (chlorpromazine), leukotriene inhibitors (montelukast)	**Increased:** Inflammation, urticarial, pain **Decreased:** Drowsiness
Nitric oxide**	**Increases** vasodilation,	PD5 inhibitors (sildenafil), Citrus, pomegranate, beets	SNRIs, amphetamines, cocaine, pseudoephedrine	**Increased:** Edema

MAOIs, monoamine oxidase inhibitors; SNRIs, serotonin-norepinephrine reuptake inhibitor ***Endocannabinoids:** Synthesized in the postsynaptic neurons, transported by retrograde neurotransmission or diffusion ****Nitric oxide:** Synthesized in the postsynaptic neurons. Transported by retrograde neurotransmission or diffusion

NEUROIMAGING

- **Electroencephalogram (EEG):** Depicts electrical activity on the surface of the brain as waveforms that vary in frequency and amplitude and/or measured in micro voltage. The waveforms are classified according to their frequency, amplitude, and shape, as well as the sites on the scalp at which they are recorded (Bazanova & Vernon, 2014).
- **Magnetic resonance imaging (MRI):** Nonradioactive imaging; uses powerful magnets and radio waves to provide a detailed image of structures; commonly performed for many patients in the psychiatric setting despite evidence to the contrary with respect to clinically relevant or significant findings (Bazanova & Vernon, 2014).
  - **Contraindications:** Pacemakers or any metallic implant such as stents, automated internal cardiac defibrillator (AICD), unmanaged claustrophobia
    - **MRI of the brain:** Can be used to evaluate cerebellopontine pathology, cranial nerves, and dysfunctions of the inner ear.
      - It is essential to indicate the indication and symptoms that are precipitating the request for MRI (Zakhari, 2014).
        - **Variables that affect results:**
          - Smoking status
          - Head motion
          - Bodyweight
          - Psychoactive drugs
          - Alcohol use
          - Mental state
- **Positron emission tomography (PET); fluorodeoxyglucose (FDG)-PET:** A nuclear medicine test that measures the uptake of sugar in the brain or body part of interest. Commonly used in psychiatry to distinguish dementia. Findings include slow metabolic uptake. Results must be correlated with clinical findings and provide more utility when repeated for comparison (Berti, Pupi, & Mosconi, 2011).

GENETICS

- **Gene:** A sequence of DNA that cause characteristics to be passed to the next generation
- **DNA:** Deoxynucleic acid, helical chain structure of amino acids in pairs, linked by four nucleotides (A) adenine, (T) thymine, (C) cytosine, (G) guanine. Note: A is always paired with T, and C is always paired with G
- **Chromosomes:** DNA structures contained in the gamete cell nucleus. Normally developed human beings have 46 total chromosomes (23 pairs from each parent)
  - **Gamete cell:** Sex cells, female is ova, male is sperm, each carries one pair of chromosomes (23)
- **Phenotype:** The observable characteristics of a specific genetic trait (allele) (e.g., CYP 450). Drug metabolism varies based on specific phenotype. Some individuals are not able to metabolize certain drugs and may have no therapeutic effect increasing the likelihood of toxicity

- **Allele:** Genetic variant (e.g., eye color, hair color); a visible expression of the allele is called phenotype. When a person has two copies of the same allele, the condition is termed homozygous, and one copy is termed heterozygous
- **Genomics**
  - Unmodifiable risk factors that contribute to the development of disease state and response to treatment
    - **Family history:** Counsel patients on becoming familiar with their personal history, including diseases and conditions, medication response, age of onset, death before age 50, substance use disorders, and suicides
- **Genogram pedigree**
  - Begin with the identified patient and regress to grandparents
  - Indicate males, females, marriages, divorces, adoptions, twins, pregnancy, consanguinity (relatives having children)
  - Autosomal dominant conditions may be present in up to 50% of offspring when a first-degree relative is affected and may exist in multiple generations
  - Recessive gene expression appears only in one generation and affects the individual who has inherited both alleles (e.g., cystic fibrosis, hemochromatosis). Refer to Table 4.3, for example, of a Punnet square
    - X linked disorders are caused by mutations on the X chromosome, which is why they are said to be transmitted through the maternal line (color blindness, fragile X syndrome)
- **Genetic counseling:** A communication process by a trained professional employed when there is concern regarding genetic risks, specific testing to help stratify the risk and to provide anticipatory guidance for expectant parents
- **First-degree relatives:** Mother, father, sibling from a shared mother or father
- **Second-degree relatives:** Maternal or paternal grandparents, siblings, and offspring
  - **Twin studies:** Monozygotic (identical), dizygotic (fraternal) influence on the incidence heritability based on rate of concordance
  - **Risk factors:** 40% to 90% heritability for psychiatric conditions, including schizophrenia (50%), bipolar disorder (70%), ADHD (70%) (Barnett & Smoller, 2009; Brikell, Kuja-Halkola, & Larsson, 2015; Gejman, Sanders, & Duan, 2010)
- **Epigenetics:** Environmental stressors that act on a gene (switch on or off) which effect the expression rather than the underlying genetic code

Table 4.3 Punnet Square

PUNNETT SQUARE	XX (Mother)	XY (Father)
	D	d
D	DD	Dd
d	Dd	dd (recessive gene expressed)

- Nutrition
- Aging
- Emotional stress
- Coping mechanisms
- Psychological reserves
- Sociological factors
- Education and new learning
- Nurturance and bonding
- Access to critical components

SELECTED NEUROPSYCHOLOGICAL TESTS (MOST COMMONLY USED)

- **Abnormal Involuntary Movement Scale (AIMS):** Clinician administered 12-item tool with a 0–4 points rating scale for seven body areas where tardive dyskinesia commonly manifests (Petzinger et al., 2001).
  - Serial testing every 3 to 6 months for all patients taking antipsychotics
  - Must consider impact on function and daily living
  - Tardive dyskinesia is diagnosed if rating mildly abnormal (2 on the 0–4 scale) in at least two body areas or moderately abnormal (rating of 3 or greater) in one body area
- **Barnes Akathisia Rating Scale (BARS):** A clinician-administered tool to assess the objective and subjective symptoms of akathisia (a syndrome of motor restlessness, subjective experience of mental unease) in patients receiving psychotropic medications (Petzinger et al., 2001).
  - Assess after patients begin psychotropic medications
  - http://www.medafile.com/zyweb/Barnes.htm
- **Connors Rating Scales—Revised (CRS-R):** A two-question survey tool administered to parents and teachers to quantify symptoms of ADHD. Scores between 60 and 70 are considered mild; greater than 70 are considered markedly atypical.
  - Children aged 3–17 years
  - Parents' Scale: http://www.pediatricenter.com/assets/forms/Conners_Parent_Rating.pdf
  - Teachers' Scale: http://www.kangospediatrics.com/docs/teacher_add_adhd_short.pdf
- **Alcohol use disorder (CAGE-AID):** Short-form clinician-administered screening tool with 79% sensitivity and 77% specificity for a score of 1; a score of 2 increases sensitivity to 93% or alcohol use disorder.
  - Questions relate to whether an individual feels they've tried to Cut down, feel Annoyed, feel Guilty, or needed an Eye opener in relation to alcohol or substance used for coping
  - https://www.integration.samhsa.gov/images/res/CAGEAID.pdfm
- **Saint Louis University Mental Status (SLUMS):** A screening test for cognitive function, currently in the public domain, comparable to the Mini-Mental Status Exam (no longer in the public domain), tests for orientation, memory, attention, and executive function (Petzinger et al., 2001).

- 30 items; scores are differentiated based on educational attainment
- Includes clock test
- http://medschool.slu.edu/agingsuccessfully/pdfsurveys/slumsexam_05.pdf
- If the patient has a high school education >26 is normal; if the patient has less than a high school education >24 is normal
- **Montreal Cognitive Assessment (MOCA):** Developed to detect early mild cognitive impairment with higher sensitivity, as it assesses across broader domains and is better suited to those with higher educational attainment (Trzepacz, Hochstetler, Wang, Walker, & Saykin, 2015).
  - Cognitive impairment by proxy of attention, concentration, executive function, visuospatial recognition, naming, memory, attention, language, calculation, orientation, delayed recall, and conceptual thinking
  - Score >26 is normal regardless of education
  - Available at: https://consultgeri.org/try-this/general-assessment/issue-3.2.pdf
- **Geriatric Depression Scale (GDS):** A 30-item self-report binary questionnaire to measure depressive symptoms (concentration, self-image, agitation, losses, motivation, obsessive traits) in older adults. The short form contains 15 questions, and both are highly correlated (Marc, Raue, & Bruce, 2008).
  - 5 to 7 minutes to complete
  - Scoring 0 to 9 normal, 10 to 19 mild, 20 to 30 severe depression
  - Ignores somatic complaints
  - Major depressive disorder (MDD) sensitivity 84%, specificity 95%
  - Available at: https://consultgeri.org/try-this/general-assessment/issue-4.pdf
- **Hamilton Rating Scale for Depression (HAM-D):** Self-report or clinician-assisted measure of depressive symptoms comprised of 17 to 21 questions, commonly used at baseline and to measure the progress of treatment (Mottram, Wilson, & Copeland, 2000).
  - Insensitive to somatic complaints
  - Scores 0 to 7 no depression, 8 to 13 mild, 14 to 18 moderate, 19 to 22 severe depression
  - Available at: https://dcf.psychiatry.ufl.edu/files/2011/05/HAMILTON-DEPRESSION.pdf
- **Patient Health Questionnaire (PHQ-2/9):** A self-administered depression screening tool commonly used in primary care settings as a reliable measure of the severity of depressive symptoms (Kroenke, Spitzer, & Williams, 2001).
  - Sensitivity 88% and specificity 88%
  - Scores range in increments of 5 (5, 10, 15, 20), indicating mild, moderate, moderately severe, and severe depression
  - Tool testing included obstetric patients
  - Available at: https://www.uspreventiveservicestaskforce.org/Home/GetFileByID/218
- **Quick Inventory of Depressive Symptomatology (QIDS):** A 16-item self-report survey assessing the severity of depressive symptoms (Lamoureux et al., 2010)
  - Sensitivity 76% and specificity 81%
  - Best used in someone who is diagnosed rather than to diagnose depression
  - Available at: https://www.mdcalc.com/quick-inventory-depressive-symptomatology-qids

- **Young Mania Rating Scale (YMRS):** A self-report/clinician observation tool to assess severity of manic symptoms in those already diagnosed with mania. Domains assessed include: mood, motor activity, social interest, sexual interest, sleep, irritability, speech, language, thought, aggression, appearance, and insight (Park & Choi, 2016)
  - **Adults:** Score over 12 consistent with mania
  - **Children:** Score over 25 consistent with mania, 20 hypomania, >13 further evaluation with more specific tools or several tools
  - Available at: https://dcf.psychiatry.ufl.edu/files/2011/05/Young-Mania-Rating-Scale-Measure-with-background.pdf
- **Children's Yale-Brown Obsessive Compulsive Scale (CY-BOCS):** A self-report/clinician-administered 10-item scale to evaluate severity of obsessions or compulsions in previously diagnosed children with obsessive compulsive disorder (Wu et al., 2014).
  - Ages 6 to 14
  - Rating 0 to 4, the higher the score, the more severe the symptoms
  - Can be used to monitor treatment progress.
  - Available at: https://iocdf.org/wp-content/uploads/2016/04/05-CYBOCS-complete.pdf
- **Yale-Brown Obsessive Compulsive Scale (YBOCS):** A self-report 10-item scale for people older than 14 years of age, each question is rated separately, and a composite score is tallied, indicating the higher the score the more severe the symptoms. This is not a diagnostic tool and is intended to measure progress in previously diagnosed patients with obsessive compulsive disorder (Abramowitz, Tolin, & Diefenbach, 2005).
  - Patient is asked to choose the top three most distressing to focus on
  - Gold standard test for assessment of obsessive-compulsive symptoms
  - Available at: https://psychology-tools.com/yale-brown-obsessive-compulsive-scale
- **Clinical Institute Withdrawal Assessment of Alcohol Scale – Revised (CIWA-Ar):** A nine-item clinician-administered/observed rating scale to quantify the severity of alcohol withdrawal symptoms. It is used to guide medication dosing and monitor response to treatment over time (Bird & Makela, 1994; Daeppen et al., 2002; Jaeger, Lohr, & Pankratz, 2001; Kitchens, 1994; Mayo-Smith, 1997; Ng, Dahri, Chow, & Legal, 2011; Nuss, Elnicki, Dunsworth, & Makela, n.d.; Rastegar et al., 2017; Reoux & Miller, 2000; Roffman & Stern, 2006).
  - Comorbid medical conditions can mask withdrawal symptoms
  - Medications may mask withdrawal symptoms
  - Symptoms may be present and not due to alcohol withdrawal
  - Not a diagnostic tool
  - Scores <8 do not require interventions, 9–19 mild to moderate withdrawal, >20 severe withdrawal
  - Available: https://www.mdcalc.com/ciwa-ar-alcohol-withdrawal#evidence
- **Clinical Opiate Withdrawal Scale (COWS):** A clinician-administered/observed tool to quantify the severity of opioid withdrawal symptoms to guide medication management. Commonly used in medically assisted treatment during induction of buprenorphine.

- Scores >10 indicate sufficient withdrawal to begin buprenorphine
- Must be mindful of symptoms due to medical comorbidities or other substance use disorder
- Medications for comorbid conditions can mask or exacerbate symptoms
- Available at: https://www.drugabuse.gov/sites/default/files/files/ClinicalOpiateWithdrawalScale.pdf

Study tip: Reviewing the content of the clinical tools will help you as a clinician, and test-taker to become familiar with the symptoms associated with the various disorders.

PSYCHOPHARMACOLOGY

- **Pharmacokinetics:** The study of what the body does to a drug concerning absorption, distribution, metabolism, and excretion (ADME)
  - **Absorption:** The movement of the drug into the bloodstream. With oral agents, this typically occurs in the small intestines
  - **Distribution:** The movement of the drug through the bloodstream to target receptors. The chemicals (substrates) bind to the protein for transport. The unbound (free) portion of the drug is considered active. If the patient is significantly malnourished or protein deficient (prealbumin <16 mg/dL), toxicity can be achieved with relatively low doses of medication. Further complicating the principle of distribution is the fat-to-lean muscle mass ratio (as in the elderly). This can lead to variable amounts of the active drug in circulation at any one time.
  - **Metabolism:** The transformation or breakdown of the drug in preparation for elimination from the body.
  - **Excretion:** The process by which substances (drugs, substrates, toxins) leave the body (feces, urine, skin).
    - **Half-life:** The time needed to clear 50% of the drug from the plasma.
- Determines dosing interval (once per half-life).
- Five half-lives are required to achieve steady state. Clearing the drug from circulation requires five half-lives.
  - Variables that can alter pharmacokinetics:
- Substrate interactions can change (induce or inhibit) CYP450 metabolism, which changes (decreases or increases) volume distribution (concentration).
- **Inducing:** Speeds up the metabolic rate, decreasing serum level of the drug
- **Inhibiting:** Slows down the metabolic rate, increasing the serum level of the drug
- **Age:** Young children, especially during periods of rapid growth and development, metabolize (CYP450, 2C9, 2C19, 2D6, and 3A4) more rapidly, thereby causing lower drug concentrations (available free drug) in the systemic circulation (subtherapeutic dose)
- Elderly patients metabolize (CYP450, 1A2) more slowly, thereby causing higher concentrations (available free drug) in the systemic circulation (increased risk of toxicity)
- Racial variations can also lead to variable concentration-response relationships (efficacy)

- **Physiological integrity:** Liver disease affecting enzyme activity (first-pass effect) can have an inhibitory effect, increasing the risk of drug toxicity. Renal insufficiency (or acute kidney injuries) can also lead to increased serum concentrations due to reduced glomerular filtration rate (GFR)
- **Nutritional status:** Low muscle mass, reduced protein, and increased fat stores can lead to increased drug concentrations and risk of toxicity (most common in the elderly)
- **Intracellular volume:** Reduced in the elderly but increased in pregnancy; can also alter drug concentrations and necessitate dose adjustment
  - **Pharmacodynamics** is the study of drug action on the body, specifically the relationship between drug concentration and effect (dose and response). Factors that can affect the action of the drug on the body include the individual's physiological profile (age, pregnancy, and genetics), nutritional status, other chemicals in circulation, disease process, drug potency, and receptor desensitization.
    - **Side effects:** A usually undesired but foreseeable effect that occurs regardless of dose and often resolves after continued therapy without intervention.
    - **Adverse effects:** Properly administered medication causing unintended and undesirable effects. The severity of the impact may be dose-dependent.
    - **Treatment failure:** Insufficiently mitigated symptoms.
      - **Tolerance:** The process of becoming desensitized and therefore less responsive to a particular dose of medication over time, necessitating increases; it may eventually lead to "poop-out" effect.
      - **Tachyphylaxis:** Rapidly diminishing responsiveness to increasing doses of the medication, known as "poop-out" effect.
    - **Therapeutic index (TI):** A ratio describing the toxic dose (TD) to effective dose (ED)
      - Drugs with a narrow TI (the therapeutic dose and TD ranges are close together) pose a higher risk for a toxicity; for example, lithium, which has a therapeutic window of 0.6 to 1.2 mEQ/L
    - Drugs with high TI have a wider safety margin

Medications generally exert their effects in one of seven ways. Medications can be:
- **Agonist:** The activation of a receptor by a chemical to produce a biological response.
- **Partial agonist:** A chemical that binds to a receptor but does not fully activate the receptor, and the biological response may be muted (e.g., buprenorphine, buspirone, aripiprazole, and norclozapine). In this case, the drug may block pain or dopamine but causes less sedation.
- **Inverse agonist:** An agent that binds to the same receptor as an agonist but induces an opposite biological response.
- **Antagonist effects:** The blocking of the receptor to inhibit the biological response. This also blocks endogenous agonists from binding.
- **Ion channel blockers:** The substrate may block the various ion channels (potassium, sodium, calcium, chloride) rather than receptor sites and exert either an inhibitory or an excitatory effect across the cell membrane.
  - **Depolarization:** Requires a cellular influx of sodium and calcium through the cell membrane, causing an excitatory response (firing).

- **Repolarization:** Requires an outflow of chloride and potassium to induce an inhibitory effect. For example, when serum potassium is elevated sufficiently, myocardial contractility will be inhibited.
- **Enzyme inhibitors:** The catalytic action of the enzyme is slowed or stopped, allowing for a neurotransmitter to remain in circulation; for example, monoamine oxidase inhibitors reduce the breakdown and eventual removal of serotonin, norepinephrine, and dopamine from circulation.
- **Reuptake inhibitors:** Hindering the absorption of a neurotransmitter by the synapse by blocking the transport protein, allowing for higher concentrations of the neurotransmitter in the synaptic cleft.

▶ PSYCHOTROPIC CLASSIFICATIONS

- **Antipsychotics:** First-generation antipsychotics (FGAs) are also known as typical antipsychotics or dopamine antagonists (Table 4.4). In treating schizophrenia, there is moderate-quality evidence that haloperidol and low-potency antipsychotics are approximately equal in their effectiveness, but there is lower-quality evidence that

Table 4.4 Neurotransmitters: Effect, Agonist, Antagonist, and Associated Pathology

Typical Antipsychotics (First-Generation Antipsychotics)	Starting Dose*; Maximum Daily Dose**	Half-life (Hours) if Given PO	Formulations	Specific Monitoring (Assuming Normal Hepatic and Renal Function)
Chlorpromazine (Thorazine)	25–200 mg/day to start; MDD 400–600 mg/day	30	Tab, IM	Class effects include sedation, orthostasis, anticholinergic effects, QTc prolongation, EPS, TD, agranulocytosis
Fluphenazine (Prolixin)	2–10 mg to start; MDD 15 mg/day	33	Tab, oral solution, IM, LAI	
Haloperidol (Haldol)	2–10 mg to start; MDD 30 mg/day; doses of up to 100 mg per day are FDA approved but uncommon	20	Tab, oral solution, IM, LAI	Class effects, + QTc prolongation, not recommended for IV use, but has been used. This further heightens the risk of QTc prolongation

Typical Antipsychotics (First-Generation Antipsychotics)	Starting Dose*; Maximum Daily Dose**	Half-life (Hours) if Given PO	Formulations	Specific Monitoring (Assuming Normal Hepatic and Renal Function)
Perphenazine (Trilafon)	8–16 mg to start; MDD 24 mg/day; doses of up to 64 mg/day may be acceptable in certain circumstances	9–19	Tab	Class effects include sedation, orthostasis, anticholinergic effects, QTc prolongation, EPS, TD, agranulocytosis
Thioridazine (Mellaril)	150 mg to start; MDD 600 mg/day	4–25	Tab	
Trifluoperazine (Stelazine)	4–10 mg/d to start; MDD 40 mg/day	3–22	Tab	

EPS, extrapyramidal side effects; ER, extended release; FDA, Food and Drug Administration; IM, intramuscular; IV, intravenous; LAI, long-acting injectable; MDD, maximum daily dose; ODT, orally disintegrating tablet; sl, sublingual; Tab, tablet; TD, tardive dyskinesia. *Elderly persons and those with impaired renal and hepatic function require lower starting dosages. **Doses listed are total daily doses intended to be divided over a 24-hour period.

they clearly differ in side effects (such as weight gain and movement disorders; Tardy, Huhn, Kissling, Engel, & Leucht, 2014).
- FGAs and second-generation antipsychotics (SGAs, or atypical antipsychotics; Table 4.5) are equally efficacious in the treatment of psychosis. However, the side-effect profiles for the SGAs may be more acceptable in the short term.
- SGAs (specifically olanzapine, risperidone, and clozapine) are often associated with weight gain, elevated prolactin levels, dyslipidemia, and insulin resistance.
- **Mood stabilizers:** Used to treat bipolar disorder but require drug-level monitoring during titration and maintenance. General considerations when selecting mood-stabilizing medications include:
  - If renal disease, avoid lithium
  - If hepatic disease or female of child-bearing age, avoid valproate
  - If history of extrapyramidal side effects, avoid aripiprazole and risperidone
  - If obese, avoid olanzapine, quetiapine, and risperidone
    - **Valproic acid (Depakene):** 60 mg/kg/day in divided doses, serum trough level 12 hours from the previous dose, half-life 13 hours, during titration check twice weekly, then monthly.
    - Therapeutic range: 50 to 125 mcg/mL (evaluate for signs of toxicity and improvement of manic symptoms).
    - If patient develops altered mental status, evaluate for hyperammonemia. Do not treat if asymptomatic (Patorno et al., 2017).
    - FDA-approved in children for seizure disorders
    - Associated with teratogenic effects in pregnancy, excreted in breast milk

TABLE 4.5 Atypical Antipsychotics

Second-Generation Antipsychotics	Starting Dose* and Usual Dose Range mg/day**	Half-life if Given PO (Hours)	Formulations	Specific Monitoring (Assuming Normal Hepatic and Renal Function)
Aripiprazole (Abilify)	2 mg/day to start; MDD 30 mg/day	75–94	Tab, ODT, oral solution, LAI	Least likely to exhibit class effects: sedation, orthostasis, anticholinergic effects, EPS, TD, agranulocytosis
Asenapine (Saphris)	10 mg/day; MDD 20 mg/day	24	SL	Class effects include sedation, orthostasis is often the limiting factor in titration, anticholinergic effects, EPS, TD, and agranulocytosis (most likely with clozapine)
Brexpiprazole (Rexulti)	0.5–1 mg/day; MDD 4 mg/day			
Cariprazine (Vraylar)	1.5 mg/day; 6 mg/day		Capsule	
Clozapine (Clozaril)	25–50 mg/day; MDD 900 mg/day		Tab, ODT, oral suspension	
Iloperidone (Fanapt)	2 mg/day; 24 mg/day		Tab	
Lurasidone (Latuda)	20–40 mg/day; 160 mg/day		Tab	
Olanzapine (Zyprexa)	5 mg/day; 30 mg/day		Tab, ODT, IM, LAI	
Paliperidone (Invega)	6 mg/day; 12 mg/day		ER tab, LAI	
Pimavanserin (Nuplazid)	34 mg/day; 34 mg/day		Tab	
Quetiapine (Seroquel)	50 mg/day; 800 mg/day		Tab, ER tab	
Risperidone (Risperdal)	1–2 mg/day; MDD 8 mg/day		Tab, ODT, oral solution, LAI	
Ziprasidone (Geodon)	40 mg/day; MDD 20 mg/day		Capsule, IM	

EPS, extrapyramidal side effects; ER, extended release; IM, intramuscular; LAI, long-acting injectable; MDD, maximum daily dose; ODT, orally disintegrating tablet; sl, sublingual; Tab, tablet; TD, tardive dyskinesia. *Elderly persons and those with impaired renal and hepatic function require lower starting dosages; see full prescribing information for specific drugs. **Doses listed are total daily doses intended to be divided over a 24-hour period.

- Monitoring includes mental status changes, complete blood count (thrombocytopenia), and liver function (transaminitis)
- **Lithium (Eskalith):** 900 to 1800 mg/day in divided doses, serum lithium trough level 12 hours from the previous dose, half-life 20 hours, during titration check twice weekly, then every 1 to 2 months when stable.
  - **Initial anti-mania:** 5 to 7 days, full effect 10 to 21 days.
  - Before initiating, evaluate renal function, electrolytes, thyroid function, EKG, negative pregnancy test (contraindicated in the first trimester, associated with Ebstein's anomaly: rightventricular outflow tract obstruction in the fetus; Patorno et al., 2017). Excreted in breast milk.
  - Narrow TI 0.6 mEq/L in elderly, 0.8 to 1.2 mEq/L.
  - FDA approved in children >7 years of age.
- **Lamotrigine (Lamictal):** 25 mg/day × 2 weeks, then 50 mg/day × 2 weeks, then 100 mg/day × 1 week to a maximum daily dose of 400 mg/day.
  - Adverse severe reaction is Stevens–Johnson syndrome (SJS; risk is increased when used in conjunction with valproic acid)
  - Cautiously used in pregnancy if the benefit outweighs risks. Excreted in breast milk; monitor infant for poor sucking, drowsiness, apnea
  - Half-life 30 hours (half-life is doubled when used in conjunction with valproic acid), smoking induces metabolism and reduces half-life by 50% (Patorno et al., 2017)
- **Carbamazepine (Tegretol):** 200 mg q12h, increase by 200 mg/day weekly to a maximum daily dose 1,200 mg/day in divided doses
  - Target dose is based on symptom abatement
  - Half-life shortens while on maintenance due to auto-metabolic effect
  - Available in tablet, chewable, liquid, and IV formulations
- **Oxcarbazepine (Trileptal; off-label, but standard):** 300 mg q12 initially and increase at weekly intervals by 600 mg/day up to 1,200 mg/day in divided doses
  - Pregnant patients should enroll in the Antiepileptic Drug Pregnancy Registry: 888-233-2334 (www.aedpregnancyregistry.org)
  - Insufficient evidence for maintenance treatment for bipolar (Patorno et al., 2017)
- **Tricyclics (TCAs; Table 4.6):** Less commonly used to treat melancholic depression that is characterized by psychomotor retardation, dysphoria, hopelessness, diurnal variation, and fatigue. Also, used less commonly for generalized anxiety disorder, panic attacks, posttraumatic stress disorder, and bulimia nervosa

TABLE 4.6 Less Commonly Used Antidepressants

Tricyclic Antidepressants (TCAs)	Monoamine Oxidase Inhibitors (MAOIs)
Clomipramine (Anafranil)	Phenelzine (Nardil)
Desipramine (Norpramin)	Tranylcypromine sulfate (Parnate)
Amitriptyline (Elavil)	Selegiline transdermal (Emsam)
Doxepin (Sinequan)	
Imipramine (Tofranil)	

- Side effects common to the class include xerostomia, blurry vision, diaphoresis, orthostatic tachycardia, drowsiness, restlessness, and palpitations.
- **Monoamine oxidase inhibitors (MAOIs; see Table 4.6):** Used to treat resistant and refractory depression
  - Not recommended for first- or second-line treatment due to the extensive side-effect profile: hypotension, dizziness, falls, dry mouth, dyspepsia, and urinary hesitancy, headache, and myoclonic jerks
  - Numerous drug–drug interactions
  - Dietary (tyramine) restrictions include aged cheese, cured meat, smoked meat, fermented foods, fish sauce, alcohol, and soy products
- **SSRIs (Table 4.7):** Usually utilized as a first-line treatment for depression and anxiety because of tolerability and safety concerning overdose. The primary receptor target is 5-hydroxytryptamine (5-HT). In general, all SSRIs reduce the presynaptic serotonin reuptake pump increasing the duration of serotonin availability in the synaptic cleft
  - Full therapeutic effects may take up to 8 weeks (or longer) as downstream effects (increased production of brain-derived neurotrophic factor) are realized
  - Class side effects include insomnia (initially and during titration), drowsiness, nausea, dry mouth, diarrhea, restlessness, inhibited arousal (erectile dysfunction), and anorgasmia
  - Evaluate for signs and symptoms of hyponatremia in the first 2 weeks. SIADH can occur at any time while on any psychotropic medication (least likely to happen with mirtazapine and bupropion) (nausea, vomiting, confusion, fatigue, restlessness, muscle weakness, and cramps)
  - SSRIs cross the placenta to the fetal brain, and risks during pregnancy include preterm birth, low birth weight, postpartum hemorrhage, and postnatal pulmonary hypertension in the infant (these findings are not from randomized controlled trials). However, maternal health is a more significant predictor of fetal health and well-being; always consider the risk versus benefit (Bérard et al., 2016; Eke & Saccone, 2016; Weisskopf et al., 2015)

TABLE 4.7 Most Commonly Used Antidepressants and Anxiolytics

SSRIs	sSNRIs
Citalopram (Celexa)	Levomilnacipran (Fetzima)
S-Citalopram (Lexapro)	Venlafaxine (Effexor)
Sertraline (Zoloft)	Desvenlafaxine (Pristiq)
Fluoxetine (Prozac)	Duloxetine (Cymbalta)
Paroxetine (Paxil)	
Vortioxetine (Brintellix)	
Vilazodone (Viibryd)	
Nefazodone (Serzone)	
Trazodone (Desyrel)	

sSNRIs, selective serotonin–norepinephrine reuptake inhibitors; SSRIs, selective serotonin reuptake inhibitors

- Selective (serotonin) norepinephrine reuptake inhibitors (sSNRIs; see Table 4.7): Commonly used as first- or second-line treatment for depression, anxiety, and neuropathic pain syndromes. This class is a dual-agent reuptake inhibitor. The higher dose range triggers the norepinephrine reuptake. There is currently one exception with the medication desvenlafaxine (Pristiq). This particular agent comes in one therapeutic dosage of 50 mg daily and has no added benefit with titration.
  - Class side effects include hypertension, insomnia (initially and during titration), drowsiness, nausea, dry mouth, diarrhea, restlessness, inhibited arousal (erectile dysfunction), anorgasmia, and retrograde ejaculation.
    - Discontinuation and withdrawal syndromes are usually due to the short half-life of the serotonin component of the medication and occur in up to one-third of patients. Augmenting with a long-acting SSRI can mitigate many of these effects during the discontinuation process (Gelenberg et al., 2010; Ogle & Akkerman, 2013).
    - Discontinuation symptoms include dizziness, fatigue, headache, nausea, agitation, anxiety, insomnia, irritability, electric-like shocks (head zaps), and audiovisual hallucinations.
- **Benzodiazepines (Table 4.8):** Ideally, used cautiously for the short-term treatment of anxiety given the high potential for dependence and abuse. Avoid this class of medication in patients with a history of substance use disorder. Patients who become tolerant or exhibit withdrawal symptoms between doses are not good candidates for long-term use.
  - Concomitant use with opioids can lead to elevated opioid levels through the CYP450 3A4 pathway.
  - Oxazepam, lorazepam, and temazepam are preferred in patients with impaired hepatic function, as may be the case in patients with alcohol use disorder.
  - Side effects include psychomotor slowing, temporary cognitive impairment, and rebound anxiety.
  - The shorter the half-life, the more likely the patient will experience withdrawal symptoms.
  - Other commonly used medications are listed in Table 4.9.

Table 4.8 Benzodiazepines

Benzodiazepine	Half-Life (hours)
Alprazolam (Xanax)	11
Chlordiazepoxide (Librium)	30
Clonazepam (Klonopin)	50
Diazepam (Valium)	96
Lorazepam (Ativan)	14
Oxazepam (Serax)	10

Table 4.9 Other Commonly Used Medications

Class/Drug(s)	Common Use	Special Monitoring
Beta-blockers/propranolol (Inderal)	Performance anxiety	Monitor for asthma, heart rate, and blood pressure
Alpha blockers/clonidine, prazosin, doxazosin	Posttraumatic stress disorder (nightmares), symptomatic support in opioid withdrawal	Monitor blood pressure and heart rate
Stimulants/amphetamine/ dextroamphetamine (Adderall), methylphenidate (Ritalin), lisdexamfetamine (Vyvanse), clonidine (Kapvay), guanfacine (Intuniv)	Attention deficit disorder and attention deficit hyperactivity disorder	Monitor blood pressure, heart rate, EKG

▶ PSYCHOPHARMACOLOGY IN PREGNANCY

- Observe extreme caution when administering any medication during pregnancy beyond known teratogenic effects. Risks include decreased appetite, premature labor, discontinuation syndromes, increased agitation or sedation, impaired mother–infant bonding, and poor maternal self-care. Untreated mental illness poses similar dangers to the health and well-being of the mother. Maternal health is the biggest predictor of the baby's health.
- Teratogenic risks associated with certain medication classes:
  - **Antiepileptic drugs (valproic acid, carbamazepine):** Neural tube defects, cleft lip, cleft palate, atrial septal defects
  - **Lithium:** Epstein's anomaly (especially in the first trimester)
- **Benzodiazepines:** Floppy baby syndrome, cleft palate

KNOWLEDGE CHECK: CHAPTER 4

1. The psychiatric-mental health nurse is evaluating a 68-year-old man for symptoms of major depression. While assessing the appearance of the patient, an obvious left-sided ptosis is noted. Which cranial nerve is directly linked to this condition?

   a. III
   b. IV
   c. V
   d. VI

2. The psychiatric-mental health nurse is performing a medication reconciliation for a patient pending admission to the partial hospital program. In which of the following situations would benzodiazepine be appropriately prescribed?

   A. Long-term treatment of panic disorder, alcohol use disorder, or bipolar disorder
   B. Long-term treatment of posttraumatic stress disorder, seizure disorder, alcohol-induced withdrawal
   C. Short-term treatment for generalized anxiety disorder, alcohol-induced withdrawal, premedication for procedures
   D. Short-term treatment for obsessive compulsive disorder, muscle spasms, and hypertension

3. A patient with chronic pain disorder takes oxycontin extended-release 30 mg every 12 hours and is recently admitted to acute psychiatry for depression with suicidal ideations. The psychiatrist prescribes clonazepam 0.5 mg at bedtime, and citalopram 10 mg for depression and anxiety. The psychiatric-mental health nurse should monitor for which of the following conditions with respect to the current use of medications?

   A. Monitor for signs and symptoms of worsening depression and suicidal ideations
   B. Monitor for changes in mental status, diaphoresis, tachycardia, tremor, and diarrhea
   C. Monitor for dystonia and muscle rigidity
   D. Monitor for abnormal involuntary movements of the face, legs, and neck

4. The psychiatric-mental health nurse is providing psychoeducation to a medical student admitted for new diagnosis of bipolar while drawing a therapeutic drug level. The nurse tells the patient "after a drug is absorbed the substrate binds to protein for transport." The patient asks which portion of the drug is available for therapeutic effects. What is the psychiatric-mental health nurse's correct response?

   A. Bound
   B. Unbound
   C. Metabolized
   D. Excreted

(See answers next page.)

1. A) III
Oculomotor nerve (III) allows for extraocular movements, eyelid function/droop, and pupil dilation. Trochlear (IV) controls downward medial gaze. Trigeminal (V) allows for ophthalmic muscles, mandibular muscles, and mastication. Abducens (VI) allows for extraocular movements and downward lateral gaze.

2. C) Short-term treatment for generalized anxiety disorder, alcohol-induced withdrawal, premedication for procedures
Benzodiazepine should not be prescribed for long-term use and are indicated for acute generalized anxiety disorder, alcohol withdrawal, and premedication for procedures. Benzodiazepine should not be prescribed for long-term panic disorder as that is an acute event, nor should they be prescribed for long-term hypertension, obsessive compulsive disorder, or muscle spasms as they are highly addictive, and withdrawal can be fatal.

3. B) Monitor for changes in mental status, diaphoresis, tachycardia, tremor, and diarrhea
Serotonin syndrome can develop when a patient takes multiple serotoninergic medications, and symptoms include alteration in mental status, restlessness, Mayo clonus, hyper reflexes, tachycardia, diaphoresis, shivering, tremor, and diarrhea. Benzodiazepines are used to treat acute anxiety, restlessness, and insomnia associated with starting an SSRI, but the physical needs need to take priority over the psychosocial needs. Dystonia and muscle rigidity or more associated with the use of antipsychotic medication.

4. B) Unbound
Unbound drug is the portion of the drug available for therapeutic effects. Bound is the part of the drug that binds to protein and fat in preparation for excretion. Metabolization is the process in which a drug is prepared for excretion. Excretion is the process in which a substance leaves the body.

5. A 19-year-old male is in an alcohol recovery group facilitated by a psychiatric-mental health nurse. The patient states that on one occasion he passed out much sooner than he usually would with far less than he would usually drink. The patient reveals the time he passed out was during a fraternity hazing in which he was butt-chugging (receiving a beer and vodka enema). What pharmacokinetic process was bypassed by this rectal administration route?

   A. Excretion
   B. Absorption
   C. Distribution
   D. First-pass effect

6. The psychiatric-mental health nurse is scheduling the serum drug level for a medication with a 24-hour half-life. How many hours will it take to reach steady state?

   A. 48 hours
   B. 72 hours
   C. 96 hours
   D. 120 hours

7. A patient with schizophrenia was discharged from the hospital on olanzapine 5 mg twice a day. He immediately resumed smoking cigarettes and escalated to one pack per day. The patient attends a psychopharmacology group facilitated by a psychiatric-mental health nurse. The patient reports he is having trouble sleeping, and the voices have started to return. Which action should the psychiatric-mental health nurse take?

   A. Call 911 to send the patient to the emergency department for stabilization
   B. Have the patient call for an appointment within the week with his psychiatrist
   C. Have the patient see the APRN today in the interim until his scheduled outpatient appointment
   D. Tell him to stop smoking and give him a nicotine patch

8. A patient who has been stable on quetiapine (Seroquel XR) for 3 months has decided to start to drink grapefruit juice twice daily because she has heard it helps with weight loss. She calls to report that since her new diet she has been feeling fatigued and difficulty waking up in the morning. Which of the following is the best response from the psychiatric-mental health nurse?

   A. "I will put in a new prescription for a lower dose of your medication"
   B. "Stop drinking the grapefruit juice and schedule an appointment to discuss the matter further"
   C. "I will prescribe you a stimulant and see you in 2 weeks"
   D. "You should make an appointment with your primary care provider for evaluation"

(*See answers next page.*)

5. D) First-pass effect
The first-pass effect is the process of uptake and conversion by which a substrate is significantly reduced through the CYP450 pathway. Non-enteric routes of administration bypass this effect. Excretion is the process by which substances leave the body. Absorption is the movement of the drug into the bloodstream. Distribution is the movement of the drug through the bloodstream to target receptors where protein binding occurs.

6. D) 120 hours
120 hours; steady state is achieved in five half-lives of the medication (5 × 24 = 120).

7. C) Have the patient see the APRN today in the interim until his scheduled outpatient appointment
Arranging bridge care pending a definitive follow-up visit to increase his olanzapine and schedule a follow-up visit because the patient's symptoms are no longer controlled, and smoking is a known inducer of the CYP450 pathway. The patient has not indicated a threat of harm to self or others, so there is no indication for 911; waiting a week to schedule the appointment allows for further deterioration. Telling a patient to stop smoking may trigger a psychological paradox and can erode therapeutic alliance.

8. B) "Stop drinking the grapefruit juice and schedule an appointment to discuss the matter further"
Stop drinking the grapefruit juice and schedule an appointment to discuss weight gain/weight loss. Grapefruit is a known inhibitor of the CYP450 pathway; stopping this will reduce the sedation over time. It is not appropriate to prescribe this patient a stimulant as the cause has not been determined. Deferring the patient to primary care is not suitable as there is a potential psychotropic drug interaction.

9. A 79-year-old female with no past psychiatric history is admitted with new-onset auditory hallucinations. The patient states her most bothersome symptom is the voices, which have kept her from sleeping through the night for the last 3 weeks, and as a result, she is tired and irritable. Which medication is indicated to help hallucinations and may help with sleep?

   A. Olanzapine 2.5 mg PO
   B. Lorazepam 1 mg PO
   C. Chlorpromazine 50 mg PO
   D. Sertraline 50 mg PO

10. A woman in her 20th week of pregnancy has been resumed on lithium for bipolar disorder. The psychiatric-mental health nurse is providing psychoeducation informs the patient that the higher dose of medication does not mean her mental illness is worse. Which of the following reasons explains the need for a higher dosage in pregnancy?

    A. Increased blood volume
    B. Increased fetal metabolism
    C. Reduced muscle mass
    D. Reduced blood volume

11. The psychiatric-mental health nurse is supervising a nursing student and tells the student nurse the relationship between drug concentration and effect on the body is known as:

    A. Pharmacology
    B. Pharmacokinetics
    C. Pharmacodynamics
    D. Physiology

12. The psychiatric-mental health nurse is providing psychoeducation regarding psychopharmacology to therapeutic support group. A patient who had previously reported feeling much better on her antidepressant suddenly says the drug seems to have stopped working. This is known as:

    A. Tolerance
    B. Tachyphylaxis
    C. Side effect
    D. Adverse effect

13. The psychiatric-mental health nurse is reviewing the blood work of the patients admitted to in-patient psychiatry. The most common electrolyte abnormalities associated with the use of psychotropic medication is:

    A. Hyperkalemia
    B. Hypercalcemia
    C. Hyponatremia
    D. Hypernatremia

(See answers next page.)

9. A) Olanzapine 2.5 mg PO

Olanzapine is an atypical antipsychotic that can help the patient sleep. Because of the patient's age, it is essential to start at a low dose and slowly titrate as tolerated. Benzodiazepines are not preferred in the elderly as they increase risk, especially at higher starting doses. Chlorpromazine potentiates many anticholinergic effects, particularly at high starting doses. Sertraline is not sedating, and the dose should be started lower in the elderly.

10. A) Increased blood volume

Increased blood volume occurs as pregnancy progresses, and patients may need higher doses of medication to maintain concentration effects. Fetal metabolism has no impact on maternal metabolism, but caution is exercised for potential adverse effects to the fetus. Pregnant women do not have decreased muscle mass or reduced blood volume.

11. C) Pharmacodynamics

Pharmacodynamics is the study of the relationship between drug concentration and its effect on the body. Pharmacology is the study of medication uses, effects, and modes of action. Pharmacokinetics is concerned with the body's effect on the drug concerning absorption, distribution, metabolism, and excretion. Physiology is a biological branch concerned with normal functions of an organism.

12. B) Tachyphylaxis

Tachyphylaxis is the rapidly diminishing responsiveness to increasing doses of the medication, also known as the poop-out effect. Tolerance is the process of becoming desensitized and therefore less responsive to a particular dose of medication over time, thereby requiring an increase.

13. C) Hyponatremia

Hyponatremia is the most common electrolyte abnormality associated with psychotropic medication; the condition is called drug-induced syndrome of inappropriate antidiuretic hormone secretion. Hyperkalemia is related to renal insufficiency, which can be acute or chronic. Hypercalcemia is associated with neoplastic disorders and abnormal bone metabolism and resorption. Hypernatremia is related to a water deficit.

14. A patient who has been stable on his long-acting injectable medication tells the psychiatric-mental health nurse that he would like to quit smoking. Which of the following is the best response from the psychiatric-mental health nurse?

    A. "Good for you, I can prescribe you a nicotine patch to help"
    B. "Let us make an appointment as your medication dose may need to be lowered"
    C. "I will refer you to a smoking cessation support group"
    D. "I am glad you have decided to quit smoking"

15. A patient has been taking valproic acid for mood stabilization from a manic episode but is still not sleeping through the night. His last drug level was 50 mcg/mL. The psychiatric-mental health nurse notices the patient seems disoriented to time and is flapping his wrists. Which of the following orders would be expected after notifying the psychiatrist on call?

    A. Give the patient his next dose of divalproex now
    B. Draw an ammonia level
    C. Increase the dose of valproic acid at the next scheduled time
    D. Augment with an atypical antipsychotic

(See answers next page.)

14. B) "Let us make an appointment as your medication dose may need to be lowered"

Making an appointment with the patient for psychoeducation and careful medication adjustment is most appropriate as the patient may become more sedated when the inducing properties of cigarette smoke are less present in the system. Verbal reinforcement and prescribing a medication sight unseen is not the preferred response. Referring the patient to smoking cessation, while helpful, does not address the potential drug–drug interactions. Expressing encouragement for healthy behaviors would be insufficient in this case.

15. B) Draw an ammonia level

Patients can develop encephalopathy due to hyperammonemia when taking valproic acid. It is essential to check the ammonia level before treating the patient. Increasing the dose of medication would worsen the situation and adding another agent does not address the underlying problem.

REFERENCES

Bérard, A., Iessa, N., Chaabane, S., Muanda, F. T., Boukhris, T., & Zhao, J. P. (2016). The risk of major cardiac malformations associated with paroxetine use during the first trimester of pregnancy: A systematic review and meta-analysis. *British Journal of Clinical Pharmacology*, 81(4), 589–604. doi:10.1111/bcp.12849

Courtwright, D. T. (1992). A century of American narcotic policy. In H. J. Gerstein & D. R., Harwood (Eds.), *Institute of Medicine (U.S.) committee for the substance abuse coverage study*. Washington, DC: National Academies Press (U.S.). Retrieved from https://www.ncbi.nlm.nih.gov/books/NBK234755/

Eke, A., & Saccone, G. (2016). Selective serotonin reuptake inhibitor (SSRI) use during pregnancy and risk of preterm birth: A systematic review and meta analysis. *British Journal of Obstetrics and Gynaecology*, 123(12), 1900–1907. doi:10.1111/1471-0528.14144. Retrieved from https://onlinelibrary.wiley.com/doi/abs/10.1111/1471-0528.14144

Gelenberg, A. J., Marlene Freeman, C. P., Markowitz, J. C., Rosenbaum, J. F., Thase, M. E., Trivedi, M. H., … Silbersweig, D. A. (2010). *Practice guideline for the treatment of patients with major depressive disorder: Third edition work group on major depressive disorder*. Retrieved from http://www.psychiatryonline.com/pracGuide/pracGuideTopic_7.aspx

Kumar, A., Datta, S. S., Wright, S. D., Furtado, V. A., & Russell, P. S. (2013). Atypical antipsychotics for psychosis in adolescents. *Cochrane Database of Systematic Reviews*, 2013(10),CD009582. doi:10.1002/14651858.CD009582.pub2 LK - http://sfx.library.uu.nl/utrecht?sid=EMBASE&issn=1469493X&id=doi:10.1002%2F14651858.CD009582.pub2&atitle=Atypical+antipsychotics+for+psychosis+in+adolescents&stitle=Cochrane+Database+Syst.+Rev.&title=Cochrane+Database+of+Systematic+Reviews&volume=2013&issue=10&spage=&epage=&aulast=Kumar&aufirst=Ajit&auinit=A.&aufull=Kumar+A.&coden=&isbn=&pages=-&date=2013&auinit1=A&auinitm=

Leucht, S., Tardy, M., Komossa, K., Heres, S., Kissling, W., & Davis, J. M. (2012). Maintenance treatment with antipsychotic drugs for schizophrenia. *Cochrane Database of Systematic Reviews*, (5), 10–12. doi:10.1002/14651858.CD008016.pub2

Lien, H. H. (2018). Antidepressants and hyponatremia. The American Journal of Medicine, 131(1), 7–8. doi:10.1016/j.amjmed.2017.09.002

Ogle, N. R., & Akkerman, S. R. (2013). Guidance for the discontinuation or switching of antidepressant therapies in adults. *Journal of Pharmacy Practice*, 26(4), 389–396. doi:10.1177/0897190012467210

Patorno, E., Huybrechts, K. F., Bateman, B. T., Cohen, J. M., Desai, R. J., Mogun, H., … Hernandez-Diaz, S. (2017). Lithium use in pregnancy and the risk of cardiac malformations. *New England Journal of Medicine*, 376(23), 2245–2254. doi:10.1056/NEJMoa1612222

Tardy, M., Huhn, M., Kissling, W., Engel, R. R., & Leucht, S. (2014). Haloperidol versus low-potency first-generation antipsychotic drugs for schizophrenia. *Advances in Psychiatric Treatment*, 20(5), 296–296. doi:10.1192/apt.20.5.296

Weisskopf, E., Fischer, C. J., Bickle Graz, M., Morisod Harari, M., Tolsa, J. F., Claris, O., … Panchaud, A. (2015). Risk-benefit balance assessment of SSRI antidepressant use during pregnancy and lactation based on best available evidence. *Expert Opinion on Drug Safety, 14*(3), 413–427. doi:10.1517/14740338.2015.997708

Abramowitz, J. S., Tolin, D. F., & Diefenbach, G. J. (2005). Measuring Change in OCD: Sensitivity of the Obsessive-Compulsive Inventory-Revised. *Journal of Psychopathology and Behavioral Assessment, 27*(4), 317–324. https://doi.org/10.1007/s10862-005-2411-y

Barnett, J. H., & Smoller, J. W. (2009). The genetics of bipolar disorder. *Neuroscience, 164*(1), 331–43. https://doi.org/10.1016/j.neuroscience.2009.03.080

Bazanova, O. M., & Vernon, D. (2014). Interpreting EEG alpha activity. *Neuroscience & Biobehavioral Reviews, 44*, 94–110. https://doi.org/10.1016/J.NEUBIOREV.2013.05.007

Berti, V., Pupi, A., & Mosconi, L. (2011). PET/CT in diagnosis of dementia. *Annals of the New York Academy of Sciences, 1228*, 81–92. https://doi.org/10.1111/j.1749-6632.2011.06015.x

Bird, R. D., & Makela, E. H. (1994). Alcohol withdrawal: what is the benzodiazepine of choice? *The Annals of Pharmacotherapy, 28*(1), 67–71. https://doi.org/10.1177/106002809402800114

Brikell, I., Kuja-Halkola, R., & Larsson, H. (2015). Heritability of attention-deficit hyperactivity disorder in adults. *American Journal of Medical Genetics Part B: Neuropsychiatric Genetics, 168*(6), 406–413. https://doi.org/10.1002/ajmg.b.32335

Daeppen, J.-B., Gache, P., Landry, U., Sekera, E., Schweizer, V., Gloor, S., & Yersin, B. (2002). Symptom-triggered vs fixed-schedule doses of benzodiazepine for alcohol withdrawal: a randomized treatment trial. *Archives of Internal Medicine, 162*(10), 1117–21. Retrieved from http://www.ncbi.nlm.nih.gov/pubmed/12020181

Gejman, P. V, Sanders, A. R., & Duan, J. (2010). The role of genetics in the etiology of schizophrenia. *The Psychiatric Clinics of North America, 33*(1), 35–66. https://doi.org/10.1016/j.psc.2009.12.003

Jaeger, T. M., Lohr, R. H., & Pankratz, V. S. (2001). Symptom-triggered therapy for alcohol withdrawal syndrome in medical inpatients. *Mayo Clinic Proceedings, 76*(7), 695–701. https://doi.org/10.4065/76.7.695

Kitchens, J. M. (1994).*Does this patient have an alcohol problem?* JAMA, *272*(22), 1782–7. Retrieved from http://www.ncbi.nlm.nih.gov/pubmed/7966928

Kroenke, K., Spitzer, R. L., & Williams, J. B. (2001). The PHQ-9: validity of a brief depression severity measure. *Journal of General Internal Medicine, 16*(9), 606–13. https://doi.org/10.1046/J.1525-1497.2001.016009606.X

Lamoureux, B. E., Linardatos, E., Fresco, D. M., Bartko, D., Logue, E., & Milo, L. (2010). Using the QIDS-SR16 to Identify Major Depressive Disorder in Primary Care Medical Patients. *Behavior Therapy, 41*(3), 423–431. https://doi.org/10.1016/j.beth.2009.12.002

Marc, L. G., Raue, P. J., & Bruce, M. L. (2008). Screening performance of the 15-item geriatric depression scale in a diverse elderly home care population. *The American Journal of Geriatric Psychiatry: Official Journal of the American Association for Geriatric Psychiatry, 16*(11), 914–21. https://doi.org/10.1097/JGP.0b013e318186bd67

Mayo-Smith, M. F. (1997). Pharmacological management of alcohol withdrawal. *A meta-analysis and evidence-based practice guideline. American Society of Addiction Medicine Working Group on Pharmacological Management of Alcohol Withdrawal. JAMA, 278*(2), 144–51. Retrieved from http://www.ncbi.nlm.nih.gov/pubmed/9214531

Mottram, P., Wilson, K., & Copeland, J. (2000). Validation of the Hamilton Depression Rating Scale and Montgommery and Asberg Rating Scales in terms of AGECAT depression cases. *International Journal of Geriatric Psychiatry, 15*(12), 1113–9. Retrieved from http://www.ncbi.nlm.nih.gov/pubmed/11180467

MTHFR gene variant | Genetic and Rare Diseases Information Center (GARD) – an NCATS Program. (2018). Retrieved September 6, 2018, from https://rarediseases.info.nih.gov/diseases/10953/mthfr-gene-variant

Ng, K., Dahri, K., Chow, I., & Legal, M. (2011). Evaluation of an alcohol withdrawal protocol and a preprinted order set at a tertiary care hospital. *The Canadian Journal of Hospital Pharmacy, 64*(6), 436–45. Retrieved from http://www.ncbi.nlm.nih.gov/pubmed/22479099

Nuss, M. A., Elnicki, D. M., Dunsworth, T. S., & Makela, E. H. (n.d.). *Utilizing CIWA-Ar to assess use of benzodiazepines in patients vulnerable to alcohol withdrawal syndrome. The West Virginia Medical Journal, 100*(1), 21–5. Retrieved from http://www.ncbi.nlm.nih.gov/pubmed/15119493

Park, S. C., & Choi, J. (2016). Using the Young Mania Rating Scale for Identifying Manic Symptoms in Patients with Schizophrenia. *Yonsei Medical Journal, 57*(5), 1298–9. https://doi.org/10.3349/ymj.2016.57.5.1298

Petzinger, G. M., Quik, M., Ivashina, E., Jakowec, M. W., Jakubiak, M., Di Monte, D., & Langston, J. W. (2001). Reliability and validity of a new global dyskinesia rating scale in the MPTP-lesioned non-human primate. *Movement Disorders: Official Journal of the Movement Disorder Society, 16*(2), 202–7. Retrieved from http://www.ncbi.nlm.nih.gov/pubmed/11295771

Rastegar, D. A., Applewhite, D., Alvanzo, A. A. H., Welsh, C., Niessen, T., & Chen, E. S. (2017). Development and implementation of an alcohol withdrawal protocol using a 5-item scale, the Brief Alcohol Withdrawal Scale (BAWS). *Substance Abuse, 38*(4), 394–400. https://doi.org/10.1080/08897077.2017.1354119

Reoux, J. P., & Miller, K. (2000). Routine hospital alcohol detoxification practice compared to symptom triggered management with an Objective Withdrawal Scale (CIWA-Ar). *The American Journal on Addictions, 9*(2), 135–44. Retrieved from http://www.ncbi.nlm.nih.gov/pubmed/10934575

Roffman, J. L., & Stern, T. A. (2006). Alcohol withdrawal in the setting of elevated blood alcohol levels. *Primary Care Companion to the Journal of Clinical Psychiatry, 8*(3), 170–3. Retrieved from http://www.ncbi.nlm.nih.gov/pubmed/16912820

Sadock, B., Sadock, V., Ruiz, P. (2015). *Synopsis of Psychiatry* (11th ed.). New York: Wolters Kluwer| Lippincott Williams & Wilkins.

Saitz, R., Mayo-Smith, M. F., Roberts, M. S., Redmond, H. A., Bernard, D. R., & Calkins, D. R. (1994). Individualized treatment for alcohol withdrawal. *A randomized double-blind controlled trial. JAMA, 272*(7), 519–23. Retrieved from http://www.ncbi.nlm.nih.gov/pubmed/8046805

Sullivan, J. T., Sykora, K., Schneiderman, J., Naranjo, C. A., & Sellers, E. M. (1989). Assessment of alcohol withdrawal: the revised clinical institute withdrawal assessment for alcohol scale (CIWA-Ar). *British Journal of Addiction, 84*(11), 1353–7. Retrieved from http://www.ncbi.nlm.nih.gov/pubmed/2597811

Trzepacz, P. T., Hochstetler, H., Wang, S., Walker, B., & Saykin, A. J. (2015). Relationship between the Montreal Cognitive Assessment and Mini-mental State Examination for assessment of mild cognitive impairment in older adults. *BMC Geriatrics, 15*(1), 107. https://doi.org/10.1186/s12877-015-0103-3

Wartenberg, A. A., Nirenberg, T. D., Liepman, M. R., Silvia, L. Y., Begin, A. M., & Monti, P. M. (1990). Detoxification of alcoholics: improving care by symptom-triggered sedation. *Alcoholism, Clinical and Experimental Research, 14*(1), 71–5. Retrieved from http://www.ncbi.nlm.nih.gov/pubmed/2178476

Wu, M. S., McGuire, J. F., Arnold, E. B., Lewin, A. B., Murphy, T. K., & Storch, E. A. (2014). Psychometric Properties of the Children's Yale-Brown Obsessive Compulsive Scale in Youth with Autism Spectrum Disorders and Obsessive–Compulsive Symptoms. *Child Psychiatry & Human Development, 45*(2), 201–211. https://doi.org/10.1007/s10578-013-0392-8

Zakhari, R. (2014). Ethylene Glycol Poisoning: Resolution of Cranial Nerve Deficit. *The Journal for Nurse Practitioners, 10*(8), 616–619. https://doi.org/10.1016/j.nurpra.2014.07.001

Part II

Disorders

Substance Use Disorders and Addiction

> ### OBJECTIVES
> - Define substance use disorder
> - Identify predisposing factors for substance use disorder
> - Identify relapse prevention strategies
> - Describe medication-assisted treatment for addiction and nonpharmacological management
> - Identify key mental status exam findings associated with various substances
> - Identify withdrawal signs and symptoms

FAST FACTS

- **Addiction:** Persistent and increased use of a substance or behavior that, when discontinued, causes distress and an urge to resume use despite related adverse consequences; sometimes known as psychological dependence.
- **Dependence:** Repeated use of a substance for physical needs leading to increased tolerance, and, when discontinued, results in physical withdrawal symptoms.
- **Abuse:** The use of any substance that deviates from approved social or medical practice.
- **Codependence:** The learned behavior pattern characterized by enabling maladaptive coping motivated by fear of losing the relationship. Usually seen in the family members of an identified patient.
- **Neuroadaptation:** The physiological process caused by a physical change in the body due to repeated exposure to a substance.
- **Cross-tolerance:** The process by which one drug can be substituted for another drug producing the same physiological and psychological effect (e.g., benzodiazepine and phenobarbital).
- **Withdrawal:** A substance-specific cluster of signs and symptoms that occurs when reducing or stopping the consistent use of the substance.
- **Tolerance:** The condition in which repeated administration of a dosage causes a decreased effect despite increasingly larger doses, which are required to obtain the effect observed of the original dosage.
- **Dual diagnosis:** The co-occurrence of a substance use disorder with a primary mood disorder.

- Psychiatric symptoms may be primarily related to substance use, discontinuation, or withdrawal.
- Neurogensis and pruning may cause physiological changes known as neuroadaptation, potentially necessitating long-term treatment.
- The term "substances" refers to drugs, alcohol, medications, or toxins that cause changes in cognition, behavior, and perceptions.

SUBSTANCE USE DISORDER

Characterized by a pattern of use leading to clinically significant impairment or distress as manifested by two or more of the following symptoms within 12 months:

- Increased consumption of larger amounts over a longer period than was intended.
- A persistent desire or unsuccessful attempts to cut down on use.
- Significant time spent in activities necessary to obtain, use, or recover from the effects of the substance.
- Cravings or strong desires for a substance.
- Recurrent use of a substance resulting in failure to fulfill major role obligations at work, school, or home.
- Continued use despite persistent or recurrent social or interpersonal problems caused by or exacerbated by the effects of the substance.
- Important social, occupational, or recreational activities are stopped or reduced because of substance use.
- Recurrent substance use in situations in which it is physically hazardous.
- Persistent substance use despite knowledge of having persistent or recurrent physical or psychological problems that are likely caused by or exacerbated by the substance.
- Tolerance develops:
  - An increased need for more of the substance to achieve the desired effect or intoxication
  - Significantly reduced efficacy with continued use of the same amount of the substance
- Withdrawal syndrome:
  - Use of the substance to relieve or avoid withdrawal symptoms
  - After cessation or reduction of use, a manifestation of two characteristic withdrawal symptoms:
    - Palpitations
    - Sweating
    - Sleep disturbance
    - Nausea, vomiting, or diarrhea
    - Hallucinations
    - Agitation, restlessness, fidgety, irritable mood, depressed mood
    - Anxiety or nervousness
    - Seizures
    - Tremulous
    - Fever, chills, cold sweats, piloerection
    - Headache
    - Yawning
    - Muscle aches

CLINICAL VIGNETTE OF THE PROTOTYPICAL PATIENT

Dr. Greggory House is a 52-year-old man with opioid use disorder; he has required increasing amounts of prescription opioids initially prescribed for back injury. Within 6 hours of missing a dose, he begins to sweat, develops goosebumps, feels nauseated, anxious, and restless. He feels everything is fine as long as he takes his medicine. He has had to find multiple physicians in order to maintain his use and has supplemented the sedative effect with alcohol each night in order to sleep. He is spending more and more time thinking about using or acquiring opioids for use. He presents as charming and effusive in order to get his physicians to like him and trust him as he presents in an overly familiar manner. He minimizes questions by becoming condescending, dismissive, and hostile to anyone he thinks wants to thwart his plan to get and use drugs.

INCIDENCE AND PREVALENCE

- At least 50% of patients with a psychiatric disorder have a comorbid substance use disorder
  - More common in patients with psychotic disorders and bipolar disorder
- Accounts for 2 million admissions each year to detox and rehab facilities
- Marijuana, tobacco, and alcohol are the most commonly abused substances
  - More common in men than women
  - Least common in Americans of Asian descent
  - Black, Hispanic, and First Nation Americans comprise the highest rates of alcohol use disorder
- More than half of motor vehicle fatalities involve driving under the influence of alcohol
- Lifetime risk for alcohol use disorder is 15% of the U.S. population
- **Risk factors:** Various theories inform the identified risk factors for the development of a substance use disorder, including biological, psychological, and sociological; no one theory contributes more significantly, but likely a confluence of variables increases the risk in aggregate.
  - Genetic loading
    - Patients with first-degree relatives who have had a substance use disorder are more likely to manifest a substance use disorder (Yuodelis-Flores & Ries, 2015).
    - Males are more likely than females.
    - Neuroadaptation can cause structural changes in the brain and increase the likelihood of addictive behavior. The reward process is highly correlated with memory function (Moberg, Bradford, Kaye, & Curtin, 2017). The physical change can be more persistent in some people and increases the chance of relapse even after a long period of sobriety.
      - These changes lead to tolerance and withdrawal and can increase the difficulty of the detox process and sobriety maintenance.
      - The positive reinforcement is known as the "feel good" sensation that accompanies the drug use, and the "feel bad" sensation is known as the negative reinforcement that accompanies the "coming down" from the "high" and withdrawal process.

- The positive reinforcement is dopamine mediated in the ventral tegmental area and nucleus accumbens in the brain.
- The neuropeptides (enkephalins, endorphins) trigger the dopamine release, which further reduces the perception of effort needed to use the substance.
- The dopamine receptor becomes increasingly sensitized with continued and increased use, and, eventually, a similar release can occur with visualizing related paraphernalia.
  - The negative reinforcements (aversion driving) are gamma aminobutyric acid-mediated; triggers symptoms of dysphoria and anxiety.

▶ SCREENING TOOLS AND EARLY INTERVENTION

- **History**
  - The clinical interview aims to develop a global understanding of the disorder to enhance the therapeutic alliance and prescribe a treatment plan. In evaluating a patient with a substance use disorder (alcohol, illicit drugs, process addiction), the following domains must be assessed (try to use open-ended questions):
  - **Current level and history**
    - "Tell me about your current use."
    - "What substances do you currently use (prescribed and illicit)?"
    - "What would a friend or loved one say about your current use?"
    - "How would you like your current use to be different?"
  - **The pattern of use**
    - "What types and amounts of substances do you use?"
    - "What is the longest period you have gone without using?"
    - "What was the reason you stopped?"
    - "What was the trigger that caused you to resume?"
  - "How has your use now changed from when you first began?"
    - "Have you been using more and more over time?"
    - "Have you used more than you intended?"
  - "When was your last use? Have you planned your next use?"
  - "Have you taken medications in a way other than was prescribed?"
  - **Social consequences**
    - "Have you ever had any legal trouble, arrests, or mandated treatment due to use?"
    - "How have your work, school, or professional obligations been affected by use?"
    - "When using drugs, have you ever behaved in a way that you later regretted?"
  - **Relational aspects**
    - "How has your use affected your relationships with your spouse, family, friends?"
    - "Do you typically use alone or with others?"
    - "Is your use a secret or do significant people in your life know about it?"
    - "How much time do you spend thinking about using, not using, acquiring, or disposing of the substance?"

- **Physical/psychological consequences**
  - "What physical symptoms have you noticed related to using?"
  - "What physical symptoms have you noticed when you stop using?"
  - "What psychological symptoms do you notice when you stop using?"
  - "What injuries have you sustained due to use?"

ASSESSMENT AND DIAGNOSIS

- **Physical exam**
  - The purpose of the exam is to determine physiological integrity and the current state of intoxication or withdrawal and identify and mitigate any risks that may be associated with detoxification and underlying conditions. The physical exam is generally unremarkable and nonspecific but may reveal the following:
  - **Neuropsychiatric:** Dysphoria, slurred speech, anxiety, ataxia, emotional lability, irritability, hallucinations, nystagmus, new-onset seizures, tremors
- **Mental status exam**
  - Manifestations are often related to the substance ingested or reflect the withdrawal of the substance on which the patient has become dependent.
    - **Stimulants:** Agitation, restlessness, irritability, grandiosity, elatedness, euphoria, aggression, lability
    - **Depressants:** Dysphoria, impaired attention, impaired memory, disinhibition, psychomotor retardation, paranoia
    - **Hallucinogens:** Mood swings, panic, aggression, paranoia, flashbacks, tremors, impaired cognition
    - **Cannabis:** Paranoia, confusion, disorientation to time
    - **Inhalants:** Irritability, delirium, confusion, stupor
- **Eyes:** Icterus (liver failure), nystagmus (opioid use), pinpoint pupils (opioid use)
- **Cardiovascular:** Hypertension (stimulant use), tachycardia (dehydration, stimulant use)
- **Pulmonary:** Focal wheezing, scattered rhonchi, hypoxia, poor effort (aspiration pneumonia)
- **Gastrointestinal:** Hepatosplenomegaly (fatty liver disease), atypical chest pain (reflux), right upper quadrant pain with inspiratory pause (gall stones), left upper quadrant pain radiating to the back (pancreatitis), epigastric pain (gastritis, peptic ulcer disease), vomiting blood (esophageal varices)
- **Endocrine:** Gonadal atrophy (anabolic steroid use), prolactinemia (substance-induced, antagonizes testosterone), gynecomastia, hyperlipidemia
- **Dermatologic:** Diaphoresis, bruising, spider nevi, telangiectasia, angiomas, palmar erythema, localized skin infections, spider veins on the abdomen (liver disease)
- **Diagnostic tests**
  - Should be guided by the presenting signs and symptoms found in the history and physical exam
  - Complete blood count, comprehensive metabolic profile, serum magnesium, thyroid function tests; serum B12 is most commonly used, but methylmalonic acid is preferred (Vashi, Edwin, Popiel, Lammersfeld, & Gupta, 2016; Table 5.1)
  - Urine drug screen (Table 5.2)

Table 5.1 Laboratory Indicators of Alcohol Dependency

Test	Lab Results
Liver enzymes	AST elevated; ALT elevated; GGT elevated
Hemogram	MCV elevated
Coagulation studies	PT increased
Electrolytes	Sodium: hyponatremia; potassium: hyperkalemia
Lipid profile	Total cholesterol elevated; triglycerides elevated
Pancreatic enzymes	Amylase elevated, Lipase elevated (more sensitive for pancreatitis)
Blood alcohol level (affected by weight, sex, and tolerance)	Legally intoxicated 0.08%, impaired 0.8%– 0.4%, risk of death >0.4%
Nutritional metabolites	Homocysteine elevated

ALT, alanine aminotransferase; AST, aspartate aminotransferase; GGT, gamma-glutamyl transferase; MCV, mean corpuscular volume; PT, prothrombin time.

Source: From Enoch, M. A., & Goldman, D. (2002). Problem drinking and alcoholism: Diagnosis and treatment. *American Family Physician, 65*(3), 441–450.

Table 5.2 Urine Screen Toxicology Drug of Abuse

Classification	Street Names	Urine Detection
Opioids	Schoolboy, hydros, dones, vics, juice, hospital heroin, oxy-coffins, killers, percs, blues, nu-blues, biscuits, blue heaven	3 days
Synthetic opioids	Demmies, dollies, dolphies	4 days
Barbiturates	Yellow jackets, angels, downers, red birds, phennies, yellows, tootsies, goofballs, peanut butter balls	3–4 weeks
Benzodiazepines	Downs, King Kong pills, jellies, jelly, Edinburgh eccies, tams, terms, mazzies, temazies, tammies, temmies, beans, eggs, green eggs, wobbly eggs, knockouts, hardball, norries, oranges, rugby balls, ruggers, terminators, red and blue, no-gos, blackout, green devils, drunk pills, brainwash, mind erasers, tem-tems, mommy's big helper, vitamin T, bit T, TZ	3–7 days
Neuropathics	Gabby	3 days
Muscle relaxants	Dance, soma coma, Wallace 200s, Las Vegas cocktail	2–5 days
Sedative hypnotics	Ludes, A-minus, zombie pills, no-go, zims, and zimmers	2–4 days

Classification	Street Names	Urine Detection
Amphetamines	Aimies, back dex, bennies, black beauties, brain pills, bumblebees, cartwheels, dexies, marathons, minibennie, pep pills, pixies, road dope, speed, truck drivers, uppers	2–4 days
Alcohol	Booze, wine, beer, and chat with ethyl	2 days
Cathinones, piperazine (bath salts)	"Bath salts," or veiled as ecstasy, Molly, cloud 9, ivory wave, flakka	3 days
Ketamine	K, ket, special K, vitamin K, vit K, kit kat, keller, Kelly's day, green, blind squid, cat valium, purple, special la coke, super acid, super C	2–4 days
LSD	LSD, acid	1–5 days
Marijuana (THC)	Weed, pot, reefer, grass, dope, ganja, Mary Jane, hash, herb, aunt Mary, skunk, boom, chronic, cheeba, blunt, ashes, baby bhang, bammy, blanket, bomber, boom, broccoli, cripple, dagga, dinkie dow, ding, dona juana, flower, flower tops, gasper, giggle smoke, good giggles, good butt, hot stick, jay, jolly green, joy smoke, joy stick, roach, pot, reefer	3 weeks
MDMA ecstasy	X, E, XTC, Adam, beans, candy, dancing shoes, disco biscuits, doves, e-bombs, egg rolls, happy pill, hug drug, love drug, macolm, Scooby snacks, smartees, sweets, skittles, thizz, vitamin E, vitamin X, vowels	1–3 days
Methamphetamine	Crystal meth, crystal, meth, christina, Tina, cris, cristy, ice, crank, speed, geep, geeter, getgo, go fast, poor man's coke, redneck cocaine, working man's cocaine, trash, garbage, wash	1–4 days
Phencyclidine (PCP)	Hog, angel dust, loveboat, lovely	2–30 days
Synthetic cannabinoids	K2, spice, fake pot	1–3 days

LSD, lysergic acid diethylamide; MDMA, methylene-dioxy-methamphetamine.

Source: From Substance Abuse Mental Health Service Administration (SAMHSA/CST) Center for Substance Abuse Treatment. (2006). *Substance abuse: Clinical issues in intensive outpatient treatment.* Rockville, MD: Substance Abuse and Mental Health Services Administration (U.S.). Retrieved from http://www.ncbi.nlm.nih.gov/pubmed/22514853.

- **Differentials (rule out):** In addition to acute intoxication, substance withdrawal must also be considered, as well as a primary or comorbid mood, psychotic, or personality disorder as either co-occurring or predisposing. Many acute exacerbations of medical conditions can mimic the signs and symptoms of alcohol withdrawal:
  - Hypo-/hyperthyroidism
  - Cushing's disease/adrenal insufficiency
  - Seizure disorder
  - Myocardial infarction
  - Cerebral vascular accident/head trauma
  - Delirium

PLANNING

In planning the care and treatment for a patient with a substance use disorder, the following questions should be considered:

- Is the patient currently intoxicated, and do they require a detox?
- Where can the patient be safely detoxed?
- What is the history with withdrawal syndromes, and do they have comorbid conditions that will complicate the detox process?
- Are they ready for rehab, and what are they willing to do?
- Are there financial implications, and is there a social support network?
- What have they tried in the past?
- What are the barriers to change?

INTERVENTION

- **Management and plan:** Management differs depending on the syndrome exhibited by the person. The main priority is to rule out and treat underlying medical conditions that may contribute to the clinical findings because withdrawal syndrome is a diagnosis of exclusion.
- **Detoxification:** A natural process in which the liver metabolizes substances from the bloodstream to facilitate excretion. Treatment is aimed at reducing the severity of symptoms associated with the withdrawal process. This process can be supported in either an inpatient or outpatient setting, depending on risk factors and comorbid conditions.
  - Inpatient indications for detox include a history of delirium tremens, seizure disorder, pregnancy, lack of social supports, unreliable clinical information, or uncontrolled medical comorbidity
  - During the detox phase, reduce stimulation of light and noise, frequently observe, check vital signs and Clinical Institute Withdrawal Assessment for Alcohol (CIWA) scale every 4 hours, clear clutter, implement passive safety measures (night lights, fall risk factors, etc.).
    - Ensure adequate hydration and electrolyte repletion
    - Before discharge, establish aftercare and contingency plans for the first 7 days

- Opioid withdrawal is not fatal. Detox can be guided by the Clinical Opioid Withdrawal Scale (COWS) https://www.mdcalc.com/cows-score-opiate-withdrawal
  - Set patient expectations that there will be a certain amount of discomfort
  - Buprenorphine is commonly used once the patient goes into withdrawal to reduce the severity of symptoms (Tompkins et al., 2009; Wesson & Ling, 2003)
- Benzodiazepine and alcohol withdrawal can be fatal and should be guided by the revised Clinical Institute Withdrawal Assessment of Alcohol Scale – Revised (CIWA-Ar) https://www.mdcalc.com/ciwa-ar-alcohol-withdrawal#evidence
  - The primary symptom is psychomotor agitation
  - Longer-acting agents are preferred and dosed based on symptoms (Enoch & Goldman, 2002; Tompkins et al., 2009; Wesson & Ling, 2003). Alternatively, fixed dosing with a gradual taper is also acceptable with close monitoring
  - Other supportive measures are sometimes necessary, including IV hydration and nutritional support
  - Patients with liver disease should use benzodiazepines that do not produce metabolites after hepatic conjugation:
    - Lorazepam
    - Oxazepam
    - Temazepam
  - Clinical management of sobriety often requires treatment of both the substance use disorder and comorbid psychiatric disorder
    - Pharmacological aversive therapy is not common but is still an accepted practice
      - Disulfiram (Antabuse) should not be used until the patient has been alcohol-free for at least 12 hours. The client should avoid any alcohol-containing products (mouthwash, cough medicine, vinegar, extracts) for up to 14 days after the last dose
      - Monitor liver enzymes and evaluate for elevated mood in patients with bipolar disorder

Table 5.3 Medication-Assisted Treatment for Addiction

Medication	Classification	Symptoms Managed
Citalopram	Selective serotonin reuptake inhibitor	Reduces desire and substance enjoyment
Bupropion	Dopamine and norepinephrine reuptake inhibitor	Reduces cravings and withdrawal intensity
Ondansetron	Selective serotonin (5-HT3) antagonist	Reduces cravings
Naloxone	Opioid antagonist	Reverses opioid sedation
Naltrexone	Opioid antagonist	Longer acting, reduces cravings, enhances abstinence efforts by blocking reward associated with substance

(continued)

Medication	Classification	Symptoms Managed
Buprenorphine	Partial opioid agonist	Reduces opioid cravings, facilitates opioid detox, preferred for long-acting formulations
Buprenorphine/naloxone	Opioid antagonist, partial opioid agonist	Reduces cravings, facilitates opioid detox, preferred for short acting formulations
Methadone	Opioid	Long-acting opioid suppresses withdrawal, requires a government approved program
Acamprosate	May inhibit glutamate and enhance GABA	Reduces alcohol cravings and promotes abstinence-reducing tolerance effects
Disulfiram	Inhibits aldehyde dehydrogenase and causes increased acetaldehyde	Aversive therapy when alcohol is consumed: vomiting, nausea, headache, flushing

GABA, gamma-aminobenzoic acid.

Sources: From Song, J., Park, J. H., Han, D. H., Roh, S., Son, J. H., Choi, T. Y., ... Lee, Y. S. (2016). Comparative study of the effects of bupropion and escitalopram on Internet gaming disorder. *Psychiatry and Clinical Neurosciences, 70*(11), 527–535. doi:10.1111/pcn.12429; Swift, R. M. (1999). Medications and alcohol craving. *Alcohol Research & Health, 23*, 207–213. Retrieved from https://pdfs.semanticscholar.org/a266/4ac300402f3857f41a68492a647c633c4079.pdf; Swift, R. M., & Aston, E. R. (2015). Pharmacotherapy for alcohol use disorder: Current and emerging therapies. *Harvard Review of Psychiatry, 23*(2), 122–133. doi:10.1097/HRP.0000000000000079; Winslow, B. T., & Onysko, M. (2016). Medications for alcohol use disorder. *American Family Physician, 93,* 457–465. Retrieved from www.aafp.org/afp

- **Medication-assisted treatment for addiction (Table 5.3):** The use of pharmacological agents to reduce cravings and reduce rewards associated with substance use.
  - Reduces the intensity of feelings, which may trigger lapse and relapse as the patient develops adaptive coping strategies
- **Nonpharmacological treatment for the individual**
  - **Support groups:** To develop empathy, promote the use of mature defense mechanisms, and address interpersonal relationships
  - **Individual therapy:** To deal with cognitive distortions and personality disorder traits
  - **Primary care provider:** To address the chronic physiological effects of substance use disorders (anemias, cardiovascular disease, GI disease, neurological, and nutritional)
  - **Psychiatric aftercare:** To address primary or comorbid mental illness
- **Family system care**
  - Substance use education
  - Support groups
  - Group therapy: Process driven to promote self-efficacy and resilience
  - Community resources
  - Factors influencing family system involvement include:
    - Therapeutic alliance with the treatment team
    - Caregiver role strain (physical, mental, financial)
    - Shame, strife, abuse
    - Personality disorders
    - Untreated mental illness

EVALUATION

- **Relapse prevention model:** Asserts that both immediate determinants and covert antecedents increase the risk of lapse and relapse, and interventions raise self-awareness, enhance self-efficacy, challenge cognitive distortions, and develop and refine roadmaps (Larimer, Palmer, & Marlatt, 1999)
- **Immediate determinants**
  - **High-risk situations:** Negative emotional states (associated with the highest rate of relapse) can be triggered by perceived peer pressure, lack of support
  - **Coping skills:** Response to high-risk situations
  - **Outcome expectancies:** What the person expects to occur in response to substance use versus abstaining. Those who drink the most have the highest expectation of positive effects.
  - **Abstinence violation effect:** The patient's reaction to a lapse, if attributed to self-failure; negative emotions may follow. Alternatively, if the lapse is viewed as a learning opportunity, relapse is less likely to occur and the likelihood of future relapse is reduced.
- **Antecedents**
  - **Lifestyle factors:** Life balance, alternative healthful behaviors, recreational activities, social connections
  - **Urges/cravings:** Environmental cues, accessibility to substance, romanticizing use, mentally minimizing consequences, rationalization
  - **Connecting to support groups**
    - Twelve-step groups or other support groups that promote socializing and comradery
    - Individual/family therapy
    - Connect to primary care
    - Psychoeducation
    - Supportive housing
    - Avoid major life decisions
  - **Adolescence is the most common time for drug and alcohol debut**
    - 35% report consistent alcohol use
    - 15% report binge-drinking
    - 50% report at least one use of illicit drugs (including marijuana)
  - **Older adults**
    - Often with comorbid medical conditions and may require a harm reduction strategy rather than total abstinence given the physiological strain of detox; requires close collaboration with a primary care provider or inpatient facility.
    - Consider social factors for accessing care, including cost, transportation, socialization, declining senses (hearing, sight, touch, and taste)

▶ CULTURAL IMPLICATIONS

Many cultures have various implications that can affect the context of mental health and substance use disorders. The mere use of substance is insufficient to constitute a use disorder if it is bound to a cultural or religious practice. In order to constitute a disorder, the psychiatric mental health nurse should inquire as to the need to use more and more to achieve a desired effect and any consequences that are affecting daily life. Cultural implications are either by shared affiliation, ethnicity, or identity. Some cultures include:

- Generational divisions (X, Z, Baby Boomers, Silent Generation, The Greatest Generation)
- African Americans
- Hispanic/Latinx
- Southeast Asian
- Asian/Pacific Islanders
- Native Americans (First Nation or Indigenous People of North America)
- Rural populations
- Homeless populations
- Lesbian, gay, bisexual, queer/questioning, transgender

The psychiatric-mental health nurse should remain curious and respectful while inquiring as to the meaning of mental illness, substance abuse, and treatment in the patient's culture rather than make assumptions based on observable attributes because people may not subscribe to culture-bound norms.

KNOWLEDGE CHECK: CHAPTER 5

1. A 61-year-old married woman who has been sober from alcohol use disorder for 25 years relapsed 3 weeks ago. She reports drinking 1.5 L of vodka and half a liter of scotch daily. On exam, she is emotionally labile, ranging from irritable to crying, slurring her words, and exhibits a bilateral upper extremity fine tremor. Vitals: blood pressure 150/100, heart rate 110, respiratory rate 18, SpO_2 98% room air. She reports feeling nauseous, sweating, and moderately anxious. What is the primary concern for this patient?

   A. Alcohol use disorder
   B. Generalized anxiety disorder
   C. Alcohol withdrawal
   D. Delirium tremens

2. A patient who has required increasing amounts of medication to achieve the desired effect and develops withdrawal symptoms when dosing is delayed is said to be:

   A. Dependent
   B. Tolerant
   C. Addicted
   D. In withdrawal

3. A patient is complaining of chronic back pain and requests a refill of his oxycodone prescription because the pain is so bad; he becomes suicidal. As a result, his primary care provider referred him to psychiatry. The patient states he can tell if he is late taking his next dose by even 1 hour as he becomes very anxious, restless, irritable, and begins sweating. He states that he is so worried about having pain attacks that much of his day is spent waiting to take the next dose. When he runs out of his medication between visits, he buys some from his friend. Which of the following best describes the patient's condition?

   A. Dependence
   B. Addiction
   C. Tolerance
   D. Withdrawal

(See answers next page.)

1. C) Alcohol withdrawal
Alcohol withdrawal symptoms include emotional lability, bilateral upper extremity tremor, hypertension, tachycardia, nausea, sweating, and anxiety. Alcohol use disorder is characterized by a pattern of use with significant impairment with two or more *Diagnostic and Statistical Manual of Mental Disorders, Fifth Edition (DSM-5)* criteria over the previous 12-month period. Generalized anxiety disorder is characterized by excessive worrying lasting at least 6 months. Delirium tremens is a severe form of alcohol withdrawal marked by global confusion, audiovisual hallucinations, fever, hypertension, and diaphoresis, which occur within 3 to 10 days of the last alcoholic drink.

2. A) Dependent
Dependence is characterized by the repeated use of a substance for physical needs leading to increased tolerance and, when discontinued, results in physical withdrawal symptoms. Tolerance is a condition in which repeated administration of the dosage causes a decreased effect despite increasingly larger doses, which are required to obtain the effect observed in the initial dosage. Addiction is psychological dependence leading to persistent and increased use of the substance or behavior and when discontinued causes distress and urges to resume use substance use despite adverse consequences. Withdrawal is a substance-specific cluster of signs and symptoms

3. B) Addiction
Addiction is psychological dependence leading to persistent and increased use of the substance or behavior and, when discontinued, causes distress and urges to resume use despite adverse consequences. Dependence is characterized by the repeated use of a substance for physical needs leading to increased tolerance and, when discontinued, results in physical withdrawal symptoms. Tolerance is a condition in which repeated administration of the dosage causes a decreased effect despite increasingly larger doses, which are required to obtain the effect observed in the initial dosage. Withdrawal is a substance-specific cluster of signs and symptoms that occur when reducing or stopping the consistent use of the substance.

4. A 30-year-old male who was started on sertraline for generalized anxiety disorder was also started on lorazepam 1 mg for sleep during the first 2 weeks as he was adjusting to the medication. At the 2-week follow-up visit, his psychiatrist increased the sertraline, but the dose of lorazepam does not seem to be helping with sleep, and the patient is requesting a higher dose. Which of the following best describes the patient's condition?

    A. Dependence
    B. Addiction
    C. Tolerance
    D. Withdrawal

5. A patient who has been drinking a six pack of beer each night to relax after work has been having trouble staying asleep through the night. When she wakes up at 2 a.m. she takes diphenhydramine 25 mg to help her fall back asleep, but this makes her sleep through the alarm clock and late for work. She also reports having a headache through midmorning until she gets her second cup of coffee. She thinks this is related to her alcohol use and has unsuccessfully tried to cut down several times in the past year. Which of the following should the psychiatric-mental health nurse do during the detox and withdrawal process?

    A. Provide a quiet low stimulation environment
    B. Monitor intake and output
    C. Ensure the patient has coffee
    D. Encourage group attendance

6. A 45-year-old man in the emergency department has no past psychiatric history and presents with passive suicidal ideations and emotional lability. Which of the following tests is essential in helping formulate a preliminary diagnosis and treatment plan?

    A. 12-lead EKG
    B. Urine toxicology
    C. Complete blood count
    D. Liver profile

7. A 43-year-old man is requesting medication-assisted treatment for addiction with Suboxone and wants to begin immediately to "get his life back." What should the psychiatric-mental health nurse do first?

    A. Assess his current level and history of use
    B. Administer Suboxone 2 mg SL daily to start now
    C. Provide psychoeducation regarding Suboxone maintenance
    D. Refer the patient to an inpatient detox facility

(See answers next page.)

4. C) Tolerance
Tolerance is a condition in which repeated administration of the dosage causes a decreased effect despite increasingly larger doses that are required to obtain the effect observed in the initial dosage. Dependence is characterized by the repeated use of a substance for physical needs leading to increased tolerance and, when discontinued, results in physical withdrawal symptoms. Addiction is psychological dependence leading to persistent and increased use of the substance or behavior and, when discontinued, causes distress and urges to resume use despite adverse consequences. Withdrawal is a substance-specific cluster of signs and symptoms that occur when reducing or stopping the consistent use of the substance.

5. A) Provide a quiet low stimulation environment
Providing a low stimulation environment for sleep and rest reduces the risk of injury and complications. Increasing stimuli by encouraging group attendance or giving stimulants is not appropriate during detox and withdrawal. Intake and output are not the priority based on the information provided.

6. B) Urine toxicology
Urine toxicology is essential because various drugs of abuse can induce various psychopathology, and all psychiatric diagnoses are made by exclusion. A 12-lead EKG will not provide insight into the presenting signs and symptoms but may guide medication selection. A complete blood count will not help explain the presenting symptoms, and any findings will require further investigation. The liver profile results will not explain the current symptom presentation but may raise the index of suspicion for further investigation.

7. A) Assess his current level and history of use
Evaluating for substance use disorder requires an evaluation of the current level and history of use. Suboxone is not prescribed until the patient is in opioid withdrawal, otherwise a precipitated withdrawal may occur. Psychoeducation should be based on the findings from the evaluation, which must occur first. Before referring a patient for any therapy, it is important to know the extent of the problem.

8. Which of the following medications is preferred for a 21-year-old male with a history of polysubstance use disorder and difficulty with medication adherence?

   A. Naltrexone 50 mg PO only when planning to use substances
   B. Naltrexone 50 mg PO daily
   C. Naltrexone 380 mg IM monthly
   D. Methadone maintenance

9. A 34-year-old man is inattentive, dysphoric, disinhibited, with impaired memory and psychomotor retardation. All of the following drugs of abuse may cause these symptoms EXCEPT:

   A. Alcohol
   B. Opioids
   C. Cannabis
   D. Stimulants

10. Which of the following agents could cause a patient to behave restlessly, agitated, grandiose, aggressive, and emotionally labile?

    A. Amphetamines
    B. Opioids
    C. Marijuana
    D. Ketamine

11. A 43-year-old man was involved in a motor vehicle collision in which he was found to have a blood alcohol concentration of 0.200. He was observed wandering around the crash site, slurring his words, and unable to provide a clear history. Emergency Medical Services brought him to the emergency department. The nurse triaged him to psychiatry for acute alcohol intoxication. What is the first priority for the patient?

    A. C-spine stabilization and head imaging
    B. IV hydration
    C. Explore the client's willingness to enter rehab
    D. Ask the patient when he had his last drink

12. When assessing a patient's withdrawal symptoms from opioids, which evidence-based tool would be most appropriate?

    A. Clinical Institute Withdrawal Assessment of Alcohol Scale-Revised (CIWA-Ar)
    B. Minnesota Multiphasic Personality Inventory (MMPI)
    C. Clinical Opioid Withdrawal Scale (COWS)
    D. Hamilton Rating Scale for Depression (HAM-D)

(See answers next page.)

8. C) Naltrexone 380 mg IM monthly
Naltrexone 380 mg IM offers the best option for medication nonadherence and harm reduction. Oral agents used at the patient's discretion, given his history of nonadherence, are less likely to be effective. Beginning someone on methadone maintenance requires a high degree of adherence.

9. D) Stimulants
Stimulants of the central nervous system do not cause psychomotor retardation and memory impairment. Alcohol, opioids, and cannabis have central nervous system depressant properties and can cause inattention, dysphoria, disinhibition, cognitive impairment, and psychomotor retardation.

10. A) Amphetamines
Amphetamines stimulate the central nervous system and can cause restlessness, agitation, grandiosity, aggressive behavior, and emotional lability. Opioids, cannabinoids, and ketamine induce euphoric feelings and blunting of affect.

11. A) C-spine stabilization and head imaging
C-spine stabilization and head imaging are of paramount importance in this intoxicated man who was involved in a motor vehicle collision. Intoxication reduces his reliability as a historian and can impair his pain sensation. Physiological needs and safety take priority over other psychosocial needs.

12. C) Clinical Opioid Withdrawal Scale (COWS)
The Clinical Opioid Withdrawal Scale (COWS) helps quantify the symptoms of opioid withdrawal to guide symptom management or Suboxone induction. The Clinical Institute Withdrawal Assessment of Alcohol Scale-Revised (CIWA-Ar) is used for alcohol withdrawal symptom assessment. The Minnesota Multiphasic Personality Inventory (MMPI) is a personality assessment. The Hamilton Rating Scale for Depression (HAM-D) screens for depression.

13. A patient presents for a follow-up visit and has a dual diagnosis of substance use disorder and major depressive disorder. He reports that he has been feeling increasingly anxious, having difficulty sleeping. He continues to attend his Alcoholics Anonymous meetings regularly but reports he had two beers 3 days ago and feels very guilty. Which of the following best describes this patient's situation?

   A. Relapse
   B. Withdrawal
   C. Intoxication
   D. Lapse

14. A patient with familial fatty liver disease and elevated liver enzymes secondary to alcohol use disorder is admitted for detox. Which of the following benzodiazepines should not be used?

   A. Temazepam
   B. Lorazepam
   C. Oxazepam
   D. Chlordiazepoxide

15. A patient who has been sober for 7 days struggles with cravings and is fearful of relapse. He reports taking naltrexone daily. What medication is used to help reduce his cravings?

   A. Citalopram
   B. Disulfiram
   C. Buprenorphine
   D. Thiamine

(See answers next page.)

13. D) Lapse
A lapse is a brief pause in sobriety, which may or may not lead to relapse. Relapse is a reactivation of the disease or return to a behavior consistent with substance use disorder after a prolonged period of sobriety. Withdrawal is a substance-specific cluster of signs and symptoms that occur when reducing or stopping the consistent use of the substance. Intoxication is a state of near poisoning, manifesting signs of inebriation (disinhibition, impaired cognition, delayed neurological response time).

14. D) Chlordiazepoxide
Chlordiazepoxide is metabolized in the liver by cytochrome P-mediated oxidation. Temazepam, lorazepam, and oxazepam are metabolized by conjugation. They are less dependent on global liver function and are preferred in patients with liver disease.

15. A) Citalopram
Citalopram and other SSRIs have been found to decrease desirability, liking, and consumption of alcohol in alcohol-dependent drinkers. Given the patient's presentation, prescribing an SSRI will help the patient without doing harm. Disulfiram is an aversive agent. Buprenorphine has been found to reduce cravings and withdrawal symptoms in patients with opioid dependence. Thiamine is indicated to prevent and mitigate Wernicke Korsakoff syndrome associated with vitamin B1 deficiency, which is commonly found in patients with alcohol dependence.

REFERENCES

Enoch, M. A., & Goldman, D. (2002). Problem drinking and alcoholism: Diagnosis and treatment. *American Family Physician, 65*(3), 441–450.

Larimer, M. E., Palmer, R. S., & Marlatt, G. A. (1999). *Relapse prevention: An overview of Marlatt's cognitive-behavioral model*. Retrieved from https://pubs.niaaa.nih.gov/publications/arh23-2/151-160.pdf

Moberg, C. A., Bradford, D. E., Kaye, J. T., & Curtin, J. J. (2017). Increased startle potentiation to unpredictable stressors in alcohol dependence: Possible stress neuroadaptation in humans. *Journal of Abnormal Psychology, 126*(4), 441–453. doi:10.1037/abn0000265

Song, J., Park, J. H., Han, D. H., Roh, S., Son, J. H., Choi, T. Y., … Lee, Y. S. (2016). Comparative study of the effects of bupropion and escitalopram on Internet gaming disorder. *Psychiatry and Clinical Neurosciences, 70*(11), 527–535. doi:10.1111/pcn.12429

Substance Abuse Mental Health Service Administration Center for Substance Abuse Treatment. (2006). *Substance abuse: Clinical issues in intensive outpatient treatment.* Rockville, MD: Substance Abuse and Mental Health Services Administration (U.S.). Retrieved from http://www.ncbi.nlm.nih.gov/pubmed/22514853

Swift, R. M. (1999). Medications and alcohol craving. *Alcohol Research & Health, 23*, 207–213. Retrieved from https://pdfs.semanticscholar.org/a266/4ac300402f3857f41a68492a647c633c4079.pdf

Swift, R. M., & Aston, E. R. (2015). Pharmacotherapy for alcohol use disorder: Current and emerging therapies. *Harvard Review of Psychiatry, 23*(2), 122–133. doi:10.1097/HRP.0000000000000079

Tompkins, D. A., Bigelow, G. E., Harrison, J. A., Johnson, R. E., Fudala, P. J., & Strain, E. C. (2009). Concurrent validation of the Clinical Opiate Withdrawal Scale (COWS) and single-item indices against the Clinical Institute Narcotic Assessment (CINA) opioid withdrawal instrument. *Drug and Alcohol Dependence, 105*(1–2), 154–159. doi:10.1016/j.drugalcdep.2009.07.001

Vashi, P., Edwin, P., Popiel, B., Lammersfeld, C., & Gupta, D. (2016). Methylmalonic acid and homocysteine as indicators of vitamin B12 deficiency in cancer. *PloS One, 11*(1), e0147843. doi:10.1371/journal.pone.0147843

Wesson, D. R., & Ling, W. (2003). The Clinical Opiate Withdrawal Scale (COWS). *Journal of Psychoactive Drugs, 35*(2), 253–259. doi:10.1080/02791072.2003.10400007

Winslow, B. T., & Onysko, M. (2016). Medications for alcohol use disorder. *American Family Physician, 93*, 457–465. Retrieved from www.aafp.org/afp

Yuodelis-Flores, C., & Ries, R. K. (2015). Addiction and suicide: A review. *The American Journal on Addictions, 24*(2), 98–104. doi:10.1111/ajad.12185

Delirium and Dementia

> ### OBJECTIVES
> - Distinguish types of cognitive disorders and their etiologies
> - Distinguish types of dementia
> - Describe types of delirium and distinguish from dementia
> - Identify the common symptoms of traumatic brain injuries and sequelae

FAST FACTS

- The cognitive assessment relies heavily on objectively verifiable neurological signs and symptoms elicited from the patient and collateral sources (family, friends, associates).
- The primary symptom associated with cognitive deficits involves either short-term or remote memory.
- The cognitive assessment must be quantified for the significance of the changes noted from baseline. The speed of onset, the frequency of signs and symptoms, and resulting behaviors must also be evaluated to quantify the level of impairment.
- Standardized tests should be utilized during the evaluation process and repeated at subsequent intervals to quantify the rate of decline or improvement.
- Often primary cognitive disorders are not reversible in nature, whereas secondary impairments can be if the underlying cause is identified and treated.
- The goal of treatment is to reduce morbidity and mortality, provide anticipatory guidance, and ensure safety.
- Cognition is the mental process of acquiring knowledge and understanding experiences through the senses.

DELIRIUM

A constellation of symptoms marked by an acute onset (hours to days) causing short-term decline in cognition with a disturbance in consciousness and inattention. Treatment should be supportive in nature and target the underlying cause (general medical condition, substance-induced, comorbidity, polypharmacy, sleep deprivation, admission/transfer/discharge from a healthcare facility). Symptoms may take up to 6 months to resolve (Lavan & Gallagher, 2016; Lien, 2018; Maldonado, 2017). There are three subtypes of delirium:

- **Hypoactive:** Characterized by psychomotor retardation, apathy
- **Hyperactive:** Characterized by psychomotor agitation, restlessness, hypervigilance
- **Mixed:** Characterized by cycling through psychomotor agitation and retardation, from apathy to hypervigilance

▶ CLINICAL VIGNETTE OF THE PROTOTYPICAL PATIENT

A 72-year-old female was admitted for altered mental status characterized by inattentiveness, agitation, and restlessness. She has been withdrawn, apathetic, and has had poor oral intake persisting for 5 days. Her past medical history includes diabetes, hypertension, peripheral vascular disease, and coronary artery diseases. Social history includes the death of her husband 6 months ago. She has had a scotch neat every night to help her fall asleep except for the last 5 days. Her medications include Effexor, Seroquel, Metoprolol, Norvasc, Hydrochlorothiazide, Lipitor, and some other medications that she cannot recall. Most recently, she has been incontinent of urine and constipated.

▶ INCIDENCE AND PREVALENCE

- Risk factors/history
  - Sensory impairment
  - Polypharmacy
  - Substance use disorder, alcohol use disorder/withdrawal
  - Pain
  - Acute illness (e.g., infection, fever, dehydration, constipation, urinary retention, multiple comorbidities, nutritional deficiency, and changes in medication titration and taper)
    - Acute onset of the fluctuating level of consciousness throughout the day
    - Sleep–wake cycle reversal
- Prevalence (varies by age and setting)
  - More common in older adults but can occur at any age
  - Often confused with depression or dementia
    - Often assumed to be a worsening of psychotic symptoms
  - Most prevalent in hospitalized individuals
  - Poor prognosis; 40% 1-year mortality rate

▶ SCREENING TOOLS AND EARLY INTERVENTION

- **Screening**
  - Standardized assessment tool is the Confusion Assessment Methods Instrument (CAMI)
  - A high index of suspicion
  - Awareness of risk factors

- **Diagnostic reasoning**
  - Resolving the underlying medical condition is essential in resolving delirium
  - Unrecognized signs and symptoms can lead to chronic delirium (weeks to months)
  - Delirium can resolve in 3–6 months; however, subsequent physiological insults (e.g., new medications, relocation, infections, worsening of comorbidities) can start a new delirium process

ASSESSMENT AND DIAGNOSIS

- **Onset of symptoms:** Acute onset from 1 hour to a few days
- **Vital signs trend:** Usually abnormal but can normalize if the course is prolonged
- **Duration of symptoms:** Usually hours to weeks but can last up to 6 months from the resolution of the underlying cause, and inadvertent causes can be introduced along the way, which resets the resolution of symptoms clock. Other triggers include new medications, withdrawal from medication, change in environment (discharge or admission), and sleep–wake cycle reversal
- **Attentiveness:** Variable attention, characteristically waxing and waning
- **Behavior:** Rages from retarded to agitated
- **Speech pattern:** Incoherent and difficult to follow
- **Reversibility:** When the underlying cause is identified, delirium is reversible

DEMENTIA

A constellation of signs and symptoms characterized by the gradual onset of multiple cognitive impairments in executive function, intellect, impaired problem-solving, and alteration in memory with preservation of level of consciousness. The signs and symptoms of the dementias are similar; the etiology can be variable (Grossman & Irwin, 2016; Tsuboi & Dickson, 2005).

▶ CLINICAL VIGNETTE OF THE PROTOTYPICAL PATIENT

A 68-year-old man has gradually become apathetic and isolative over the course of several years with increasing cognitive impairment in both short-term and remote memory, often conflating past events as recent events. There have been increasing periods of urinary incontinence, anger outbursts, low frustration tolerance, and a change in personality.

▶ INCIDENCE AND PREVALENCE

- Dementia of the Alzheimer's type (DAT) usually occurs in the sixth decade of life (onset in the fourth–fifth decade is most likely familial) and is the most prevalent type. It is characterized by a gradual onset and progressive decline without focal neurological deficits

- Definitive diagnosis can only be made postmortem with evidence of amyloid deposits and neurofibrillary tangles
  - **Lewy body dementia:** Characterized by abnormal clumps of protein causing neuronal malfunction (commonly occurring in patients with Alzheimer's disease and Parkinson's disease), and characterized by visual hallucinations of small creatures, exacerbated by anti-psychotic medications
- **Pick's disease (frontotemporal dementia):** Onset in the fifth to sixth decades of life, more common in men, marked by personality change; cognitive decline occurs later in this disease process
  - **Klüver–Bucy syndrome:** Uninhibited cheery, hypersexual, hyperorality (carbohydrates especially)
- **Creutzfeldt–Jakob disease:** Precipitous onset prion disease, sometimes referred to as mad cow disease. Remarkable for a rapid decline that progresses to death within 6 months. It is more common in middle-aged adults and initially presents as fatigue, flu-like symptoms, and cognitive impairment. Later, it progresses with aphasia, apraxia, emotional liability, and psychosis
- **Huntington's disease:** Subcortical dementia characterized by motor abnormalities including psychomotor slowing, choreoathetoid movements, and executive dysfunction complicated by impaired language, memory, and insight later in the disease process
- **Vascular dementia:** Rare under age 65, more sudden onset than Alzheimer's (formerly known as multi-infarct dementia); the second most common type, caused by cardiovascular and cerebrovascular disease, manifests with progressive cognitive decline in a stepwise fashion, evidenced by rapid episodic deterioration with interspersed plateau phases marking new baselines. Previously lost function is not regained
  - Risk factors include signs and symptoms of cardiovascular disease (hypertension with funduscopic abnormalities, cardiomyopathy, dyslipidemia, smoking, carotid bruits, and diabetes)
- Dementia in HIV is an indication of poor prognosis and likely death within 6 months. In late stages of the decline, psychotic symptoms may manifest (Sacktor et al., 2016; Tan & McArthur, 2012). Other indicators of advanced dementia in HIV include:
  - HIV dementia is a more severe form of HIV-associated neurocognitive deficits (HAND) syndrome: subcortical dementia with parenchymal abnormalities, visualized on MRI.
  - The decline is progressive in nature with motoric and behavioral abnormalities.
    - Secondary psychiatric disorders (obsessive-compulsive disorders, posttraumatic stress disorders, generalized anxiety disorder, depression, and mania) can develop
    - Accompanying symptomatology (mania, mutism, global cognitive impairment, seizure disorder, delusions, hallucinations, apathy, and self-neglect) can raise the index of suspicion for an organic etiology

▶ SCREENING TOOLS AND EARLY INTERVENTION

- Dementia-specific history includes reports of a gradual onset of cognitive decline, impaired executive function (e.g., impaired organization, problem-solving difficulty, difficulty learning new information), losing valuables, wandering/getting easily lost, and a decline in activities of daily living
  - Impaired remote memory is the most prominent symptom

ASSESSMENT AND DIAGNOSIS

- **Mental State Exam (Table 6.1):** Significant overlap of dementia and delirium with the distinguishing feature being duration of onset
  - **Delirium neurological findings:** Psychomotor agitation/restlessness, purposeless, random actions, uncoordinated, tremor, myoclonus, nystagmus, asterixis
  - **Appearance:** Disheveled, inattentive, apathetic
  - **Speech:** Dysarthric, incoherent rambling, disorganized, impoverished
  - **Affect:** Labile, constricted, nonreactive
  - **Mood:** Difficult to elicit
  - **Thought process:** Distractible, disorganized, +/− perceptual disturbance
  - **Thought content:** Disorganized, with delusions and hallucinations
  - **Orientation:** Varies; disorientation is common
  - **Memory:** Immediately impaired
  - **Concentration:** Limited to impaired
  - **Abstraction:** Impaired
  - **Insight:** Poor to fair but can be difficult to elicit
  - **Judgment:** Impaired, may inadvertently self-harm or lash out to caregivers
- **Diagnostic tests:** Guided by the signs and symptoms, risk factors, and incidence and prevalence of the disorder based on age and sex
  - Complete blood count
  - Comprehensive metabolic profile
  - Infectious diseases (syphilis, HIV)
  - Chest x-ray
  - Urinalysis +/− culture
  - Toxicology screen
  - EKG
  - Head imaging (commonly used but not evidence-based)
- Etiologies for delirium include:
  - Nutritional deficiencies
  - Anemia enough to cause poor perfusion symptoms
  - Electrolyte abnormalities
  - Fever
  - Dehydration
  - Infection (urinary tract, pneumonia, sepsis)
  - Constipation
  - Toxicity
  - Poor perfusion
- Dementia differentials:
  - Parkinson's disease
  - Primary mood disorder
  - Anxiety
  - Intoxication
  - Stroke
  - Hearing loss
  - Head injury
- Differences between dementia and delirium can be found in Table 6.2.

TABLE 6.1 Mental State Exam Corresponding to Brain Region and Impairment

Test/Function	Corresponding Brain Area	Dementia	Delirium
Orientation: Person, place, time	Temporal, frontal, cingulate cortex	Impaired late phase	Acutely impaired due to level of consciousness
Immediate recall	Wernicke, Broca	FTD > AD	Acutely impaired inattentiveness
Delayed recall > 2 min	Hippocampus, medial temporal lobe	AD > FTD	
Attention: spelling, calculation, preservation task shifting, three-step command	Prefrontal, frontal, cingulate gyrus		
Language: naming, repetition, reading and comprehension, writing	Left temporal, left parietal, Wernicke, Broca	VASC > AD > FTD	
Intersecting pentagon	Right parietal, basal ganglia, prefrontal cortex		
Abstract thinking: proverb interpretation and conceptualization	Frontal, prefrontal	FTD > AD	
Trail making test A	Right-sided frontal and parietal		
MoCA (trail B)	Left-sided frontal and parietal		
Verbal fluency	Frontal, prefrontal		Acutely impaired with variable findings complicated by inattentiveness
Right-left orientation	Left parietal	VASC > AD > FTD	
Comprehension	Temporal lobe	AD > VASC	
Planning and sequencing	Frontal lobe		
Constructional ability, spatial relationships, left-side attentiveness	Right parietal		
Performing learned functions, writing	Left parietal		
Visual processing	Occipital		Hallucinations

AD, Alzheimer's disease; FTD, frontotemporal dementia; VASC, vascular dementia

Source: From Grossman, M., & Irwin, D. J. (2016). The mental status examination in patients with suspected dementia. Continuum, 22(2), 385–403. doi:10.1212/CON.0000000000000298; Schwartz, E. (2010). Mental status examination. In C. Nemeroff & W. E. Craighead (Eds.), The Corsini encyclopedia of psychology (pp. 1–2). Hoboken, NJ: John Wiley & Sons, Inc. doi:10.1002/9780470479216.corpsy0541

TABLE 6.2 Differences Between Dementia and Delirium

Dementia	Delirium
Symptoms usually start gradually, are fairly constant on a day-to-day basis, and slowly and steadily become worse over the course of about a decade	Symptoms usually appear over a few hours to a few days, and may fluctuate on and off during the day, and often occur at night
Memory loss	Memory loss
Difficulty speaking and communicating	Difficulty speaking and communicating
Difficulty with complex tasks	Rambling or nonsense speech
Difficulty planning and organizing	Difficulty reading and writing
Disorientation	Disorientation
Loss of coordination	Wandering attention
Personality changes	Becoming easily distracted
Inability to reason	Becoming withdrawn
Fear	Inability to focus
Anxiety	Inability to reason
Inappropriate behavior	Reduced awareness of the environment
Paranoia	Agitation
Agitation	Hallucinations
Hallucinations	Disturbed sleep
Anger or depression	

PLANNING

The use of antipsychotic medications in people with dementia should only occur if the benefit greatly outweighs the risk.

INTERVENTION

Pharmacological management
- **Cholinesterase inhibitors:** Believed to slow the loss of function and reduce agitated behaviors; however, they do not prevent the pathological progression of disease
  - Gradually titrate. Adverse reaction is nausea, diarrhea, vomiting, weight loss, insomnia, vertigo.
    - Donepezil from 5 to 23 mg/day
    - Rivastigmine 1.5 to 6 mg twice daily or 4.5 to 13.3 mg daily transdermal patch
- **N-Methyl D-aspartate glutamate receptor antagonists:** Believed to enhance cognition, preventing overexciting glutamate receptors. Stalling the neurodegenerative process and promote synaptic plasticity
  - Adverse effects include nausea and vomiting; titrate gradually
  - Memantine 10 to 20 mg/day

- **Medical foods:** Believed to provide essential nutrients (medium-chain fatty acids) by introducing sufficiently high concentration of ketones to cross the blood–brain barrier (Chintapenta, Spence, Kwon, & Blaszczyk, 2017; Thaipisuttikul & Galvin, 2012)
  - Axona 40 g packet contains 20 g of medium-chain triglycerides to be mixed into 4 to 8 oz. water; drink immediately. Adverse effects include bloating, nausea, and diarrhea during acclimation. Symptomatic support is indicated. If adverse effects persist, reduce the dose in half and gradually titrate as tolerated
    - Metabolized into ketone bodies for energy with impaired glucose metabolism
- **Psychosis and agitation**
  - Nonpharmacological therapies are first-line
    - Psychoeducation of patient, family, and caregivers regarding progression of anticipated cognitive decline, long-term care needs
    - Safety planning regarding wandering, driving, fire safety, falls risk
    - Routine predictable patterns in daily living, anticipating needs, diversion, recreational therapy to normalize behaviors
  - While antipsychotics are not recommended and have a black-box warning, they can be used at the lowest effective dose with attempts at weaning periodically
    - Adverse effects include extrapyramidal symptoms, sedation, orthostasis, and anticholinergic side effects
- **Depression:** Commonly co-occurring in patients with dementia
  - Treat depressive symptoms targeting insomnia first, followed by loss of appetite, irritability, and depressed mood
  - Least amount of most effective doses for 6 to 12 months and attempt to taper, although usually chronic and may require lifelong treatment
  - Depressive symptoms may be less severe as dementia progress and as awareness of circumstances diminishes

EVALUATION

- Many antiretroviral medications and protease inhibitors are metabolized via the CYP450 pathway leading to many drug–drug interactions
- Observe for signs of toxicity, mixed chronic delirium, or encephalopathy if symptoms fail to improve or decline in an unexpected manner

▶ CULTURAL IMPLICATIONS

- The psychiatric-mental health nurse should remain curious and respectful while inquiring as to the meaning and role of elderly persons in the cultural context. Caring for a patient with dementia requires care for the family, friends, and loved ones as well. Interpretation of the patient's culture must be considered in building a care alliance. Avoid making assumptions based on observable attributes because people may not subscribe to cultural norms.

Many cultures have various implications that can affect the understanding of neurocognitive disorders. The decline in mental abilities may be minimized and expected. Families may not seek formal care until a very late stage in the disease course.

TRAUMATIC BRAIN INJURY

Traumatic brain injuries can arise from a single event or, more commonly, as a series of events: Chronic traumatic encephalopathy (CTE) triggers a cascade of symptoms similar to other neurocognitive disorders. This condition can occur at any age, have lasting effects, and may not be reversible.

▶ CLINICAL VIGNETTE OF THE PROTOTYPICAL PATIENT

A 48-year-old male veteran who sustained a closed head injury 2 years ago continues to experience poor frustration tolerance, impulsivity, irritability, disrupted sleep, inattentiveness, and finds it difficult to sustain motivation to get through his workday. He has become increasingly isolative and shows no interest in activities he enjoyed before his deployment. His partner is bothered by his dramatic increase in sexual desire, leading to various anonymous sexual encounters.

▶ INCIDENCE AND PREVALENCE

- Severity is characterized by duration of associated loss of consciousness at the time of injury, effect on verbal and motor skills, and posttraumatic amnesia
- Impairment can be lifelong, including limitations in emotional regulation, cognition, and behavioral regulation
- Results when the brain accelerates and decelerates inside the cranium, triggering the inflammatory cascade. The injury can occur in a cumulative nature over time as in repeated exposures:
  - Blasts, vehicle accidents, falls, head strikes
- Symptoms may include photosensitivity, memory impairment, headaches, vertigo, irritability, circadian rhythm disturbance, increased or decreased sexual desire, sensory deficits
- Increased risk for suicide

▶ SCREENING TOOLS AND EARLY INTERVENTION

ASSESSMENT AND DIAGNOSIS

- No diagnostic studies can determine previous mild TBI. Neuropsychiatric testing may help distinguish posttraumatic disorder, depression, anxiety, and dementia
  - **Management:** Pharmacology is symptom-focused, and benefits should outweigh risks
  - **Nonpharmacological:** Safety planning for suicidality, support network enhancement, avoid central nervous system suppressants, occupational therapy for vestibular dysfunction, and motor accommodations

- Teach caregivers and family members to allow for increased time to perform tasks to enhance autonomy
- Reduce distractions
- Teach environmental cuing to compensate for cognitive impairment
- Treat anger and irritability with redirection, diversion, and appeasement
- Mild TBI should recover fully in 3 months; residual symptoms may take up to 6 months

PLANNING

Care is planned according to the functional deficits identified and expected decline, with actual problems taking priority over potential problems.
- Disturbed thought process
- Chronic confusion
- Impaired verbal communication
- **Self-care deficits:** Bathing/hygiene, dressing, grooming, and toileting
- Impaired physical mobility
- Disturbed sleep pattern
- Disturbed sensory perception
- Social isolation
- Compromised family coping
- Wandering
- Risk for injury

INTERVENTION

- Assess patient's thought processing ability on every shift.
  - Observe patient for cognitive functioning, memory changes, disorientation, difficulty with communication, or changes in thinking patterns.
  - Changes in status may indicate progression of deterioration or improvement in condition.
- Orient patient to environment as needed if patient's short-term memory is intact. Use of calendars, radio, newspapers, television, and so forth, are also appropriate.
  - Reality orientation techniques help improve patient's awareness of self and environment only for patients with confusion related to delirium or with depression. It may be reassuring for patients in the very early stage of dementia who are aware that they are losing their sense of reality.
    - **Caveat:** Reality orientation is not effective when dementia becomes irreversible because the patient can no longer understand reality. Television and radio programs may be overstimulating, can increase agitation, and can be disorientating to patients who cannot distinguish between reality and fantasy or what they may view on television.

- Maintain a regular daily schedule and routine to prevent problems that may result from thirst, hunger, poor sleep, or inadequate physical activity.
  - If basic physiological and psychological needs are not met, the therapeutic alliance can be eroded. The patient can become agitated and anxious. Routines can be reassuring. Predictable behavior is less threatening to the patient and does not tax limited ability to function and understand the environment.
- Label drawers, use written reminders and notes, pictures, and color-coding tools to assist patients.
- Expose patients to natural light during the earlier part of the day and dimmer lighting in the evening to reinforce the circadian rhythm and maintain adequate sleep.
- Allowing hoarding and wandering in a secure environment can increase a patient's sense of safety and security.
- Limit decision-making, provide support and encouragement with positive reinforcement for desired behaviors, allow for socialization without the expectation to engage.
  - Socialization helps to reduce isolation. Forcing interaction usually results in confusion, agitation, and hostility.
- Provide anticipatory guidance to family members and caregivers to reduce frustration on the part of both parties (e.g., normal findings for the stage of the disease, expected aspects of decline, expectation that function will not be restored).
- Keep the immediate area free from clutter and reduce safety hazards.

EVALUATION

- Evaluate the patient for the rate of expected decline associated with dementia and supporting care deficits accordingly.
- Look for signs of elder abuse and neglect due to caregiver role strain.
  - Assess family's knowledge of patient's disease, erratic behaviors, and possible violent reactions.
  - Provide opportunity for family to express concerns and lack of control over situation.
  - Assist family in identifying patient's reactions and behaviors and reasons for them.
  - Instruct caregivers regarding the need to maintain their own health and social contacts.
  - Consult with social workers as appropriate to identify community support resources and potential respite care options.

KNOWLEDGE CHECK: CHAPTER 6

1. A 66-year-old woman employed as a federal appeals lawyer is being seen by the psychiatric-mental health nurse accompanied by her son, who has been concerned about progressive memory problems. Which of the following would be most helpful in distinguishing between common forgetfulness and cognitive impairment?

    A. Brain MRI with and without contrast
    B. Montreal Cognitive Assessment (MoCA)
    C. Family history
    D. Hamilton Depression Scale (HAM-D)

2. A 70-year-old retired male with a history of hypertension controlled with amlodipine, metoprolol, valsartan, and furosemide has been referred from his primary care provider for depression. Formerly an avid reader, the patient has lost interest in reading and has become increasingly isolative as he has been spilling things during his lunch club meetings and finds this embarrassing, which makes him feel self-conscious and anxious. In which portion of the mental status exam would the psychiatric-mental health nurse expect to find a deficit?

    A. Orientation to person, time, and place
    B. Delayed recall
    C. Abstract thinking
    D. Intersecting pentagon

3. A 53-year-old man presents to the emergency department with complaint of sore throat progressively worsening for 3 days with intermittent fever. In triage, he tells the RN that he took ibuprofen 400 mg 4 hours ago for the pain, and currently his vital signs are blood pressure 120/80, heart rate 88, respiratory rate 12, SPO_2 96% on room air. While waiting for the results of the rapid strep test, the patient becomes agitated, restless, confused, and increasingly difficult to redirect. He is transferred to the Psychiatric Emergency Department because it is a locked unit. Which of the following conditions most likely explains these findings?

    A. Presenile dementia
    B. Personality disorder
    C. Mixed delirium
    D. Mood disorder

(See answers next page.)

1. B) Montreal Cognitive Assessment (MoCA)

The Montreal Cognitive Assessment is a psychometrically validated screening tool for mild cognitive impairment, including visuospatial abilities, short-term recall, trail making, attention, concentration, language, and orientation. A brain MRI is helpful in identifying structural changes that may account for behavior if the affected brain region correlates with the impairment. Family history is important for stratifying risk factors and genetic predisposition but does not confirm a current diagnosis. The Hamilton Depression Scale is used to screen for major depressive disorder, which can affect cognition, but the chief complaint was related to cognition.

2. D) Intersecting pentagon

Intersecting pentagons are used to assess visuospatial impairment, which reflects the function of the right parietal lobe, basal ganglia, and prefrontal cortex. Orientation to person, place, and time reflects the temporal lobe, frontal lobe, and cingulate cortex and is impaired in late phases of dementia. Delayed recall reflects the function of the hippocampus and the medial temporal lobe and is more common in Alzheimer's dementia than frontotemporal dementia. Abstract thinking reflects the function of the frontal and prefrontal regions of the brain.

3. C) Mixed delirium

Mixed delirium is characterized by a cyclical manifestation of psychomotor retardation and agitation with a disturbance in consciousness; risk factors include infectious process, fever, and relocation. Dementia is a slowly progressive process that impairs cognition with the preservation of level of consciousness. Personality disorder is characterized by a historical pattern of rigid maladaptive coping mechanisms that cause distress. Mood disorder is a diagnosis of exclusion in which there is an insufficient number of symptoms to meet full criteria for major depressive disorder, bipolar disorder, or generalized anxiety disorder.

4. The psychiatric-mental health nurse evaluates a 70-year-old female who was admitted to the skilled nursing facility 3 days ago from the hospital, where she was treated for urinary tract infection, pneumonia, and dehydration. The staff reports that the patient is restless and agitated, awake most of the night, intermittently sleeping during the day, and has poor PO intake. Which of the following actions should the psychiatric-mental health nurse take first?

   A. Administer quetiapine 12.5 mg PO at bedtime and every 6 hours as needed for agitation as ordered
   B. Physical exam including vital signs and call the physician to report findings
   C. Transfer the patient to the emergency department
   D. Call family members for collateral information on her baseline functioning

5. Karen is a 68-year-old former legal secretary who enjoys an active social life with her husband. She feels she has something wrong with her medically and has seen many specialists over the year who have found nothing wrong with her. Her husband reports that she continually repeats the same five stories over and over again as if she is telling them for the first time. On two occasions in the last year, she has gotten lost coming home from the supermarket and was found by the police a half-mile from her former place of employment. Which of the following conditions might best explain these symptoms?

   A. Vascular dementia
   B. Huntington's disease
   C. Creutzfeldt–Jakob disease
   D. Mixed delirium

6. Which type of dementia is characterized by a gradual onset and progressive decline without focal neurological deficits?

   A. Alzheimer's disease
   B. Pick's disease
   C. Vascular dementia
   D. Huntington's disease

(See answers next page.)

4. B) Physical exam including vital signs and call the physician to report findings

Physical exam including vital signs and notify the physician to rule out delirium given the patient's history, age, and clinical presentation. Prescribing medication can worsen delirium and mask symptoms of an underlying cause. Transferring the patient to the emergency department may worsen or trigger delirium. Obtaining collateral information is helpful in helping to establish a baseline pattern of function, but the acute problem of delirium must be addressed and ruled out first.

5. A) Vascular dementia

Vascular dementia is the second most common dementia and is caused by progressive cardio/cerebrovascular disease and manifests in cognitive decline and plateau phases in which previously lost function is not regained. Huntington's dementia is a subcortical disease characterized by motor abnormalities including psychomotor slowing, choreoathetoid movements, and executive dysfunction complicated by impaired language, memory, and insight later in the disease process. Pick's disease is also known as frontotemporal dementia and is characterized by a change in personality and cognitive decline; a subtype is Klüver–Bucy syndrome, which is manifested by uninhibited cheerfulness, hypersexuality, and hyperorality. Creutzfeldt–Jakob disease is a precipitous onset cognitive decline that rapidly progress to death; symptoms include fatigue and cognitive impairment and eventually aphasia, apraxia, emotional lability, and psychosis. Mixed delirium is characterized by a cyclical manifestation of psychomotor retardation and agitation with a disturbance in consciousness; risk factors include infectious process, fever, and relocation.

6. A) Alzheimer's disease

Alzheimer's disease is the most prevalent type of dementia and is characterized by a gradual onset and progressive decline without focal neurological deficit. Pick's disease is also known as frontotemporal dementia and is characterized by a change in personality and cognitive decline; a subtype is Klüver–Bucy syndrome, which is manifested by uninhibited cheerfulness, hypersexuality, and hyperorality. Vascular dementia is the second most common dementia and is caused by progressive cardio-/cerebrovascular disease and manifests in cognitive decline and plateau phases in which previously lost function is not regained. Huntington's dementia is a subcortical disease characterized by motor abnormalities including psychomotor slowing, choreoathetoid movements, and executive dysfunction complicated by impaired language, memory, and insight later in the disease process.

7. A 50-year-old man with a diagnosis of Parkinson's disease is admitted to the hospital after tripping and falling and breaking his hip while on a business trip, where he was inspecting a slaughterhouse. The third day after surgery, the patient is having tremors, intermittent slurred speech, dysarthria, and dysgraphia. The orthopedist is attributing his symptoms to slow postoperative progression complicated by having not taken his antiparkinsonian medications for 2 days and the effects of narcotics. Psychiatry was asked to see the patient for mood disorder and possible delirium to aid in planning discharge to subacute rehab. On exam, the patient is unable to name the day, month, or year; he has poor three-object registration and recall, scoring 12 of 30 on a mental state exam; his speech fluency and attention span are incongruent with his baseline; he has no decline in his level of consciousness. What support services might the patient and/or family require?

A. Partial Hospital Program
B. Physical therapy
C. Vocational rehabilitation
D. Grief counseling and palliative care

8. A 68-year-old man with no past psychiatric history but with a history of polysubstance use disorder is admitted for psychosis (disorganized thoughts, rapid pressured speech, persistent rumination, paranoid delusions, and apathy). Which of the following tests would be most important in determining the etiology of his new-onset symptoms?

A. Urine toxicology screening
B. HIV testing
C. Mental state exam
D. Urine culture

9. When evaluating a 78-year-old man, the psychiatric-mental health nurse notices the patient frequently leans in with the right side of his head and frequently asks for things to be repeated. His daughter is very worried that he has dementia or depression because he has also become increasingly isolated, as well as increasingly irritable as he believes people are yelling at him out of frustration of not being heard. The daughter is tearful, anxious, and frustrated. What should the psychiatric-mental health nurse do first?

A. Separate the patient from the daughter and interview him alone
B. Examine the patient's ear canals
C. Order a CT scan of the head
D. Provide anticipatory guidance regarding aging parents to the daughter

10. When providing anticipatory guidance to the loved ones of a 68-year-old woman who has been diagnosed with dementia, what is the most important information to convey?

A. The importance of taking medications exactly as prescribed
B. Safety planning regarding wandering, driving, and fire and fall risk
C. Implementing advance directives for end-of-life care
D. Encouraging the patient's autonomy in expressing their wishes

(See answers next page.)

7. D) Grief counseling and palliative care
Palliative care and hospice findings are most consistent with Creutzfeldt–Jakob disease characterized by precipitous onset cognitive decline that rapidly progresses to death; symptoms include fatigue and cognitive impairment and eventually aphasia, apraxia, emotional lability, and psychosis. Partial hospital program is most helpful for major depressive disorder identified by five of nine symptoms lasting for 2 weeks, with more than one of the nine symptoms being either depressed mood or anhedonia. Other symptoms can include a change in appetite with weight gain or weight loss, impaired cognition, fatigue, feelings of low self-worth, inattention, and recurrent thoughts of death. Movement disorders such as Parkinson's disease can benefit from physical therapy, which can provide neuromuscular education and slow the decline of executive function. Vocational rehab is to help compensate for deficits that are due to physical or mental disabilities that are expected to allow for meaningful work.

8. B) HIV testing
HIV-associated dementia, a neurocognitive disorder with parenchymal abnormalities visualized on MRI, manifests a progressive decline with associated symptoms including obsessive-compulsive disorder, generalized anxiety disorder, depression, and mania. Urine toxicology, while essential in the initial evaluation of a person with altered mental status, is of low yield in this case as polysubstance use disorder is known. A mental state exam has at least partially been completed, given the clinical findings identified in the question. Urine culture is important in the evaluation of delirium, but given the high-risk lifestyle factors, HIV must be ruled out as the treatment requires antiretroviral therapy.

9. B) Examine the patient's ear canals
The patient is leaning in to hear and asking for things to be repeated, but there are no signs and symptoms to indicate dementia or depression. Separating the patient from his daughter may be appropriate but physical needs need to be evaluated first. Head CT scan is not indicated based on the presenting symptoms and increases the risk of incidental findings. Anticipatory guidance should be based on actual problems to help provide for future care needs.

10. B) Safety planning regarding wandering, driving, and fire and fall risk
Safety planning regarding wandering, driving, and fire and fall risk is warranted. Medication adherence is important but a lesser priority in this case. Advance directives for end-of-life care is an important discussion but less priority than attending to immediate safety needs. Helping the patient retain autonomy is an important ethical principle to govern care, but the current healthcare system puts priority on safety planning.

11. Which of the following conditions frequently occurs in patients with dementia but may improve as the condition declines?

    A. Psychosis
    B. Personality disorders
    C. Depression
    D. Delirium

12. Jose is a 48-year-old veteran of Operation Iraqi Freedom, during which he sustained a traumatic brain injury that left him unconscious for 7 days. He has progressively regained function and is able to perform his instrumental activities of daily living most days. His wife is worried because he has periods where she does not recognize him as he becomes irritable, fails to remember important dates and events, and gets headaches so bad that he says he wishes he had died in the war. What is the priority action for the psychiatric-mental health nurse to take during this office visit?

    A. Provide anticipatory guidance and coping mechanisms to the patient and his wife
    B. Refer the patient to the emergency department for suicidal ideation
    C. Prescribe antipsychotic medications to be used when the patient becomes irritable
    D. Refer the patient to a neurologist

13. The husband of a 68-year-old woman with major depressive episodes is concerned about cognitive decline in his wife. Which of the following statements best addresses his concern regarding this symptom?

    A. The cognitive decline is reversible once the depression is treated
    B. It will be important to plan for her long-term care needs
    C. I can prescribe a medication to enhance her memory
    D. It is normal for you to be worried about your wife

14. The primary distinguishing feature between dementia and delirium is:

    A. Onset of symptoms and duration
    B. Disturbance in consciousness
    C. Age of the patient
    D. Comorbid conditions

15. The primary treatment for delirium is:

    A. Antipsychotic medications
    B. Mood stabilizing medications
    C. Identifying and treating the underlying cause
    D. Anticipatory guidance and psychoeducation

(See answers next page.)

11. C) Depression
Depression commonly occurs in patients with dementia, but the symptoms are reduced as the patient loses self-awareness. Psychosis is more common in patients with HIV-associated dementia and can worsen as dementia progresses. Personality disorder is characterized by a historical pattern of rigid maladaptive coping mechanisms that cause distress. Delirium is characterized by a cyclical manifestation of psychomotor retardation and agitation with a disturbance in consciousness; risk factors include infectious process, fever, and relocation. Psychosis is characterized by the onset of delusions, hallucinations, or disorganized thinking and speech, or grossly disorganized or catatonic behavior.

12. A) Provide anticipatory guidance and coping mechanisms to the patient and his wife
Providing anticipatory guidance and coping mechanisms to the patient and his wife regarding traumatic brain injuries can help mitigate the impact of some of the symptoms. Referring the patient to the emergency department for suicidal ideations is inappropriate as the patient is not acutely suicidal. Prescribing antipsychotic medication to be used when the patient becomes irritable may be appropriate, but nonpharmacological measures as firstline are preferred. Referring the patient to a neurologist is not warranted as the primary problem is the sequelae of a traumatic brain injury and family system involvement for ongoing care.

13. A) The cognitive decline is reversible once the depression is treated
The cognitive decline associated with depression is reversible once the depression is treated. Long-term care planning for cognitive impairment secondary to a mood disorder is not eminently indicated. Prescribing medication to enhance memory is not indicated in a patient with a primary mood disorder that is insufficiently treated. Placating the family member without sufficient psychoeducation is not the best answer.

14. B) Disturbance in consciousness
Disturbance in consciousness is the primary distinguishing feature between dementia and delirium. All delirium is traditionally acute onset and dementia is chronic onset; certain dementias can be more precipitous. Patients of any age can have either delirium or dementia. Patients with both dementia and delirium can have comorbid conditions.

15. C) Identifying and treating the underlying cause
Identifying and treating the underlying cause is the primary treatment for dementia. Adding medications to a patient with delirium with an unknown underlying cause may worsen or compound the delirium as polypharmacy is another causative factor. Anticipatory guidance and psychoeducation are appropriate when tailored to a specific condition.

REFERENCES

Chintapenta, M., Spence, J., Kwon, H. I., & Blaszczyk, A. T. (2017). A brief review of caprylidene (Axona) and coconut oil as alternative fuels in the fight against Alzheimer's disease. *The Consultant Pharmacist, 32*(12), 748–751. doi:10.4140/TCP.n.2017.748

Grossman, M., & Irwin, D. J. (2016). The mental status examination in patients with suspected dementia. *Continuum, 22*(2), 385–403. doi:10.1212/CON.0000000000000298

Lavan, Ac. H., & Gallagher, P. (2016). Predicting risk of adverse drug reactions in older adults. *Therapeutic Advances in Drug Safety, 7*(1), 11–22. doi:10.1177/2042098615615472

Lien, H. H. (2018). Antidepressants and hyponatremia. *The American Journal of Medicine, 131*, 7–8. doi:10.1016/ j.amjmed.2017.09.002

Maldonado, J. R. (2017). Psychiatric aspects of critical care medicine: Update. *Critical Care Clinics, 33*(3), xiii–xv. doi:10.1016/j.ccc.2017.04.001

Sacktor, N., Skolasky, R., Seaberg, E., Munro, C., Becker, J. T., Martin, E., … Miller, E. (2016). Prevalence of HIV-associated neurocognitive disorders in the Multicenter AIDS Cohort Study. *Neurology, 86*, 334–340. doi:10.1212/ WNL.0000000000002277. Retrieved from http://n.neurology.org/content/86/4/334.short

Schwartz, E. (2010). *Mental status examination*. In C. Nemeroff & W. E. Craighead (Eds.), *The Corsini encyclopedia of psychology* (pp. 1–2). Hoboken, NJ: John Wiley & Sons, Inc. doi:10.1002/9780470479216.corpsy0541

Tan, I. L., & McArthur, J. C. (2012). HIV-associated neurological disorders. *CNS Drugs, 26*(2), 123–134. doi:10.2165/11597770-000000000-00000

Thaipisuttikul, P., & Galvin, J. E. (2012). Use of medical foods and nutritional approaches in the treatment of Alzheimer's disease. *Clinical Practice, 9*(2), 199–209. doi:10.2217/cpr.12.3

Tsuboi, Y., & Dickson, D. W. (2005). Dementia with Lewy bodies and Parkinson's disease with dementia: Are they different? *Parkinsonism & Related Disorders, 11*, S47–S51. doi:10.1016/j.parkreldis.2004.10.014

Psychotic Disorders

▶ OBJECTIVES

- Define delusional disorder
- Describe diagnostic distinctions of psychosis and schizophrenia
- Distinguish delusional disorder from psychosis
- Distinguish delusion from hallucination
- Describe various subtypes of delusions

FAST FACTS

- Positive symptoms are the most obvious in patients with psychotic disorders and often cause the client to encounter the healthcare system. Some examples include talking out loud self, auditory and visual hallucinations, and grandiosity.
- Negative symptoms offer a worse prognosis for people with schizophrenia, and other psychotic disorders symptoms include anhedonia, apathy, alogia, and can also manifest as isolation, withdrawal, and emotional shut down (blunted affect).
- A psychotic disorder must cause dysfunction for a specific duration with specific symptoms including cognitive and social deficits in someone who should have achieved the developmental milestone.
- Psychosis is generally defined as disorganized behavior accompanied by at least one of the following signs or symptoms: delusions, hallucinations, and/or disorganized speech (marked by frequent derailment or incoherence) lasting <1 day. The following timelines distinguish the classification of psychotic disorders according to the *DSM 5*:
  - **Lasting 1 day to <1 month:** Brief psychotic disorder
  - **Lasting >1 month but <6 months:** Schizophreniform disorder
  - **Lasting >6 months:** Schizophrenia

SCHIZOPHRENIA

Symptoms must be present for a significant portion of time during a 1-month period (or less if treatment is successful) (American Psychiatric Association, 2013). Symptoms must include either delusions, hallucinations, or disorganized speech *with* either grossly disorganized or catatonic behavior *or* negative symptoms (affect blunting, avolition, anhedonia, apathy, alexithymia).

- **Etiology theories:** Based on speculation and correlation, and not clearly defined.
  - **Genetic predisposition:** No specific gene identified as causative but, based on the work of twin studies, incidence increases from 1% risk of illness in the general population to 50% risk of illness in identical twins if one person has schizophrenia
    - 15% increased risk in fraternal twins of a person with schizophrenia
    - 40% increased risk if both parents have schizophrenia
  - **Neurodevelopmental**
    - Oxygen deprivation, maternal malnutrition, substance use disorder, or other infectious illness and/or exposure to toxins
    - Corollary (not causative) radiological findings include enlarged ventricles, smaller frontal and temporal lobes, cortical atrophy, decreased cerebral blood flow, smaller hippocampus, and amygdala (Sadock, Sadock, & Ruiz, 2015)
      - Reduced serotonin, gamma-aminobutyric acid, dopamine in the mesocortical pathway
      - Excess glutamate, dopamine in the mesolimbic pathway

▶ CLINICAL VIGNETTE OF THE PROTOTYPICAL PATIENT

A 22-year-old male presents with pressured speech and bizarre delusions that he cannot move his body because if he does the color will leave him. He talks back to himself in an argumentative fashion. His affect is labile, shifting from laughing to crying to hostile with episodes of grandiosity. He was brought in by the ambulance in a state of undress wearing a blue feather boa demanding an appointment with Mr. Chase, the owner of the bank whom he insists owes him money.

▶ INCIDENCE AND PREVALENCE

- More common in males than females
- More common in firstborn, lower socioeconomic status, urban areas
- Male onset ages 18 to 25 years, more prevalent negative symptoms than women, worse prognosis, more hospitalizations, less responsive to medication
- Female age of onset 25 to 35 years, more associated dysphoria and paranoid delusions with comorbid hallucinations, less prodromal symptoms than men
- Community education to reduce stigma and promote socialization and support services
- Genuine hallucinations coincide with a delusion

▶ SCREENING TOOLS AND EARLY INTERVENTION

- Psychosis and schizophrenia are diagnoses of exclusion; the first step to diagnosing the condition is to:
  - Rule out malingering and factitious disorders
  - Requires a high index of suspicion, and has been found in 30% of disability evaluations, 29% of personal injury evaluations, 19% of criminal evaluations (Docherty et al., 2015; Tracy & Rix, 2017)
  - 66% to 88% of auditory hallucinations are reported as voices coming from outside the patient's head
    - **Hallucinations:** A perceptual disturbance involving one of the five senses (auditory, visual, tactile, olfactory, gustatory; Ilyas, Chesney, & Patel, 2017)
  - 7% of hallucinations are vague and inaudible
  - Auditory hallucinations are usually intermittent in nature rather than continuous
  - 33% of patients reporting auditory hallucinations describe them as commanding
  - >50% of patients with commanding auditory hallucinations do not follow the commands
    - 10% rate of suicide
    - 20% to 40% rate of attempted suicide
  - 30% of auditory hallucinations are in the form of questions, but the majority are chastising or commenting on what the patient is doing rather than seeking information
- Rule out substance-induced disorder
- Rule out underlying medical condition and delirium
- Rule out an adjustment disorder
- Rule out simply oddly related (eccentric)/no mental disorder
- Determine specific primary disorder
  - **Delusional disorder:** A deeply held belief despite evidence to the contrary lasting at least 1 month without prominent hallucinations. Functional impairment relates to the delusional system and, to a lesser degree, the overt psychotic symptoms
    - **Delusions:** A well-organized, sometimes plausible belief despite evidence to the contrary or a lack of evidence to substantiate the deeply held belief. Usually, a manifestation of perceived loss of control over the mind or body, bizarre in nature, and may involve thought broadcasting, thought insertion, and thought withdrawal; subtypes include:
      - **Somatic:** Content is focused on bodily functions, perceived physical ailments, malodorous, malformed, or infected
      - **Persecutory:** Content is focused on being targeted or victimized by law enforcement, people are out to get them; the patient is often irritable, angry, or hostile; collects injustices as proof of persecution
      - **Jealous:** Content is focused on the belief of infidelity and attempts to control the behavior of the partner in an effort to prevent imagined infidelity
      - **Grandiose:** Content is focused on the client's great talent, knowledge, or skill
      - **Erotomaniac:** Content is focused on the belief that someone is in love with the client, the love is idealized, may contain sexual content, often the perceived lover is a famous, powerful, or authoritative individual who may not even know the client

- **Brief psychotic disorder:** The client has characteristic features of schizophrenia (hallucinations, delusions, disorganization) lasting at least 1 day but <1 month. Usually characterized by an acute onset, the client manifests disorganized speech and behavior and possible catatonia. Client returns to baseline normal self after 1 month or sooner.
- **Schizophreniform disorder:** The client has characteristic features of schizophrenia (hallucinations, delusions, disorganization) lasting at least 1 month but <6 months.
- **Schizoaffective disorder:** The client has characteristic features of schizophrenia (hallucinations, delusions, disorganization) >2 weeks without prominent mood symptoms, *and* manic or depressive features are present most of the time when not in psychosis.
- **Schizophrenia:** Characterized by at least two of the following symptoms persisting longer than 6 months: hallucinations, delusions, disorganized thoughts, disorganized behavior, negative symptoms, disorganized speech, and catatonia, and persisting at least 6 months.
  - **Prodrome:** Characterized by odd beliefs, ideas of reference, unusual perceptual experiences, negative symptoms, and deterioration of function prior to the onset of active psychosis.
  - **Active psychosis:** Symptoms include delusions, hallucinations, disorganized speech, grossly disorganized behavior, and negative symptoms.
  - **Residual phase:** Persistent functional impairment, abnormalities in affect, impaired cognition, and impaired communication.

ASSESSMENT AND DIAGNOSIS

- **Assessment**
  - Behavioral and cognitive symptoms
  - Impaired social and occupational functioning: Underemployed or unemployed, lower academic achievement, limited intellectual capacity
  - Limited interpersonal relationships and increasing isolation
  - **Impaired self-care:** Poor grooming and hygiene, and inappropriately dressed for the season
  - Disorganized speech and behavior
  - Negative symptoms occur earlier in the disease process; positive symptoms tend to decrease over time
- **Mental State Exam:** An oddly related individual in their mid-20s, with disorganized speech, tangential and circumstantial with ideas of reference, pressured to the point of word salad, flat or blunted affect, anxious mood, with paranoid delusions and commanded auditory hallucinations, disorganized thoughts, concrete thought pattern, difficulty with abstraction, oriented to person only, poor insight, and poor judgment
- No specific diagnostic tests
- Differentials include seizure disorder, toxicity, substance-induced psychosis, neurosyphilis, Wilson's disease, Wernicke–Korsakoff syndrome, auto-immune encephalitis, thyrotoxicosis encephalitis.

PLANNING

- Develop an individualized care plan in collaboration with other members of the healthcare team that considers the social and cultural context of the client.
- Identify priorities of care in accordance with Maslow's hierarchy of needs (physiological needs must take precedent over psychological needs).
- Initially, basic physiologic and safety needs may need to be met in a hospital setting while medications are titrated and diagnostic tests are completed.
- Arranging for psychoeducation along the continuum of care allows for timely information and builds engagement and therapeutic alliance, reducing isolation as a common complication of psychosis.

INTERVENTION

- Clinical management
  - Safety in low stimulation environment
  - Basic needs for nutrition, hydration, and hygiene
  - Antipsychotic medications: Provide D2 blockade in the mesolimbic (reduces positive symptoms), mesocortical (reduces negative symptoms), nigrostriatal (causes extrapyramidal symptoms [EPS]), and tuberoinfundibular (causes prolactinemia, galactorrhea, and gynecomastia) dopamine pathways
    - Rapidly identify and stabilize psychotic symptoms
      - Often requires medications and hospitalizations
      - Criteria for hospitalization include potential self-harm, including neglect, impulsivity, and manifestations of poor judgment
    - Class effects include the following to varying degrees:
      - Metabolic syndrome
        - Impaired glucose tolerance/diabetes/insulin resistance
        - Obesity
        - Dyslipidemia
        - Hypertension
      - QTc prolongation except for aripiprazole (shown to shorten QTc)
      - Agranulocytosis
      - Secondary Parkinson's symptoms (quetiapine is the least offensive)
      - Extrapyramidal side effects (EPSE)
        - Monitor Abnormal Involuntary Movement Scale (AIMS)
    - Most patients will require lifelong medication
    - Psychoeducation is essential to client and support system
  - Nonpharmacological management of psychosis
    - **Individual therapy:** Supportive versus insight-oriented, focusing on helping reality testing, building life skills, goal setting and coping skills, distress tolerance, and cognitive behavioral therapy have shown some benefit
      - Help client develop a psychiatric advance directive
    - **Group therapy:** Collaborative problem-solving, psychoeducation, anticipatory guidance, life skills practice, and medication management
      - Identifying symptom triggers
      - Early identification of relapse
      - Reflect on past patterns of behavior in times of crisis

- When to seek professional help
- Identify support network and build relationships
- Identify community resources
- Provides daily structure
- Reduces stigma and isolation
- Promotes independence
- Alert to risk of relapse and comorbidity related to substance use disorders
- Review risk factors for suicidality and self-harm
  - Substance use disorder is comorbid in 20% to 40% of patients with psychotic conditions
  - **Tobacco use disorder ranges up to 90%:** Clients report improved cognition; however, smoking induces the CYP450 pathway and reduces antipsychotic efficacy, necessitating increased dosages
- May need to reduce antipsychotic dosage if client reduces or quits smoking
- Assertive community treatment (ACT)
  - Intensive care management with a multidisciplinary team includes home visits and the use of long-acting injectable medications
    - Best for clients with medication nonadherence
    - Frequent recidivism
    - Failing to go to outpatient appointments
- Movement disorders/adverse effects
  - **Akathisia:** Inability to remain still, motor restlessness, often mistaken for anxiety
  - **Akinesia:** Absent movement, difficulty starting, flat affect, and avolition, often mistaken for disinterest
  - **Dystonia:** Involuntary muscle spasm
  - **Pseudo-Parkinson's:** Shuffling gait, motor slowing, masked flat facial expression, tremor, and cogwheel rigidity
  - **Tardive dyskinesia:** Abnormal involuntary movements in a rhythmic pattern affecting face, mouth, tongue, jaw (potentially irreversible)
  - **Neuroleptic malignant syndrome:** Rare life-threatening condition that can occur at any time in a client receiving antipsychotic medication (Stroup & Gray, 2018). It most commonly occurs with typical versus atypical antipsychotics within the first 2 weeks of starting treatment.
    - Manifestations
      - Increased creatinine phosphokinase (CPK)
      - Leukocytosis
      - Hyperactive reflexes
      - Delirium
      - Hypertension
      - Hyperthermia
      - Tachycardia
      - Tachypnea
      - Muscle rigidity (lead pipe rigidity)
    - Risk factors for neuroleptic malignant syndrome
      - Rapid dose escalation
      - Parental route of administration
      - Higher potency (higher affinity for D2 blockade) typical antipsychotics

- **Treatment:** Emergent and focuses on cardiopulmonary support (Chung et al., 2013; Pawar, Rosenberg, Adamson, LaRosa, & Chamberlain, 2015; Ward & Schwartz, 2013)
  - Stop the offending agent
  - Antipyretic treatment: Acetaminophen and cooling blanket
  - IV hydration
  - Benzodiazepine
  - Dantrolene: Interferes with calcium release from skeletal muscle cells, used to reduce muscle rigidity (commonly used off-label for neuroleptic malignant syndrome, not Food and Drug Administration approved; Strawn, Keck, & Caroff, 2007)
  - Parlodel (bromocriptine): Dopamine receptor agonist
- Treatment for adverse effects
  - Reduce dosages to the least amount of most effective antipsychotic medication.
  - Pharmacological treatment for adverse effects: Aimed at dopamine receptor (D2) antagonism (allowing more dopamine). When dopamine is blocked from the receptor site, acetylcholine (Ach) is increased, triggering extrapyramidal side effects. The following agents are known to cause delirium, especially in the elderly:
    - Cogentin (benztropine) or Artane (trihexyphenidyl): Anticholinergic used in akinesia, akathisia, dystonia, pseudo-Parkinson's
    - Benadryl (diphenhydramine): Antihistamine used in akinesia, dystonia, pseudo-Parkinson's
    - Symmetrel (amantadine): Dopamine agonist used in akinesia and pseudo-Parkinson's
    - Inderal (propranolol): Beta-blocker used in akathisia
    - Catapres (clonidine): Alpha-blocker used in akathisia
    - Klonopin (clonazepam) or Ativan (lorazepam): Benzodiazepine used in akathisia and dystonia

EVALUATION

- Good prognostic indicators include:
  - Level of educational attainment
  - Later onset of symptoms
  - Clear precipitant/substance-induced
  - Married and good social support network
  - No family history
  - Rapid treatment of psychotic symptoms
- Ongoing care/follow-up visits:
  - Review medication compliance
  - Adverse effects of medication
  - Attention to nutrition, hydration, elimination, socialization, daily structure
  - Attention to upcoming life stressors

- Attention to coping mechanisms
- Screen for suicidality/homicidal ideations
  - Screen for sense of purpose versus hopelessness
  - Protective factors
  - Attempts at suicide
  - Hospitalizations between visits
  - Emergency department visits
- Vital signs, specifically weight and body mass index
- Assess for ongoing primary care provider relationship and screening labs for metabolic syndrome
  - Encourage primary care relationship for age-appropriate disease screenings.
  - Clients with schizophrenia and psychotic disorders have a reduced life expectancy of approximately 20 years (Ilyas et al., 2017).

▶ CULTURAL IMPLICATIONS

- People of various cultures may underutilize the healthcare system due to language barriers and cultural beliefs about health and treatment options. Language translators and cultural brokers may be effective strategies in reducing trans cultural barriers to healthcare.
- Culturally competent care extends beyond awareness by providing for the client's needs in accordance with their identity.
- A heightened sense of awareness can enhance therapeutic alliance by reducing feelings of alienation and inadvertent offensiveness.

KNOWLEDGE CHECK: CHAPTER 7

1. A 19-year-old male is attending his post-hospital discharge appointment where he was diagnosed with psychosis. He has been taking risperidone 4 mg by mouth twice daily. Which of the following is the top priority during this first encounter with outpatient mental healthcare services?

    A. Baseline EKG, weight, hemoglobin A1C
    B. Establish a therapeutic alliance
    C. Draw a prolactin level
    D. Administer a long-acting injectable

2. The psychiatric-mental health nurse is evaluating a 30-year-old female who reports intermittent auditory hallucinations in which a familiar female voice is commenting on her as she eats. In an effort to deal with the voices, she has been using headphones and listens to podcasts and music all the time, but it is interfering with her ability to do her work. Which of the following questions would help in understanding her symptoms?

    A. "How long have you been experiencing the voices?"
    B. "Do the voices bother you?"
    C. "Are you able to ignore the voices?"
    D. "What has helped you deal with the voices?"

3. A couple presents with their 18-year-old son who was referred by his primary care provider for evaluation of symptoms related to perceptual disturbances, oddly related interpersonal communication, neglect of basic hygiene, and increasing isolative behaviors. These symptoms are most consistent with:

    A. Active psychosis
    B. Schizophrenia prodrome
    C. Residual psychosis
    D. Schizophrenia

4. A 28-year-old female is referred from her employee assistance program from a tech company for poor hygiene and erratic behaviors interfering with her work. The client states her company is spying on her and setting her up to fail for the last 9 months. While speaking she stops herself and begins to talk back to someone who is not present. These symptoms are most consistent with:

    A. Psychosis
    B. Delusions
    C. Hallucinations
    D. Depression

(See answers next page.)

1. B) Establish a therapeutic alliance
Establishing a therapeutic alliance is the top priority in order to proceed with any further care for this patient. Baseline EKG, weight, and hemoglobin A1C, while essential, may not be completed unless the patient therapeutic alliance is established. Prolactin level is expected to be elevated in a patient taking risperidone and other long-acting injectables and may provide insight into compliance, but other factors can cause this level to rise. Administering a long-acting injectable is preferred in clients who are medication nonadherent.

2. A) "How long have you been experiencing the voices?"
Asking how long the client has been experiencing the voices helps to determine a more accurate diagnosis and can inform long-term care options. Asking if the voices are bothersome may further inform the assessment. Asking if the client is able to ignore the voices informs what specific coping strategies have been successful or unhelpful in the past. Inquiring of past helpful coping strategies is beneficial in empowering clients to problem solve.

3. B) Schizophrenia prodrome
Schizophrenia prodrome is characterized by odd beliefs, ideas of reference, unusual perceptual experience, negative symptoms, and deterioration of function prior to the onset of active psychosis. Active psychosis is characterized by delusions, hallucinations, disorganized speech, disorganized behavior, and/or pervasive negative symptoms. Residual phase psychosis is characterized by persistent functional impairment, abnormalities of affect, impaired cognition, and impaired communication.

4. A) Psychosis
Psychosis is characterized by paranoid delusions, poor self-care, erratic behavior, and auditory hallucinations persisting for >6 months. Delusions are deeply held beliefs despite evidence to the contrary. Hallucinations are perceptual disturbances involving one of the five senses. Depression is a mood disorder that can cause psychotic symptoms, including hallucinations, delusions, and cognitive impairment, but there is no mention of a primary mood disorder in this question.

5. A 55-year-old female recently accepted a severance package for early retirement from her job as a fashion buyer for a major retail store. Over the past 6 months, she has increasingly become isolated, neglecting her self-care and collecting various things of no real value. Her appearance is unkempt, and her affect is flat. Before being called back to the consultation room, the psychiatric mental health nurse notices that the client seems to be talking to herself audibly. During the consultation, the client makes poor eye contact and wants frequent reassurance that no one is listening in. Which of the following would be the best action for the nurse to take?

   A. Send the client to the Psychiatric Emergency Department
   B. Speak in a calm, reassuring voice and evaluate for comorbid conditions
   C. Administer an antipsychotic medication for atypical psychosis
   D. Psychoeducation regarding MRI of the brain

6. When providing anticipatory guidance for the parents of a 23-year-old male with schizophrenia, which of the following statements is most accurate?

   A. Medications are most effective for the anhedonia, apathy, and lack of motivation
   B. Medications are most effective for hallucinations, disorganization, and delusions
   C. Schizophrenia is caused by the use of marijuana
   D. Most clients with schizophrenia can live a normal life without medication

7. A 61-year-old female is referred to the psychiatric emergency department with complaints of abdominal pain, nausea, and bloody stools. Despite an extensive evaluation, no underlying cause for her symptoms can be identified, and her hemoglobin is normal. The client insists there is something physically wrong with her. Which of the following best describes her condition?

   A. Persecutory delusion
   B. Grandiose delusion
   C. Jealous delusion
   D. Somatic delusion

(See answers next page.)

5. B) Speak in a calm, reassuring voice and evaluate for comorbid conditions

Speaking in a calm, reassuring voice and evaluating for comorbid conditions can help build a therapeutic alliance and gather essential information to formulate an accurate assessment and plan. Sending the client to the emergency department may rupture the therapeutic alliance, and in this case, there is no indication of an imminent threat to self or others. Prescribing an antipsychotic may be appropriate, but the diagnosis of atypical psychosis is not definitive. Head imaging studies are often low yield and should be reserved for atypical presentations that require further assessment.

6. B) Medications are most effective for hallucinations, disorganization, and delusions

Medications are most effective for positive symptoms. Medications are the least effective for negative symptoms. Schizophrenia is not caused by marijuana, but marijuana can induce psychosis, paranoia, and disorganized behavior, which should resolve when the substance is cleared from the body. Most clients with schizophrenia are on lifelong medication, and life is often difficult despite the best treatment.

7. D) Somatic delusion

With somatic delusion, content is focused on bodily functions and perceived ailments despite evidence to the contrary or absence of evidence for the physical complaint. With persecutory delusions, content is focused on feeling targeted, victimized, and/or singled out by authority figures. Grandiose delusions are focused on the client's great talent, status, skills, or knowledge. Jealous delusions are focused on infidelity with attempts to control the behavior of others they believe are being unfaithful.

8. A 33-year-old female with history of schizoaffective disorder was brought to the emergency department by police for disruptive behavior, auditory hallucinations, and self-neglect. The client screams that she had stopped taking her medication. The psychiatrist orders Haldol 5 mg PO, which the client willingly accepts. An hour later, the client demonstrates an involuntary upward deviation of the eyes and hiccoughs. Which of the following interventions should the psychiatric-mental health nurse do first?

   A. Draw stat labs for complete blood count, creatinine phosphokinase
   B. Stat EKG
   C. Haldol 5 mg IM stat
   D. Benadryl 25 mg IV push

9. A 45-year-old man who takes olanzapine 5 mg twice daily for psychosis reports a perpetual sense of restlessness and an inability to sit still. He says, "sometimes it gets so bad I want to jump out of my own skin." Which of the following is the most likely explanation?

   A. Dystonia
   B. Akinesia
   C. Akathisia
   D. Tardive dyskinesia

10. The psychiatric-mental health nurse is evaluating a 37-year-old man who takes a long-acting injectable paliperidone palmitate and reports that he is glad to not have to take a pill every day. He reports that often, for the first few days after he gets his injection, he notices that he walks slower than usual and, with a shuffling gait, feels stiffness in his joints, and people think he is depressed, but the symptoms dissipate as the month progresses. Which of the following best describes this condition?

    A. Dystonia
    B. Akinesia
    C. Akathisia
    D. Pseudo-Parkinson's

11. A condition characterized by abnormal involuntary movements in a rhythmic pattern often affecting the mouth, tongue, and jaw that is potentially irreversible is known as:

    A. Tardive dyskinesia
    B. Neuroleptic malignant syndrome
    C. Pseudo-Parkinson's
    D. Dystonia

(See answers next page.)

8. D) Benadryl 25 mg IV push
Benadryl 25 mg IV push is an antihistamine used for anticholinergic effect, indicated for use in acute extrapyramidal symptoms, such as dystonia, oculogyric crisis, and diaphragm spasm. Stat labs are not the priority in this client with an oculogyric crisis as they will not change the management or solve the problem. Stat EKG does not address the presenting problem. Haldol may worsen the problem and is likely the cause of the problem.

9. C) Akathisia
Akathisia is the inability to remain still, includes motor restlessness, and is often mistaken for anxiety but described in similar terms. Dystonia is an involuntary muscle spasm due to dopamine blocking agents such as antipsychotic medication. Akinesia is the absence of movement or the difficulty in starting movements with associated flat affect and apathy and is related to dopamine-blocking agents such as antipsychotic medications. Tardive dyskinesia is a constellation of involuntary movements in a rhythmic pattern that is potentially irreversible due to dopamine blocking agents.

10. D) Pseudo-Parkinson's
Pseudo-Parkinson's is a movement disorder exhibited by a shuffling gait, motor slowing (bradykinesia), masked faces, and low-frequency tremor at rest. Akathisia is characterized by the inability to remain still and motor restlessness and is often mistaken for anxiety but described in similar terms. Dystonia is an involuntary muscle spasm due to dopamine blocking agents such as antipsychotic medication. Akinesia is the absence of movement or the difficulty in starting movements with associated flat affect and apathy and is related to dopamine-blocking agents such as antipsychotic medications.

11. A) Tardive dyskinesia
Tardive dyskinesia is a constellation of involuntary movements in a rhythmic pattern that is potentially irreversible due to dopamine-blocking agents. Neuroleptic malignant syndrome is a rare life-threatening reaction to neuroleptic antipsychotic medication and is associated with high fever, delirium, muscle rigidity, autonomic instability, and diaphoresis. Pseudo-Parkinson's is a movement disorder exhibited by a shuffling gait, motor slowing (bradykinesia), masked faces, and low-frequency tremor at rest. Akathisia is characterized by the inability to remain still and motor restlessness and is often mistaken for anxiety but described in similar terms. Dystonia is an involuntary muscle spasm due to dopamine blocking agents such as antipsychotic medication.

12. An uninsured client who was discharged from the hospital on haloperidol 10 mg twice daily presents to the walk-in mental health clinic. The psychiatric-mental health nurse notes on exam the client has tachypnea, tachycardia, and tremors, the skin is hot to the touch, and is overall very rigid. What should the psychiatric-mental health nurse do first?

    A. Administer Benadryl 25 mg PO stat
    B. Call 911 for transfer to the emergency department
    C. Discontinue the Haldol
    D. Attempt to establish peripheral IV access

13. When providing psychoeducation to the parents of a 20-year-old male with psychosis, which of the following is considered a good prognostic indicator?

    A. Early onset
    B. Substance-induced
    C. First degree family member with schizophrenia
    D. Delayed treatment with antipsychotics

14. A 37-year-old homeless man admitted with the diagnosis of psychosis insists that his legs are infested with parasites. Which intervention should the psychiatric-mental health nurse take first?

    A. Examine the client for infestation
    B. Tell the client he is experiencing somatic delusion
    C. Tell the client he is having a paranoid delusion
    D. Give report to the inpatient psych unit and continue with admitting the patient

15. A client states "I see dead people walking the halls at night." Which of the following responses is most appropriate?

    A. "What makes you think there are dead people walking?"
    B. "Let's think about this, a dead person would not be able to walk down the hallway"
    C. "That must be scary for you. I realize that it's real to you, but no dead people are walking"
    D. "I do not see the dead people you're talking about"

(See answers next page.)

12. B) Call 911 for transfer to the emergency department

Call 911; the client is in acute physiological distress with a high index of suspicion for neuroleptic malignant syndrome and is in need of acute medical attention. Prescribing medication should not take priority over advanced life support. Stopping Haldol is correct but does not take priority over getting the client to the hospital. Attempting to establish IV access can occur after 911 has been called.

13. B) Substance-induced

Substance-induced psychosis offers the best prognosis because often, when the substance is stopped and cleared from the body, the client can return to baseline. Early-onset, first-degree relative, and delayed treatment of psychotic symptoms are all poor prognostic indicators.

14. A) Examine the client for infestation

Before assuming that the client is having a delusion, the psychiatric-mental health nurse should first rule out a physical cause for the client's symptoms. Attempting to reorient the client without investigating physical causes can be counterproductive and corrupt therapeutic alliance. If the patient has an infestation, he may need to go through a decontamination process prior to admission to inpatient psychiatry.

15. C) "That must be scary for you. I realize that's real to you, but no dead people are walking"

Empathizing with the client is the most therapeutic response regarding his altered perception and promotes therapeutic alliance. Challenging the delusion can reduce therapeutic alliance and generate hostility, as can failing to validate what seems real to the client.

REFERENCES

American Psychiatric Association. Task Force on DSM-5. (2013). *Diagnostic and statistical manual of mental disorders (DSM-5)* (5th ed.). Washington, DC: Author.

Chung, D. T., Ryan, C. J., Hadzi-Pavlovic, D., Singh, S. P., Stanton, C., & Large, M. M. (2017). Suicide rates after discharge from psychiatric facilities: A systematic review and meta-analysis. *JAMA Psychiatry, 74*(7), 694. doi:10.1001/JAMAPSYCHIATRY.2017.1044

Chung, I., Weber, G. M., Cuffy, M. C., Vedula, G., Samstein, B., & Moitra, V. K. (2013). A 59-year-old woman who is awake yet unresponsive and stuporous after liver transplantation. *Chest, 143*(4), 1163–1165. doi:10.1378/chest.12-1498

Docherty, N. M., Dinzeo, T. J., McCleery, A., Bell, E. K., Shakeel, M. K., & Moe, A. (2015). Internal versus external auditory hallucinations in schizophrenia: Symptom and course correlates. *Cognitive Neuropsychiatry, 20*(3), 187–197. doi:10.1080/13546805.2014.991387

Ilyas, A., Chesney, E., & Patel, R. (2017). Improving life expectancy in people with serious mental illness: Should we place more emphasis on primary prevention? *The British Journal of Psychiatry: The Journal of Mental Science, 211*(4), 194–197. doi:10.1192/bjp.bp.117.203240

Pawar, S. C., Rosenberg, H., Adamson, R., LaRosa, J. A., & Chamberlain, R. (2015). Dantrolene in the treatment of refractory hyperthermic conditions in critical care: A multicenter retrospective study. *Open Journal of Anesthesiology, 5*(4), 63–71. doi:10.4236/ojanes.2015.54013

Sadock, B., Sadock, V., & Ruiz, P. (2015). *Synopsis of psychiatry* (11th ed.). New York, NY: Wolters Kluwer| Lippincott Williams & Wilkins.

Strawn, J. R., Keck, P. E., & Caroff, S. N. (2007). Neuroleptic malignant syndrome. *American Journal of Psychiatry, 164*(6), 870–876. doi:10.1176/ajp.2007.164.6.870

Stroup, T. S., & Gray, N. (2018). Management of common adverse effects of antipsychotic medications. *World Psychiatry, 17*(3), 341–356. doi:10.1002/wps.20567

Tracy, D. K., & Rix, K. J. (2017). Malingering mental disorders: Clinical assessment. *British Journal of Psychiatric Advances, 23,* 27–35. doi:10.1192/apt.bp.116.015958

Ward, M., & Schwartz, A. (2013). Challenges in pharmacologic management of the hospitalized patient with psychiatric comorbidity. *Journal of Hospital Medicine, 8*(9), 523–529. doi:10.1002/jhm.2059

Sleep Disorders

> **OBJECTIVES**
> - Identify insomnia workup and diagnostic criteria
> - Identify common etiologies for insomnia, including obstructive sleep apnea and restless legs syndrome
> - Distinguish types of insomnia
> - Review narcolepsy
> - Identify nonpharmacological insomnia treatment
> - Identify common pharmacological interventions for insomnia

FAST FACTS

- Poor sleep can often mimic the symptoms of depression, inattentiveness, irritability, and cognitive impairment.
- Obstructive sleep apnea is often caused by mechanical problems such as obesity, enlarged tonsils, deviated septum, or other partial airway obstruction.
- Central sleep apnea is often due to neurological etiology, can occur in partial seizure disorders, nerve conduction defects, and does not include snoring.
- The most commonly reported symptoms associated with sleep disorders include chronic fatigue and exhaustion, insomnia, hypersomnia, inattention, irritability, and moodiness.

HYPERSOMNOLENCE

A diagnosis of exclusion characterized by persistent sleepiness despite getting at least 7 hours of sleep overnight. Symptoms include a strong sleep drive, difficulty waking up from sleep, accompanied by feelings of confusion, combativeness, or irritability (Vadnie & McClung, 2017).

▸ CLINICAL VIGNETTE OF THE PROTOTYPICAL PATIENT

A 25-year-old recently married man presents at the prompting of his new wife. He reports excessive daytime sleepiness despite sleeping 8 hours at night and is anxious to drive out of fear of falling asleep while driving. He has been going to bed earlier and earlier to get enough sleep, but his wife insists that he is depressed because he is less engaged and sleeping so much.

▸ INCIDENCE AND PREVALENCE

- Risk factors include:
  - Acute daily and persistent stress
  - Excessive alcohol consumption
  - Remote history of viral infection
  - History of head trauma in the previous 2 years
  - Family history
  - Dementia
  - Parkinson's disease

▸ SCREENING TOOLS AND EARLY INTERVENTION

The patient's perception of sleep disturbance may differ from what is objectively measured.

- 2-week sleep diary
- History and physical exam
- Inquiring about sleep hygiene and bedtime rituals

ASSESSMENT AND DIAGNOSIS

- Specifically inquire about several episodes of daytime sleepiness
- Frequency of naps and feeling refreshed upon waking
- Difficulty waking up from sleep
- Feelings of confusion and combativeness while trying to wake up
- Extraneous movements when attempting to fall asleep
- Difficulty falling asleep staying asleep or early morning rising (terminal insomnia)
- Frequency and consistency of symptoms
- Experiencing nightmares, vivid dreams, sleepwalking, eating, or having sex while sleeping
- Headaches when waking up in the morning, persistent grogginess, confusion, mood swings, inappropriate laughing or crying, or personality changes
- Abnormal physiological symptoms (e.g., hypoxia, dyspnea, neurological dysfunction)
- Varied needs for sleep associated with normal aging

- Anxiety
- Chronic stress
- Depression
- Physical discomfort
- Environmental variations
- Excessive stimulation
- Medications
- Pain
- Substance abuse
- Awakening earlier or later than desired
- Increased frequency of illness
- Persistent fatigue
- Interrupted sleep
- Irritability
- Problems with concentration and memory
- Sleepiness during the day
- Who is reporting the sleep difficulty?

PLANNING

- Identify specific short-term goals to address sleep disturbance
- Identify priority needs to enhance safety while sleeping and while awake
- Identify key behavioral factors that are influencing the client's sleep pattern

INTERVENTION

- Nonpharmacological interventions (Table 8.1)
- **Light control:** Exposure to full spectrum blue light during the day and avoiding blue lights within 4 hours of going to bed
- Avoiding alcohol consumption within 2 hours of bedtime
- Administer prescribed medications to habituate and regulate the sleep–wake cycle
- **Cognitive behavioral therapy:** Prescribing the problem, structured time to worry or let go, consciousness raising, enhance self-efficacy regarding the ability to sleep, cognitive therapy relaxation therapy, and stimulus control and sleep restriction

Table 8.1: Nonpharmacological Interventions for Insomnia

Treatment	Goal	Special Considerations
Sleep diary	- Establish baseline pattern, track progress, remind of sleep hygiene practices	
Psychoeducation	- Teach how sleep is regulated and sleep stages	- Review normal age-related changes (rapid growth and development, menopause, elderly) - Review comorbidity impact on sleep

(continued)

Table 8.1: Nonpharmacological Interventions for Insomnia (*continued*)

Treatment	Goal	Special Considerations
Sleep restriction	■ Enhance continuity of sleep and sleep efficiency	■ Explore why extra time is spent in bed (other than sleep and sex) ■ Explore activities to be done outside of bed ■ Identify other places for nonsleep resting ■ Eliminate daytime naps (or limit to 30 minutes with alarm clock) ■ Delay bedtime if napping more than 30 minutes (within 4 hours of bedtime)
Control stimuli	■ Teach that the bed is only for sleep and sexual activity ■ Move all nonsleep activities out of the bedroom ■ Get out of bed if not asleep within 30 minutes	■ Encourage the use of nightlights and assistive devices at night ■ Consider fall risk with all nighttime interventions ■ If patient requires assistance to mobilize at night, use stimuli control during the daytime only so patient remains in bed at night
Sleep hygiene education	■ Focus on daytime habits and sleep environment that interferes with sleep	■ Ensure daily physical activity ■ Void before going to bed and take bedtime medications with sips of water
Cognitive behavioral therapy	■ Challenge automatic thought patterns and dysfunctional beliefs about sleep	■ Help set realistic expectations
Allocated worry time	■ Rumination often occurs at bedtime; schedule time to worry and problem solve during the day	■ Distinguish worry from introspection ■ Use content of worry to inform treatment planning
Relaxation training	■ Reduce physiological and cognitive arousal starting 2 hours before bedtime. Teach progressive muscle relaxation, meditation, prayer, guided imagery, biofeedback	■ Elicit activities patient is already doing and is willing to do ■ Consider preferences in strategizing

EVALUATION

- Assess the potential barriers to healthy sleep hygiene
- Attend to the onset and duration of sleep aides
- Evaluate the reduction in collateral symptoms (e.g., improved attentiveness, less daytime sleepiness, less avoidant behaviors)

▶ CULTURAL IMPLICATIONS

- Regardless of culture, the physiological and psychological need for consistent sleep is universal to health and well-being. Situations and circumstances can alter adequate sleep temporarily, but restorative sleep must be obtained for optimal health.

INSOMNIA

- Characterized by difficulty falling asleep, staying asleep, or waking up too early (given the opportunity for sleep) with excessive daytime sleepiness (EDS).
  - **Chronic:** Symptoms should be present at least three times per week for 3 months.
  - **Short-term:** Symptoms should be present at least three times per week for less than 3 months.
- Functional impairment is characterized by an inability to get enough restorative sleep at night to allow for efficient daytime functioning.
- Increased risk for poor occupational performance, mood disorder, sexual dysfunction, binge eating disorder, cardiovascular disease, reduced immunity, and impaired cognition.

▶ CLINICAL VIGNETTE OF THE PROTOTYPICAL PATIENT

A 68-year-old female reports feeling tired by lunchtime due to waking up at 3 a.m. and being unable to fall back to sleep. She at times takes a 2-hour afternoon nap and finds it difficult to go to bed until midnight. She reports increasing her coffee intake after lunch in order to try and make it through the day.

▶ INCIDENCE AND PREVALENCE

- 70 million adults in the United States have a sleep disorder. Insomnia is the most common sleep disorder affecting 30% of adults
- 10% have chronic insomnia
- 40% of people report accidentally falling asleep during the day
- 5% of adults report falling asleep while driving
- 35% of the population gets less than 7 hours per sleep each night

▶ SCREENING TOOLS AND EARLY INTERVENTION

The patient's perception of sleep disturbance may differ from what is objectively measured.
- 2-week sleep diary
- History and physical exam
- Inquiring about sleep hygiene and bedtime rituals

ASSESSMENT AND DIAGNOSIS

- Specifically inquire about several episodes of daytime sleepiness
- Frequency of naps and feeling refreshed upon waking
- Difficulty waking up from sleep
- Feelings of confusion and combativeness while trying to wake up
- Extraneous movements when attempting to fall asleep
- Difficulty falling asleep staying asleep or early morning rising (terminal insomnia)
- Frequency and consistency of symptoms
- Experiencing nightmares, vivid dreams, sleepwalking, eating, or having sex while sleeping
- Headaches when waking up in the morning, persistent grogginess, confusion, mood swings, inappropriate laughing or crying, or personality changes
- Abnormal physiological symptoms (e.g., hypoxia, dyspnea, neurological dysfunction)
- Varied needs for sleep associated with normal aging
- Anxiety
- Chronic stress
- Depression
- Physical discomfort
- Environmental variations
- Excessive stimulation
- Medications
- Pain
- Substance abuse
- Awakening earlier or later than desired
- Increased frequency of illness
- Persistent fatigue
- Interrupted sleep
- Irritability
- Problems with concentration and memory
- Sleepiness during the day
- Who is reporting the sleep difficulty?

PLANNING

- Identify specific short-term goals to address sleep disturbance
- Identify priority needs to enhance safety while sleeping and while awake
- Identify key behavioral factors that are influencing the client's sleep pattern

INTERVENTION

- Nonpharmacological interventions (Table 8.1)
- **Light control:** Exposing to full spectrum blue light during the day and avoiding blue lights within 4 hours of going to bed
- Avoiding alcohol consumption within 2 hours of bedtime
- Administer prescribed medications to habituate and regulate the sleep–wake cycle
- **Cognitive behavioral therapy:** Prescribing the problem, structured time to worry or let go, conscienceless raising, enhance self-efficacy regarding the ability to sleep, Cognitive therapy relaxation therapy, stimulus control, and sleep restriction

EVALUATION

- Assess the potential barriers to healthy sleep hygiene
- Attend to the onset and duration of sleep aides
- Evaluate the reduction in collateral symptoms (e.g., improved attentiveness, less daytime sleepiness, less avoidant behaviors)

▶ CULTURAL IMPLICATIONS

- Regardless of culture, the physiological and psychological need for consistent sleep is universal to health and well-being. Situations and circumstances can alter adequate sleep temporarily, but restorative sleep must be obtained for optimal health.

NARCOLEPSY

Two or more episodes of sleep latency less than 8 minutes and or two or more episodes of sleep with rapid eye movement periods (Vadnie & McClung, 2017).

- **Overnight polysomnography (PSG):** Completed the night before the MULTIPLE SLEEP LATENCY TESTING (MSLT) in order to document at least 6 hours of sleep and to rule out obstructive sleep apnea (OSA)
  - **MSLT:** Monitor daytime napping to determine sleep latency
- **Cerebrospinal fluid testing:** Hypocretin (orexin) level <109 pg/mL

▶ CLINICAL VIGNETTE OF THE PROTOTYPICAL PATIENT

A 16-year-old girl with episodic passes out throughout the day with persistent fatigue despite sleeping 16 hours some nights. She goes days without having "spells," but notices that when she is sleep deprived at night the episodes become more frequent. Early mornings are very difficult to wake.

INCIDENCE AND PREVALENCE

- A rare sleep disorder affecting one in 2,000 adults
- Most patients who have narcolepsy remain undiagnosed (25% of people who have narcolepsy have been diagnosed and received treatment)

SCREENING TOOLS AND EARLY INTERVENTION

The patient's perception of sleep disturbance may differ from what is objectively measured.
- 2-week sleep diary
- History and physical exam
- Inquiring about sleep hygiene and bedtime rituals

ASSESSMENT AND DIAGNOSIS

- Specifically inquire about several episodes of daytime sleepiness consistently
- Frequency of naps and feeling refreshed upon waking
- Difficulty waking up from sleep
- Feelings of confusion and combativeness while trying to wake up
- Extraneous movements when attempting to fall asleep
- Difficulty falling asleep staying asleep or early morning rising (terminal insomnia)
- Frequency and consistency of symptoms
- Experiencing nightmares, vivid dreams, sleepwalking, eating, or having sex while sleeping
- Headaches when waking up in the morning, persistent grogginess, confusion, mood swings, inappropriate laughing or crying, or personality changes
- Abnormal physiological symptoms (e.g., hypoxia, dyspnea, neurological dysfunction)
- Varied needs for sleep associated with normal aging
- Anxiety
- Chronic stress
- Depression
- Physical discomfort
- Environmental variations
- Excessive stimulation
- Medications
- Pain
- Substance abuse
- Awakening earlier or later than desired
- Increased frequency of illness
- Persistent fatigue
- Interrupted sleep
- Irritability
- Problems with concentration and memory
- Sleepiness during the day
- Who is reporting the sleep difficulty?

PLANNING

- Identify specific short-term goals to address sleep disturbance
- Identify priority needs to enhance safety while sleeping and while awake
- Identify key behavioral factors that are influencing the client's sleep pattern

INTERVENTION

- Nonpharmacological interventions (Table 8.1)
- **Light control:** Exposing to full spectrum blue light during the day and avoiding blue lights within 4 hours of going to bed.
- Avoiding alcohol consumption within 2 hours of bedtime
- Administer prescribed medications to habituate and regulate the sleep–wake cycle

EVALUATION

- Assess the potential barriers to healthy sleep hygiene
- Attend to the onset and duration of sleep aides
- Evaluate the reduction in collateral symptoms (e.g., improved attentiveness, less daytime sleepiness, less avoidant behaviors)

▶ CULTURAL IMPLICATIONS

- Regardless of culture, the physiological and psychological need for consistent sleep is universal to health and well-being. Situations and circumstances can alter adequate sleep temporarily, but restorative sleep must be obtained for optimal health.

OBSTRUCTIVE SLEEP APNEA (OSA)

Sleep disorder characterized by multiple episodes of apnea and waking during the night.

▶ CLINICAL VIGNETTE OF THE PROTOTYPICAL PATIENT

A 36-year-old obese male presents with pre-diabetes and hypertension whose bed partner reports very loud snoring after what seems like a very long period of breath holding. At times he awakes drenched in sweat and always falls asleep if he sits still for more than 10 minutes; on several occasions he has veered onto the shoulder of the road while driving.

▶ INCIDENCE AND PREVALENCE

- Can occur in 2% of children and 20% of adults and is associated with:
  - Impaired school and work performance
  - Impaired coordination and increased risk of accidents (driving and heavy machinery)
- Etiology:
- Narrow naso/oropharyngeal anatomy, obesity

▶ SCREENING TOOLS AND EARLY INTERVENTION

- Assessment of daytime sleepiness with persistent falling asleep due to sleep deprivation
- Morning headaches

ASSESSMENT AND DIAGNOSIS

- PSG, electroencephalogram (EEG) for definitive diagnosis
- Common complaint is snoring with gasps while sleeping
- Frequently misdiagnosed as a mood disorder or attention deficit hyperactivity disorder.
- Major risk factor for poor glycemic control and type 2 diabetes, congestive heart failure, hypertension, sexual dysfunction, and obesity

PLANNING

- Identify specific short-term goals to address sleep disturbance
- Identify priority needs to enhance safety while sleeping and while awake
- Identify key behavioral factors that are influencing the client's sleep pattern

INTERVENTION

- Nonpharmacological interventions (Table 8.1)
  - **Light control:** Exposing to full spectrum blue light during the day and avoiding blue lights within 4 hours of going to bed
  - Avoiding alcohol consumption within 2 hours of bedtime
  - **Cognitive behavioral therapy:** Prescribing the problem, structured time to worry or let go, conscienceless raising, enhance self-efficacy regarding the ability to sleep, cognitive therapy, relaxation therapy, stimulus control, and sleep restriction
- Pharmacological interventions:
  - **Benzodiazepines:** Highly addictive, used as a last resort, use the least amount of most effective medication, avoid in patients with OSA or chronic obstructive pulmonary disease (COPD)
    - May cause residual drowsiness
    - Increases fall risk among the elderly

- Sedative hypnotics
  - Zolpidem (Ambien, Ambien CR, Intermezzo)
  - Short half-life (less residual drowsiness)
  - Given on an empty stomach
  - Rapid onset
- Eszopiclone (Lunesta)
  - Intermediate half-life
  - Residual drowsiness
  - Melatonin receptor agonist:
- Ramelteon (Rozerem)
  - Low bioavailability
  - Variable efficacy
  - Low incidence of adverse effects
  - Low incidence of residual drowsiness
- Orexin receptor antagonist
  - Suvorexant (Belsomra): Suppresses wakefulness
    - Very long half-life
    - Residual drowsiness (hungover feeling)
- Antidepressants used for insomnia
  - Tricyclic antidepressants
  - Mirtazapine (off label)
  - Trazodone (off label)

EVALUATION

- Assess the potential barriers to healthy sleep hygiene
- Attend to the onset and duration of sleep aides
- Evaluate the reduction in collateral symptoms (e.g., improved attentiveness, less daytime sleepiness, less avoidant behaviors)

▶ CULTURAL IMPLICATIONS

- Regardless of culture, the physiological and psychological need for consistent sleep is universal to health and well-being. Situations and circumstances can alter adequate sleep temporarily, but restorative sleep must be obtained for optimal health.

RESTLESS LEGS SYNDROME

A movement disorder of the lower limbs is triggered at the moment of falling asleep, creating an irresistible urge to move the legs that disrupts the initiation of sleep. Symptoms may arise also in the upper extremities (Ford et al., 2014). Highly correlated with brain iron deficiency; however, it can be present in people with normal iron saturation.

▶ CLINICAL VIGNETTE OF THE PROTOTYPICAL PATIENT

A 43-year-old man reports daytime sleepiness caused by poor sleep at night. He reports a vague sensation in the legs, which he describes as a deep itching, sometimes "pins and needles," or as if something is crawling up his leg. The symptom is relieved by moving his legs; however, his bed partner wakes up as a result. There has been increasing interpersonal conflict as a result.

▶ INCIDENCE AND PREVALENCE

- 4% to 14% in the general population
- More common in advancing age
- Signs and symptoms
  - Any unpleasant sensation of the legs noted with lying down or sitting down
  - The discomfort is alleviated by movement
  - Symptoms are not accounted for by other conditions such as myalgia, venous stasis, leg edema, arthritis, leg cramps, positional discomfort, or habitual foot tapping
- Demographics
  - 5% to 15% of the general population
  - 30% onset of symptoms before 20 years of age
  - Symptoms gradually progress over time and begin to disrupt sleep after 50 years of age.
- Comorbidity and risks
  - Associated with increased risk of hypertension
  - Headaches, cognitive impairment, irritability (due to disrupted sleep cycle)

▶ SCREENING TOOLS AND EARLY INTERVENTION

- History and physical
  - Complaints of pins and needles, internal itching, tactile sensation
  - Difficulty falling asleep
  - EDS

ASSESSMENT AND DIAGNOSIS

- Specifically inquire about several episodes of daytime sleepiness
- Frequency of naps and feeling refreshed upon waking
- Difficulty waking up from sleep
- Feelings of confusion and combativeness while trying to wake up
- Extraneous movements when attempting to fall asleep
- Difficulty falling asleep staying asleep or early morning rising (terminal insomnia)
- Frequency and consistency of symptoms

- Experiencing nightmares, vivid dreams, sleepwalking, eating, or having sex while sleeping
- Headaches when waking up in the morning, persistent grogginess, confusion, mood swings, inappropriate laughing or crying, or personality changes
- Abnormal physiological symptoms (e.g., hypoxia, dyspnea, neurological dysfunction)
- Varied needs for sleep associated with normal aging
- Anxiety
- Chronic stress
- Depression
- Physical discomfort
- Environmental variations
- Excessive stimulation
- Medications
- Pain
- Substance abuse
- Awakening earlier or later than desired
- Increased frequency of illness
- Persistent fatigue
- Interrupted sleep
- Irritability
- Problems with concentration and memory
- Sleepiness during the day
- Who is reporting the sleep difficulty?

PLANNING

- Identify specific short-term goals to address sleep disturbance
- Identify priority needs to enhance safety while sleeping and while awake
- Identify key behavioral factors that are influencing the client's sleep pattern

INTERVENTION

- **Psychoeducation:** Management tailored to the most bothersome symptom
- Dopaminergic agents
  - Pramipexole
  - Bromocriptine
  - Levodopa/carbidopa
- Antiepileptic drugs
  - Gabapentin
  - Pregabalin
- Alpha-blocker
  - Clonidine
- Nutritional supplementation
  - Ferrous gluconate or ferrous sulfate
  - Magnesium oxide

EVALUATION

- Assess the potential barriers to healthy sleep hygiene
- Attend to the onset and duration of sleep aides
- Evaluate the reduction in collateral symptoms (e.g., improved attentiveness, less daytime sleepiness, less avoidant behaviors)

▶ CULTURAL IMPLICATIONS

- Regardless of culture, the physiological and psychological need for consistent sleep is universal to health and well-being. Situations and circumstances can alter adequate sleep temporarily, but restorative sleep must be obtained for optimal health.

KNOWLEDGE CHECK: CHAPTER 8

1. A 38-year-old male reports excessive daytime sleepiness for the last 2 weeks in the setting of restructuring at his job. He is unable to tell if he is having more trouble falling asleep or staying asleep. Sometimes he wakes up at 4 a.m. and is unable to fall back asleep. Which of the following is the best action for the psychiatric-mental health nurse to take?

   A. Have him raise the temperature in his bedroom
   B. Advise him to take melatonin
   C. Request the patient complete a sleep log
   D. Add an extra blanket to his bed covers

2. A 45-year-old female reports that she has difficulty falling back asleep after she wakes up at 4 a.m. for the last month. She understands that it is better to get out of bed rather than lay in bed awake. She uses this time to catch up on her reading but as a result is very sleepy during the day. What intervention should the psychiatric-mental health nurse recommend?

   A. Melatonin when she wakes at 4 a.m.
   B. Mop the kitchen floor as soon as she wakes up at 4 a.m.
   C. Diphenhydramine 25 mg at bedtime
   D. Sleep diary for 2 weeks

3. A 44-year-old male with type 2 diabetes is evaluated in the partial hospital program for mood disorder. He is becoming increasingly irritable, inattentive, and forgetful, and frequently falls asleep in front of his computer at work. He is worried he will get fired and lose his benefits, which he needs to cover his diabetic supplies. He says, "I am so worried that my blood sugars are as high as 300 and on occasion have wet the bed." Which of the following should the psychiatric-mental health nurse do first?

   A. Psychoeducation regarding Provigil 100 mg daily
   B. Coordinating an outpatient sleep study
   C. Psychoeducation regarding Mirtazapine 15 mg at bedtime
   D. Coordinate a referral back to primary care for glycemic control

4. A 25-year-old woman reports frequently falling asleep during the day for the last 6 months. This has been affecting her work as a computer help desk agent, noting she sometimes nods off during calls but also during times of high volume. When her head hits the back of the chair, she wakes up and realizes what has happened. She insists she consistently sleeps 8 hours each night. This is most consistent with which of the following?

   A. Narcolepsy
   B. Circadian rhythm sleep disorder
   C. Hypersomnia
   D. Night terrors

(See answers next page.)

1. C) Request the patient complete a sleep log
Request the patient complete a sleep log to gather more information regarding sleep latency, sleep efficiency, and sleep maintenance in order to make appropriate recommendations. Prior to advising any intervention, an assessment must be completed. Environmental factors conducive to sleep include reducing the temperature of the environment and adding a blanket warmer.

2. B) Mop the kitchen floor as soon as she wakes up at 4 a.m.
Recommending a paradoxical intervention to address the sleep maintenance problem helps the patient realize a sense of control over her insomnia. Nonpharmacological interventions are preferred to pharmacological interventions. A sleep diary is used to gather information and to help clearly identify the type of insomnia.

3. B) Coordinating an outpatient sleep study
A sleep study would help to diagnose if the underlying cause is obstructive sleep apnea (OSA), which is known to have symptoms of irritability, cognitive impairment, and excessive daytime sleepiness, and poor glycemic control. Provigil is indicated for OSA, but a diagnosis has yet to be made. Mirtazapine is indicated for depression and anxiety, but an underlying medical condition must be ruled out first.

4. A) Narcolepsy
Narcolepsy is characterized by two or more episodes of sleep latency lasting less than 8 minutes and/or two or more episodes of rapid eye movement (REM) sleep; it commonly occurs in the late teens and 20s. Circadian rhythm sleep disorder is often caused by changes in scheduling (shift work, jet lag) and requires a period of acclimation. Primary hypersomnia is excessive daytime drowsiness not due to an environmental sleep disturbance, underlying medical condition, substance-induced disorder, or mood disorder, and is not associated with sleep paralysis (cataplexy). Night terrors are episodes of screaming or intense fear and flailing 2 to 3 hours after falling asleep and are often paired with sleepwalking, unlike nightmares, which are not remembered and are most common in children between the ages of 2 to 12.

5. John is a 22-year-old RN who has started his first job in the cardiothoracic ICU. After his orientation, he began his full-time position working three 12-hour night shifts per week. On his days off, he reports excessive fatigue during the day with periods of falling asleep while driving. He also reports difficulty staying awake at work during his first night back to work. Which of the following is the most likely diagnosis?

   A. Narcolepsy
   B. Circadian rhythm sleep disorder
   C. Hypersomnia
   D. Night terrors

6. Ella is trying to help her 3-year-old son sleep through the night but reports recently he has had three episodes of waking up within 3 hours of falling asleep with inconsolable screaming and crying. He then falls back asleep on his own and has no memory of what happened. What would be the best intervention?

   A. Recommend diphenhydramine 12.5 mg at bedtime
   B. Create and maintain bedtime routine and reduce stimuli
   C. Order polysomnography and EEG
   D. Prescribe desmopressin nasal spray

7. A 52-year-old obese man with type 2 diabetes reports dozing off while driving, watching TV, or reading, with increased apathy and fatigue. The psychiatric-mental health nurse practitioner ordered a sleep study, which revealed ten episodes of apnea lasting 15 to 20 seconds each per hour of sleep. Which of the following interventions should the psychiatric-mental health nurse provide psychoeducation?

   A. Antidepressant medications
   B. Referral to otolaryngology
   C. Referral to otolaryngology for rhinoplasty
   D. Continuous positive airway pressure

8. A father brings his 6-year-old son to integrative family practice clinic because he is worried that the son sits up in bed shortly after falling asleep and screams. He says he is inconsolable and unable to be awakened during these episodes, but eventually he falls back asleep. The father states he is not able to fall back asleep after those episodes and is exhausted and lately falling asleep at work during the day. The child is energetic and playful during the day and has no memory of the episodes. Which of the following is the best response from the psychiatric-mental health nurse?

   A. "Are you worried you are doing something wrong?"
   B. "I can see you're upset, but really you are overreacting."
   C. "I can see this is upsetting for you."
   D. "Tell me why you can't fall back asleep after your son does?"

(See answers next page.)

5. B) Circadian rhythm sleep disorder

Circadian rhythm sleep disorder is often caused by changes in scheduling (shift work, jet lag) and requires a period of acclimation. Primary hypersomnia is excessive daytime drowsiness not due to an environmental sleep disturbance, underlying medical condition, substance-induced disorder, or mood disorder, and is not associated with sleep paralysis (cataplexy). Night terrors are episodes of screaming or intense fear and flailing 2 to 3 hours after falling asleep and are often paired with sleepwalking, unlike nightmares, which are not remembered and are most common in children between the ages of 2 and 12. Narcolepsy is characterized by two or more episodes of sleep latency lasting less than 8 minutes and/or two or more episodes of rapid eye movement (REM) sleep; it commonly occurs in the late teens and 20s.

6. B) Create and maintain bedtime routine and reduce stimuli

Creating and maintaining a bedtime routine, reducing stress, preventing the child from becoming over tired, and avoiding staying up too late are all appropriate interventions for night terrors. Prescribing diphenhydramine is not indicated for night terrors and can have paradoxical effects. Polysomnography and EEG are indicated for diagnosing obstructive sleep apnea, narcolepsy, and seizure disorders and are not indicated in this case. Desmopressin is indicated for nocturnal enuresis in children older than 6 years old.

7. D) Continuous positive airway pressure

Continuous positive airway pressure (CPAP) is the treatment of choice for obstructive sleep apnea. Antidepressant medications are not known to normalize the sleep pattern in patients with obstructive sleep apnea. Referral for surgery is reserved for CPAP treatment failure.

8. C) "I can see this is upsetting for you."

"I can see this is upsetting for you" is a simple nonjudgmental statement that communicates empathy and serves as an open-ended prompt to efficiently elicit the most important information. The father may be troubled by something other than the son's night terrors and his own excessive daytime sleepiness. Specifically directed statements such as "Why can't you fall back asleep?" or "Are you worried you are doing something wrong?" are less likely to garner complete essential information. Avoid using statements that contain a "but" in your initial response to a patient, as it may be construed as a minimizing of their problems and feelings and will inhibit a therapeutic alliance.

9. The psychiatric-mental health nurse is providing psychoeducation and anticipatory guidance to the concerned parent regarding night terrors. At which stage of sleep is this most likely to occur?

   A. Any stage of sleep
   B. Stage 1
   C. Stage 2
   D. Stage 3 to 4

10. The psychiatric-mental health nurse is leading a sleep disorders group. Which type of sleep disturbance is most consistent with major depressive disorder?

    A. Early morning awakening
    B. Sleeping too deeply
    C. Easily awakened/sleeping too lightly
    D. Decreased effect of trazodone

11. A patient recently diagnosed with major depression and early morning awakening is likely to have which of the following hormonal states accounting for his symptoms?

    A. Elevated testosterone
    B. Elevated cortisol
    C. Elevated catecholamine
    D. Decreased cortisol

12. A 30-year-old man has been started on sertraline 50 mg daily for major depression 1 week ago. He presents for follow-up. Which of the following sleep patterns is he expected to report?

    A. No change in sleep pattern
    B. Increased sleep latency
    C. Decreased sleep latency
    D. Increased sleepiness earlier in the evening

13. A 56-year-old woman with depressed mood reports a decrease in weight, libido, and ability to sleep. In addition, she reports intermittent episodes of constipation. Which neurovegetative symptom should be addressed first?

    A. Constipation
    B. Sleep
    C. Weight loss
    D. Depressed mood

(See answers next page.)

9. D) Stage 3 to 4
Stage 3 to 4 is when night terrors and parasomnia occur (usually within 3 hours of falling asleep). Sleep terrors do not occur in stages 1, 2, or rapid eye movement (REM) sleep.

10. B) Sleeping too deeply
Early-morning awakening is most consistently associated with major depression; sleeping too deeply is associated with oversedation. Easily awakened/sleeping too lightly can be associated with hypervigilance in the setting of posttraumatic stress disorder (PTSD). The decreased effect of trazodone is not associated with a diagnosis of major depression and may indicate a need for titration.

11. B) Elevated cortisol
An elevated cortisol level is observed in patients with depression and early-morning awakening. Catecholamine and testosterone are decreased in patients with major depression.

12. A) No change in sleep pattern
Increased sleep latency (difficulty falling asleep) is a common adverse effect associated with selective serotonin reuptake inhibitors (SSRIs) and is especially pronounced during initiation and titration of dosage. No change in sleep pattern. SSRIs are clinically activating, and the patient may perceive less need for sleep initially.

13. B) Sleep
Sleep should be the first symptom targeted, and a primary sleep disorder should be ruled out as it can account for many of the symptoms associated with major depression. Many psychotropic medications can make constipation worse, as can a disrupted sleep cycle.

14. A 79-year-old female is in a long-term care facility with history of hypertension, coronary artery disease, and atrial fibrillation. The patient is having difficulty sleeping and was started on lorazepam 2 mg at bedtime. The patient has become increasingly agitated and wandering and has been further prescribed lorazepam 2 mg every 6 hours. The patient is also prescribed hydrochlorothiazide 25 mg daily, digoxin 0.125 mg every other day, diltiazem sustained release 360 mg daily, and isosorbide 30 mg daily. What should the psychiatric-mental health nurse do first?

    A. Call the physician and arrange for a hospital transfer
    B. Orthostatic vital signs, review intake and output, and call the physician
    C. Call the physician for an antipsychotic medication
    D. Hold the Ativan and call the physician

15. A 68-year-old man presents with his wife for evaluation of his sleep disorder. The wife reports he does not sleep well at night and wanders around the house. He then sleeps much of the day. Which of the following medications would have the desired effect?

    A. Chlorpromazine
    B. Haloperidol
    C. Trazodone
    D. Lorazepam

14. B) Orthostatic vital signs, review intake and output, and call the physician

A delirium workup is indicated and should include orthostatic vital signs; review the bowel log, the intake and output record, and the most recent blood work—these symptoms are consistent with agitated delirium. Delirium can alter sleep patterns. Adding other medications may make delirium worse. Once an underlying cause is considered, weaning the lorazepam would be appropriate as the dose is quite high (8 mg/24 hours).

15. C) Trazodone

Trazodone is a serotonergic agent commonly used to help with sleep latency and maintenance, which can reduce wandering at night. It is also associated with increased bleeding and orthostatic changes, so starting low is preferred. Benzodiazepines should be avoided in the elderly as they can disinhibit and make behaviors worse and trigger delirium. Antipsychotics should be avoided in the elderly as they are associated with increased extrapyramidal symptoms and tardive dyskinesia. These medications are also anticholinergic and can lead to urinary retention and confusion.

REFERENCES

Fiorentino, L., & Martin, J. L. (2010). Awake at 4 AM: Treatment of insomnia with early morning awakenings among older adults. *Journal of Clinical Psychology*, *66*(11), 1161–1174. doi:10.1002/jclp.20734

Ford, E. S., Wheaton, A. G., Cunningham, T. J., Giles, W. H., Chapman, D. P., & Croft, J. B. (2014). Trends in outpatient visits for insomnia, sleep apnea, and prescriptions for sleep medications among U.S. adults: Findings from the National Ambulatory Medical Care Survey 1999–2010. *Sleep*, *37*(8), 1283–1293. doi:10.5665/sleep.3914

Pace-Schott, E. F., & Spencer, R. M. C. (2014). Sleep loss in older adults: Effects on waking performance and sleep-dependent memory consolidation with healthy aging and insomnia. In M. T. Bianchi (Ed.), *Sleep deprivation and disease* (pp. 185–197). New York, NY: Springer. doi:10.1007/978-1-4614-9087-6_14

Pigeon, W. R., Hegel, M., Unützer, J., Fan, M.-Y., Sateia, M. J., Lyness, J. M., … Perlis, M. L. (2008). Is insomnia a perpetuating factor for late-life depression in the IMPACT cohort? *Sleep*, *31*(4), 481–488. doi:10.1093/sleep/31.4.481. Retrieved from http://www.ncbi.nlm.nih.gov/pubmed/18457235

Vadnie, C. A., & McClung, C. A. (2017). Circadian rhythm disturbances in mood disorders: Insights into the role of the suprachiasmatic nucleus. *Neural Plasticity*, *2017*, 1504507. doi:10.1155/2017/1504507

Wickwire, E. M., Shaya, F. T., & Scharf, S. M. (2016). Health economics of insomnia treatments: The return on investment for a good night's sleep. *Sleep Medicine Reviews*, *30*, 72–82. doi:10.1016/j.smrv.2015.11.004

Wilt, T. J., MacDonald, R., Brasure, M., Olson, C. M., Carlyle, M., Fuchs, E., … Kane, R. L. (2016). Pharmacologic treatment of insomnia disorder: An evidence report for a clinical practice guideline by the American College of Physicians. *Annals of Internal Medicine*, *165*(2), 103. doi:10.7326/M15-1781

Mood Disorders

OBJECTIVES

- Distinguish among mood disorders
- Identify comorbid conditions associated with mood disorders
- Review atypical presentations of depression
- Describe nonpharmacological treatments for mood disorders
- Identify adverse effects associated with psychopharmacological agents
- Review criteria for hospitalization

FAST FACTS

- Most common mental illness
- Most major depression will affect 1 in 6 men or 1 in 4 women in their lifetime
- Most cases of major depression will resolve with or without treatment in one year; 50% of people will have a subsequent recurrence of depression in their lifetime; 80% of people who have had two episodes of depression will have a third episode
- Mood disorders are among the most treatable mental illnesses

DEPRESSIVE DISORDERS

Characterized by a constellation of symptoms with an overarching theme of melancholy. The severity of symptoms can constitute various conditions ranging from dysthymia to major depression with psychotic features.

- Cultural differences can affect the manifestations of depression and sadness
- Nonpathological expected reaction to a particular life stressor
  - **No longer exclusions for grief reaction:** If the patient meets criteria for the major depressive disorder, the condition can be diagnosed and treated
- Pathological characteristics of depression
  - Disproportionate (subjectively defined) to events
  - **Impairs function:** The patient is unable to meet Maslow's hierarchy of needs: physiological, psychosocial, safety, and belonging

- Symptoms of depressive disorder without precipitant
■ Etiological theories
    - Biological theories
        ■ **Genetic:** Assumes a genetic cause linked to single nucleotide polymorphism disorder.
            – Usually the patient has a depressed first-degree relative
    - Children of depressed parents are three times more likely to experience a major depressive disorder (MDD) and have a 40% chance of having the first episode before age 18
        ■ It is unclear if this is a biological predisposition versus learned behavior
        ■ The earlier the onset age of symptoms, the stronger the assumed genetic load
    - **Endocrine dysfunction:** Common neurovegetative symptoms associated with MDD (e.g., sleep disturbance, appetite dysregulation, libidinal drive, fatigue, and anhedonia) are associated with hypothalamic and pituitary hormones
        ■ Postpartum mood disturbances are correlated with endocrine-mediated functions
        ■ Dysregulation of the hypothalamic-pituitary axis (HPA) is also another theory of endocrine dysfunction-induced mood disorder
    - The stress response triggers a cascade of various hormones in an effort to maintain homeostasis, which, over time, can become taxed and inefficient, leading to neurovegetative symptoms of depression and anxiety, primarily due to cortisol toxicity and eventually causing structural changes in the brain
        ■ **Growth hormone:** Nutrient metabolism (lipids, carbohydrates, protein)
        ■ **Thyroid stimulating hormone:** Metabolism and all bodily functions
        ■ **Adrenocorticotropic hormone:** Stress response
        ■ **Prolactin:** Lactation and antagonizes testosterone (inhibits libido)
        ■ **Follicle stimulating hormone:** Reproductive function
        ■ **Antidiuretic hormone:** Water regulation
        ■ **Oxytocin:** Feelings of well-being, love, and belonging
    - **Structural brain abnormalities:** Neuroimaging has shown various brain structures that are linked to symptoms of chronic and severe depression
        ■ It is unclear if the structural changes preceded the symptoms or the persistence of symptoms caused the structural changes
    - Hypovolemic hippocampus
    - Hypovolemic prefrontal cortex and limbic regions
    - Symptoms of depression are common in people who have experienced traumatic brain injuries and stroke
    - **Neurotransmitter theory:** Also known as the biogenic amine or bioamine theory implicating a deficiency in dopamine, serotonin, and norepinephrine. This theory remains popular largely due to its simplicity to communicate and understand despite numerous studies to the contrary (Delgado et al., 1999)
        ■ Difference in certain chemicals may contribute to symptoms of depression (not causal)
    - Circadian rhythm (chronobiologic)
    - Psychodynamic theories
    - Aggression-turned inward (Sigmund Freud) and object loss (Ronald Fairbairn, D.W. Winnocott, and Harry Guntrip)

- A real or perceived psychological trauma occurred during the first 5 years of life during the psychosexual development phase (Carveth Toronto, 2007; Haddad et al., 2008)
  - The mother is lost due to illness, death, emotional unavailability, postpartum depression, a second child, or other major responsibility (return to work)
  - The child experiences anxiety, despair, grief, and mourning
  - The child feels unsafe and expresses emotions outwardly for fear of causing further separation, as it has been imagined that the child is the cause of the trauma (Sigmund Freud).
  - The child uses immature defense mechanisms to cope and develops a love/hate relationship with the love object (mother)
    - The child develops self-anger as a safer alternative and excessive guilt
    - The person may manifest low self-esteem, excessive guilt, an inability to cope with anger, or self-destructive tendencies, which manifest as an adult whenever a loss or perceived loss is experienced
  - Cognitive theory (Aaron Beck) and learned helplessness-hopelessness (M. Seligman; Boysan, 2019; Bredemeier, Beck, & Grant, 2018)
    - A person learns over time from as early as the psychosexual development phase or throughout their life to respond to stressful life events in a depressed victim-like manner. The person comes to believe that random bad things are happening to them and they lack control over their life
    - Lack of control perception leads to maladaptive coping or nonreactive coping where behavior becomes passive because of reinforced perceptions of hopelessness, helplessness, and powerlessness
    - The person develops an automatic tendency toward negativistic interpretations of life and self-pity, and many cognitive distortions arise as a means of reinforcing pessimistic delusions and generalizing this perception to every aspect of life
    - **Personality:** People with low self-esteem are easily overwhelmed by stress, are more pessimistic in nature, and are also more likely to experience depressive symptoms
  - **Environmental:** Continuous exposure to violence, neglect, abuse, or poverty may increase already vulnerable people's likelihood of developing depressive symptoms (Connolly & Beaver, 2016).
- Risk factors for postpartum depression include (Ghaedrahmati, Kazemi, Kheirabadi, Ebrahimi, & Bahrami, 2017):
  - Poor marital relationship
  - Stressful life events
  - Negative attitude toward pregnancy
  - Lack of social support

▶ CLINICAL VIGNETTE OF THE PROTOTYPICAL PATIENT

A 26-year-old man reports poor sleep, diminished interest in new things, excessive guilt, low energy, difficulty concentrating, no longer finding pleasure in things he once enjoyed, and no interest in sex.

▶ INCIDENCE AND PREVALENCE

- Demographics, incidence, and prevalence
  - 10 million adults affected each year; the leading cause of disability claims
  - 50% of people with MDD never receive treatment
  - Average age of onset is in the second decade of life
  - More prevalent in women than men during reproductive years—25% female, 12% males; equivocal before puberty
  - Primary driver of increased morbidity, associated with higher mortality (four times greater than the population at large); 15% die by suicide
  - Untreated symptoms last approximately 4 months or more, median duration approximately 3 months, majority of patients recover in 12 months, approximately 20% fail to recover in 24 months (high risk for chronicity; Spijker et al., 2002)
  - MDD is a chronic and recurrent disorder; 40% of patients meet full *DSM-5* criteria, 20% do not meet full criteria but have significant impairment
  - Prior depressive episodes predict future episodes (60% risk of second episode, 70% risk of third episode given a second episode, 90% risk of a fourth episode and chronicity (Hidaka, 2012)
  - Bipolar 1 disorder 0.4%
  - Bipolar 2 disorder 0.3%
  - Bipolar not otherwise specified (NOS) 0.8%
  - Total bipolar disorder 1.5%
  - Major depressive disorder 6.0%
  - Dysthymic disorder 1.7%
- Risk factors
  - Genetic loading—first-degree relative
  - Predisposing environment
  - Acute stress
  - Singleness
  - Multiple losses or sudden success
  - Female gender
  - Postpartum period
  - Perimenopausal

▶ SCREENING TOOLS AND EARLY INTERVENTION

- Psychoeducation for at-risk family members
- Community outreach to increase awareness and reduce stigma associated with mental healthcare
- Integrated care models that include psychiatrically informed primary care services and consultation liaison psychiatric services
- Early intervention programs in elementary school, middle school, high school, college, and health and employee assistance programs

ASSESSMENT AND DIAGNOSIS

- History and physical exam
- Elicit a detailed history that includes onset and duration of symptoms (Table 9.1), severity, aggravating and alleviating factors, and current and past treatment, if any.
- Rule out mood disorders induced by substances or general medical conditions.
- Elicit a social history to include a baseline level of function, marital status, occupation, education, legal troubles, illicit drug use, history of abuse, and the current feeling of safety in the present living situation.
- Obtain a history of medications previously prescribed, currently prescribed, the reason for discontinuation, and include supplements, herbal remedies, and any other health practices.
- Inquire about past surgeries and physical traumas, pending and previous diagnostics (e.g., computed tomography [CT] scans, magnetic resonance imaging [MRI], biopsy, endoscopy, specialty consultations).
- Clarify the functional impairment attributable to mood symptoms of concern.
    - Identify skill deficits that are impeding independence, distinguish motivation from the inability.
    - Track improvement versus decompensation and rate of decline.
    - Involve support systems with psychoeducation regarding realistic expectations.
- Corroborate all information with various collateral sources.
- Assess for multiple physical complaints that are unrelated and for which no organic cause is identified.

Table 9.1 Mood Symptoms for Major Depressive and Bipolar Disorders

Major Depressive Disorder	Bipolar Disorder[a]
Sleep changes	Distractibility
Interest loss	Impulsive
Guilt	Grandiosity
Energy decreased	Flight of ideas
Cognition impaired/concentration impaired	Agitated activity
Appetite change	Sleep deficit
Psychomotor agitation/retardation	Talkativeness
Suicidal ideation or preoccupation	

[a]Mnemonic is DIGFAST.

PLANNING

- Ongoing and follow-up care goals
    - Psychoeducation, goals, risks, benefits, potential adverse effects of medication
    - Track progress and quantify the severity of symptoms
    - Assess suicidality at every visit
    - Evaluate for psychosis at every visit
        - Atypical depressive symptoms more commonly occur (but the name arises as a result of not meeting the first noted symptoms of melancholia)

- Increased appetite
- Increased sleep >10 hours
- The physical sensation of heaviness (like walking through quicksand)
- Increased interpersonal sensitivity to rejection leading to social or occupational impairment
    - Maladaptive coping strategies may include binge-eating episodes, excessive risk-taking behavior, substance use disorder, increased or abnormal use of pornography from baseline
    - Patients may be misdiagnosed with cyclothymia, bipolar 2 disorder, or attention deficit disorder with or without hyperactivity
    - **Major depressive disorder:** Characterized by episodes of depressed mood or anhedonia for at least 2 weeks with associated symptoms adversely effecting sleep, appetite, activity level, concentration, feelings of guilt, low self-worth, and suicidal thoughts or behaviors (American Psychiatric Association. Task Force on *DSM-5*, 2013).
- Symptoms can be further classified as mild, moderate, or severe.
- The course of the disorder can further be specified into partial remission, full remission, single episode, or recurrent, with or without psychotic features.
- Children manifest similar symptoms as adults; however, irritability, somatic complaints, and social withdrawal are often first recognized.
- Separation anxiety is often comorbid.
- Elderly patients will often present with somatic complaints, hypochondriacal symptoms, psychotic delusions, or ambivalence about the severity of symptoms.

INTERVENTION

- **Treatment:** Nonpharmacological treatments are preferred, and all selective serotonin reuptake inhibitors (SSRIs) carry black box warnings when used in children.
    - Exercise
    - Cognitive behavioral therapy
    - Family therapy
    - Group therapy
    - Interpersonal psychotherapy (preferred in children/adolescents)
    - Phototherapy
    - **Psychopharmacology:** Treatment is recommended for at least 1 year after the remission of symptoms. Patients with two or more episodes of depression may require lifelong medication
        - Medication selection should target specific symptoms if multiple symptoms regulate sleep first. Monotherapy is preferred. Identify measurable target symptoms. Antidepressants may induce hypomanic/manic symptoms in susceptible patients
        - Other considerations include cost, side effect profile, overdose risk, the risk for drug–drug and drug–food interactions, and CYP450 genomic variability.
        - Obtain baseline labs and electrocardiogram (EKG) before starting medications (within the diagnostic investigation)
        - Medications take 8 to 12 weeks for full effect and can stop working after a time of stability (poop out effect)

- Withdrawal syndrome is most common with medications with shorter half-lives
- SSRIs are firstline due to their safety profile and low overdose risk; effective for comorbid anxiety disorders
- Selective serotonin–norepinephrine reuptake inhibitors (SNRIs) can raise blood pressure and should be monitored
- The most common electrolyte abnormality associated with antidepressants is hyponatremia
- **Tricyclic antidepressants:** Considered a second-line option, high risk for overdose, avoid in patients with cardiac disease or conduction defects.
- Monoamine oxidase (MAOI) medications should be considered third line after electroconvulsive therapy (ECT); psychoeducation regarding dietary restrictions is essential, high risk for overdose
    - Requires 14-day wash-out from all SSRI/SNRI agents to reduce risk of serotonin syndrome
    - Symptoms of hypertensive crisis include sudden onset of worst headache ever, facial flushing, palpitations, pupillary dilation, fever, diaphoresis
        - Phentolamine 5 to 15 mg IV or IM: Blocks alpha-adrenergic receptors to briefly antagonize epinephrine and norepinephrine to reduce blood pressure
        - ED evaluation
    - **Electroconvulsive therapy (ECT):** Therapeutically induced grand mal seizure in an anesthetized (sedated and paralyzed) patient. The usual course is six to 12 treatments. Mechanism of action is unknown
        - **Indications for ECT:** Patient preference, nihilistic delusions (Dobek, Blumberger, Downar, Daskalakis, & Vila-Rodriguez, 2015) with severe neurovegetative symptoms, treatment resistance; benefit outweighs the risk of treatment and anesthesia
        - **Relative contraindications for ECT:** Cardiac disease, aortic stenosis, pulmonary insufficiency, inability to tolerate anesthesia
        - **Possible adverse effects of ECT:** Cardiovascular ischemia, headache, muscle aches, cognitive impairment
- **Transcranial magnetic stimulation:** Skin surface electrode/coil on the scalp to create a magnetic region throughout the head. Performed in an office setting, does not require anesthesia, requires five sessions per week for 6 weeks. The magnet makes noise and can cause some skin tingling. The patient may complain of headache or ear pain due to the noise (similar to an MRI machine). Mechanism of action is unknown. Rare instances of seizures in patients have been reported (Dobek et al., 2015)
- **Vagal nerve stimulation (VNS):** Indicated for treatment-resistant depression, requires a pulse generator implanted in the subclavian area (anesthesia required). Adverse effects can include voice changes, muscle spasms, dyspnea, throat or neck pain, skin tingling, and dysphagia. Mechanism of action concerning the treatment of depression is unknown
- **Dysthymia (persistent depressive disorder):** Characterized by a depressed mood most of the day for most of the days for at least 2 years
- **Premenstrual dysphoric disorder:** Characterized by an acute onset affective lability, irritability, anger, and/or increased interpersonal conflicts; may be accompanied by feelings of depressed mood, feelings of low self-worth, hopelessness, self-deprecating

thoughts, and increased anxiety, occurring in the week preceding menstruation. Symptoms improve on the second or third day of menstruation and resolve by the week after menstruation.
- **Disruptive mood dysregulation:** Characterized by severe and recurrent temper outbursts manifested verbally and/or behaviorally that are grossly out of proportion to the provocation with irritable or angry mood most of the days between the outbursts.
- **Bipolar 1 disorder:** Characterized by at least one manic episode that may have been preceded by or followed by a hypomanic or major depressive episode.
  - Mania is characterized by DIGFAST criteria
  - A distinct period of irritable mood or elevated energy lasting 7 days comprising at least three of the following symptoms:
    - Distractibility
    - Indiscretions/impulsivity
    - Grandiosity
    - Flight of ideas
    - Decreased need for sleep
    - Talkativeness (pressured/uninterruptible)
- Impairment required hospitalization for stabilization
  - **Bipolar 2 disorder:** Characterized by at least one hypomanic episode and one major depressive episode
    - **Hypomanic criteria:** Distinct period of elevated mood or irritability lasting 4 days and three DIGFAST symptoms
    - Change in mood and function is observable by others but not so severe as to warrant hospitalization
  - **Cyclothymic disorder:** Characterized by periods of hypomanic symptoms that do not exceed full criteria and depressive episodes that do not meet full criteria for major depressive disorder
- **Psychopharmacology:** Most important to regulate sleep first

EVALUATION

- Hospitalization criteria
  - Suicidality with lethality (intent, plan, means, substance use, previous attempt, family history, recent loss)
  - Lacking social supports
  - Unable to care for self (Maslow's hierarchy levels 1 and 2)

▶ CULTURAL IMPLICATIONS

- East Asian cultures tend to characterize their symptoms in terms of physical complaints, including head swelling, overwhelming and persistent fatigue, generalized weakness, and sleeplessness.
- Some Chinese people do not see depression as pathology but a way of life, a matter of fate, and there is nobility in withstanding hardship as stoic traits are valued.

KNOWLEDGE CHECK: CHAPTER 9

1. A 68-year-old man with no past psychiatric history reports that for the last 2 weeks he believes his internal organs have been removed, and that he has no mouth and therefore does not need to eat or drink. Which of the following best describes the patient's condition?

   A. Schizophrenia
   B. Capgras syndrome
   C. Cotard's syndrome
   D. Folie a deux

2. A 35-year-old woman 7 days postpartum is brought by the mobile crisis team to the emergency department at the request of the husband. The patient has no past psychiatric history and takes only prenatal vitamins. He reports that his wife has not been sleeping and has noticed her walking around their apartment in the middle of the night, crying and talking to nobody. In addition, she has been ignoring the baby, but last night she told him that it was "Lucifer's seed and it must be destroyed." Which of the following most likely explains these symptoms?

   A. Delusional disorder
   B. Depression with psychosis
   C. Schizoaffective disorder
   D. Schizophrenia

3. A 48-year-old divorced Black woman is admitted to the inpatient psychiatric unit after a serious suicide attempt by overdosing on acetaminophen. She has been admitted seven times with similar presentations after failing multiple treatments with antidepressants. She has been unable to work and has lost interest in all activities she once enjoyed. For the last 2 weeks, she has had increased sleep latency, early morning awakening, difficulty concentrating, fatigue, hopelessness, and poor appetite. Which of the following symptoms makes this person a candidate for electroconvulsive therapy (ECT)?

   A. Poor compliance with medications
   B. History of bipolar illness
   C. Melancholic depression with a history of poor response to medications
   D. Persistent depression with psychotic symptoms

1. C) Cotard's syndrome

Cotard's syndrome is a nihilistic delusion (things, including the self, do not exist) associated with psychotic depression in this case. Folie a deux is a shared delusion of one person influenced by another in which the treatment is to separate the two parties. Capgras syndrome is a delusional belief that people have been replaced by impostors and is associated with psychosis. Schizophrenia is a chronic and severe thought disorder affecting perceptions and is manifested by gross disorganization.

2. B) Depression with psychosis

Depression with psychosis in the postpartum period (because it has occurred within 4 weeks of delivery) is characterized by depression, mood lability, delusions, and hallucinations. Very psychotic disorders such as schizophrenia or schizoaffective disorder are less common in this clinical presentation and require a longer duration of time to qualify for the diagnosis.

3. C) Melancholic depression with a history of poor response to medications

Melancholic depression with a history of poor response to medications and the need for a quick antidepressant response are the universally accepted criteria that encourage ECT over medication and in major depression. Poor compliance with medication would not make a clinician choose ECT over medications as failure has not been demonstrated (treatment over objection and long-acting injectables are often preferred). A history of bipolar illness alone is not sufficient to recommend ECT over medication (lithium and valproic acid must often be stopped when ECT is begun because they alter the seizure threshold). Persistent depression with psychotic symptoms in the absence of failed medication trials would not sufficiently tip the balance in favor of ECT.

4. A patient meeting criteria for major depressive disorder is prescribed fluoxetine 20 mg daily. The psychiatric-mental health nurse is reviewing the chart for quality indicators of a near miss. Which of the following conditions should have been documented and excluded from the differentials before prescribing a selective serotonin reuptake inhibitor (SSRI)?

   A. Panic disorder
   B. Obsessive-compulsive disorder
   C. Bipolar disorder
   D. Generalized anxiety disorder

5. The mother of a 19-year-old male is convinced his bipolar condition was caused by his drinking and drug use. Which of the following statements is true regarding bipolar disorder?

   A. Patients with bipolar disorder have a better prognosis than patients with unipolar depression
   B. Patients with bipolar disorder usually do not require lifelong treatment compared to patients with major depression if they abstain from drugs and alcohol
   C. Bipolar disorder has a stronger genetic etiology than major depression
   D. Bipolar disorder is more common than depression in the United States

6. The certified nurse midwife is evaluating 29-year-old woman 2 weeks postpartum and finds her neglecting her self-care and minimally attentive to the baby and will not allow anyone else to care for the baby. During the visit, a psychiatric-mental health nurse can provide webcam consultation and liaison services. Based on the information provided, what is the priority in the management of this patient?

   A. Electronically prescribe an antipsychotic
   B. Electronically prescribe a mood stabilizer
   C. Admit the patient to the hospital
   D. Electronically prescribe an antidepressant

7. A 60-year-old man has been treated for depression for the last 2 years with a medication he cannot remember. He reports that he has had increasing urinary hesitancy, xerostomia, and intermittent lightheadedness. Which of the following medications is this patient most likely prescribed?

   A. Doxepin
   B. Fluoxetine
   C. Lithium
   D. Lamictal

(See answers next page.)

4. C) Bipolar disorder
Bipolar disorder must be ruled out prior to prescribing antidepressant medications because they are known to induce mania in susceptible patients. Antidepressants may be carefully administered to patients with bipolar disorder with predominantly depressed features (often must have a mood-stabilizing agent on board). Assess if compulsive disorder, generalized anxiety disorder, and panic disorder will all be well treated with SSRI medication.

5. C) Bipolar disorder has a stronger genetic etiology than major depression
Bipolar disorder has a stronger genetic etiology than major depression. Bipolar patients do not have a better prognosis than unipolar patients; patients with bipolar disorder usually require lifelong treatment compared to patients with depression. Bipolar disorder has no gender or geographic predilection.

6. C) Admit the patient to the hospital
Admit the patient to the hospital because, in her present condition of postpartum psychosis, the mother is an immediate danger to the infant. Prescribing medications in this instance does not consider the well-being of the child in the immediate aftermath.

7. A) Doxepin
Doxepin is a tricyclic antidepressant known for its anticholinergic properties, including dry mouth, orthostasis, urinary hesitancy, and retention leading to dysuria. Fluoxetine is a selective serotonin reuptake inhibitor mostly associated with gastrointestinal (GI) upset and sexual dysfunction. Lithium is most often associated with nephrogenic diabetes insipidus, and symptoms include polyuria, polydipsia, altered mental status, and tremor. Lamictal is an antiepileptic drug commonly used for mood stabilization associated with GI upset and, during periods of titration, Stevens-Johnson syndrome.

8. When providing psychoeducation to a patient with treatment-resistant depression about electroconvulsive therapy (ECT), you tell the patient that the most common adverse effect of treatment is which of the following?

   A. Arrhythmia
   B. Amnesia
   C. Respiratory depression
   D. Psychosis

9. A patient who is considering electroconvulsive therapy (ECT) for resistant depression inquires as to the number of sessions she would likely require. Based on the best evidence currently available, what is the best response from the psychiatric-mental health nurse?

   A. 40
   B. 20
   C. 10
   D. 4

10. A 38-year-old investment banker reveals that on weekends he visits the Delightful Dungeon and pays a dominatrix to tie him up, humiliate him, and whip him. He finds these sessions painful but very sexually arousing. He can become aroused and climax without this experience but finds this activity novel and has no desire to stop. Which of the following diagnoses is most likely?

    A. Atypical depression
    B. Sexual sadism
    C. No diagnosis
    D. Sexual masochism

11. A pregnant woman with depression is reluctant to take medication for fear of causing her baby neonatal abstinence syndrome due to selective serotonin reuptake inhibitor (SSRI) medication. Her husband states they would like to use a faith healer instead. Which of the following is most accurate regarding the prognosis of depression during pregnancy?

    A. The actual course of depression cannot be predicted
    B. If the patient does not take medication she will continue to deteriorate
    C. There is no risk of adverse effect associated with SSRIs
    D. The patient will likely require an involuntary commitment to a mental institution

(See answers next page.)

8. B) Amnesia
Amnesia is the most common adverse effect associated with ECT. Anesthesia-induced arrhythmia and respiratory depression are very rare side effects and often do not occur unless the patient is predisposed. Psychosis can often be improved rather than worsened after ECT. ECT is often preferred in cases of psychotic depression.

9. C) 10
Major depression treated with ECT usually requires between 6 and 12 sessions. Patients receiving ECT for catatonia can be treated with as little as 2 to 4 sessions. Patients with psychosis or mania may require 20 to 40 treatments for a positive therapeutic response.

10. C) No diagnosis
No diagnosis meeting *DSM-5* criteria for paraphilia is most likely for this patient. The patient does not have an occupational or social dysfunction, nor does he express any distress caused by his activities. If the patient was distressed by his behavior, he may meet the criteria for sexual masochism characterized as the arousal caused by psychological or physical punishment. Sexual sadism requires arousal caused by giving punishment. Fetishism requires the involvement of nonliving objects to cause arousal. The patient does not demonstrate symptoms of atypical depression (mood temporarily lifts in response to positive events, weight gain, excessive daytime sleepiness despite adequate sleep, hypersensitivity to criticism).

11. A) The actual course of depression cannot be predicted
The prognosis of depression cannot be predicted. It is not a foregone certainty that if the patient does not take medication she will continue to deteriorate. There is risk of neonatal abstinence syndrome associated with SSRIs, and it is not certain that the patient will require involuntary commitment if she does not take this medication.

12. A 25-year-old female is referred by her women's health nurse practitioner for evaluation. The patient reports that the week before her period, every month she feels angrier and is increasingly irritable, and has difficulty concentrating, low energy, and a desire to sleep more and eat more ice cream. These symptoms all seem to stop the week after her period. For which of the following conditions should psychoeducation be provided by the psychiatric-mental health nurse?

    A. Cyclothymic
    B. No diagnosis; normal female behavior
    C. Dysthymia
    D. Premenstrual dysphoric disorder

13. A 30-year-old man was recently terminated from his job for impulsive corporate spending. He was brought to the emergency department by the police for public nudity. The urine toxicology is negative, and all labs are normal. The patient is pressured and difficult to interrupt. He is demanding to leave and wants to speak to his lawyer, and he states that "the founding fathers declare that all men are created with the inalienable right to life and liberty, and President Trump has caused the Federal Bureau of Investigation (FBI) to trample my rights, which is a high crime and he should be impeached." What action should the psychiatric-mental health nurse take first?

    A. Call the physician for injection of Haldol
    B. Provide clothing
    C. Place the patient in four-point restraints
    D. Release the patient

14. A 70-year-old man with a history of hypertension is being evaluated for late effects of a cerebrovascular accident. Which of the following conditions is most associated with microvascular ischemia?

    A. Anxiety
    B. Obsessive compulsive disorder
    C. Depression
    D. Posttraumatic stress disorder (PTSD)

15. A patient who has been admitted for major depressive disorder has comorbid pedophilic disorder. Which of the following actions should the psychiatric-mental health nurse take first?

    A. Ask the client if he has molested children
    B. Establish a therapeutic alliance
    C. Self-reflect regarding the ability to remain non-judgmental while caring for this patient
    D. Alert all the unit patients of the patient's pedophilia diagnosis

(See answers next page.)

12. D) Premenstrual dysphoric disorder
The patient meets criteria for premenstrual dysphoric disorder; duration is not sufficiently long to qualify for major depressive disorder. Dysthymia requires the persistence of symptoms for at least 2 years. Cyclothymic disorder requires alternating between symptoms of depression and hypomania without meeting full criteria most of the time for at least 2 years, and a symptom-free period cannot exceed 2 months.

13. B) Provide clothing
Providing clothing addresses the physical need for shelter and safety while attempting to restore dignity and will enhance the therapeutic alliance. Calling for sedation or restraints is not the priority as the patient is not posing imminent harm to himself or others. The patient needs a psychiatric evaluation before he can be released.

14. C) Depression
Depression is a common comorbid condition associated with microvascular ischemia, such as cerebrovascular accident (CVA) and myocardial infarction. Anxiety and PTSD are not associated with late effects of CVA, but the patient may have hypervigilance regarding self-care and adopt obsessive compulsive behaviors regarding self-care measures.

15. C) Self-reflect regarding the ability to remain non-judgmental while caring for this patient
The psychiatric-mental health nurse should self-reflect and decide if care can be rendered non-judgmentally in the patient's best interest. Asking if the client has molested children is not a therapeutic or priority action in the acute care setting. Prior to establishing a therapeutic alliance, the psychiatric-mental health nurse must convey a non-judgmental attitude. Alerting unit patients of the pedophilia diagnosis is a violation of patient confidentiality. Also, pedophilia does not mean the patient has abused children; it only connotes an attraction to them.

REFERENCES

American Psychiatric Association. Task Force on *DSM-5*. (2013). *Diagnostic and statistical manual of mental disorders* (5th ed.). Washington, DC: American Psychiatric Publishing.

Boysan, M. (2019). An integration of quadripartite and helplessness-hopelessness models of depression using the Turkish version of the Learned Helplessness Scale (LHS). *British Journal of Guidance & Counselling*, 1–20. doi:10.1080/03069885.2019.1612033

Bredemeier, K., Beck, A. T.,& Grant, P.M. (2018). Exploring the temporal relationship between cognitive insight and neurocognition in schizophrenia: A prospective analysis. *Clinical Psychological Science*, 6(1), 76–89. doi:10.1177/2167702617734019

Carveth Toronto, D. L. (2007). Self-punishment as guilt evasion: The case of Harry Guntrip. *Canadian Journal of Psychoanalysis/Revue Canadienne de Psychanalyse*, 15. Retrieved from http://www.yorku.ca/dcarveth/guntrip

Connolly, E. J., & Beaver, K. M. (2016). Considering the genetic and environmental overlap between bullying victimization, delinquency, and symptoms of depression/anxiety. *Journal of Interpersonal Violence*, 31(7), 1230–1256. doi:10.1177/0886260514564158

Delgado, P. L., Miller, H. L., Salomon, R. M., Licinio, J., Krystal, J. H., Moreno, F. A., … Charney, D. S. (1999). Tryptophan depletion challenge in depressed patients treated with desipramine or fluoxetine: Implications for the role of serotonin in the mechanism of antidepressant action. *Biological Psychiatry*, 46(2), 212–220. Retrieved from http://www.ncbi.nlm.nih.gov/pubmed/10418696.

Dobek, C. E., Blumberger, D. M., Downar, J., Daskalakis, Z. J., & Vila-Rodriguez, F. (2015). Risk of seizures in transcranial magnetic stimulation: A clinical review to inform consent process focused on bupropion. *Neuropsychiatric Disease and Treatment*, 11, 2975–2987. doi:10.2147/NDT.S91126

Ghaedrahmati, M., Kazemi, A., Kheirabadi, G., Ebrahimi, A., & Bahrami, M. (2017). Postpartum depression risk factors: A narrative review. *Journal of Education and Health Promotion*, 6. doi:10.4103/JEHP.JEHP_9_16

Haddad, S. K., Reiss, D., Spotts, E. L., Ganiban, J., Lichtenstein, P., & Neiderhiser, J. M. (2008). Depression and internally directed aggression: Genetic and environmental contributions. *Journal of the American Psychoanalytic Association*, 56(2), 515–550. doi:10.1177/0003065108319727

Hidaka, B. H. (2012). Depression as a disease of modernity: Explanations for increasing prevalence. *Journal of Affective Disorders*, 140(3), 205–214. doi:10.1016/J.JAD.2011.12.036

Spijker, J., De Graaf, R., Bijl, R. V, Beekman, A. T. F., Ormel, J., & Nolen, W. A. (2002). Duration of major depressive episodes in the general population: Results from the Netherlands Mental Health Survey and Incidence Study (NEMESIS). *British Journal of Psychiatry*, 181(3), 208–213. doi:10.1192/bjp.181.3.208

Anxiety and Related Disorders

OBJECTIVES

- Identify the diagnostic criteria for anxiety disorders
- Distinguish among similar features of subcategories of anxiety
- Review psychopharmacological agents that are commonly used for anxiety disorders
- Identify nonpharmacological agents used to treat anxiety
- Describe the diagnostic criteria for posttraumatic stress disorder

FAST FACTS

- More common in females than males 2:1
- Characterized by excessive worries and fears, which may be rational or irrational
- Can be a learned behavioral response
- Often comorbid with mood disorders
- Most effective and enduring treatment is cognitive behavioral therapy

GENERALIZED ANXIETY DISORDER

Characterized by persistent and consistent excessive worry, apprehension regarding an impending or perceived distressing situation that is disruptive to daily functioning affecting perceptions, memory, judgment, and motor response lasting at least 6 months.

- **Signs and symptoms** (three or more of the following)
  - Restlessness
  - Fatigue
  - Irritability
  - Muscle tension
  - Sleep disturbance

▶ CLINICAL VIGNETTE OF THE PROTOTYPICAL PATIENT

A 24-year-old female reports intermittent headaches, constantly taps her foot, clicks or chews on her pen, is irritable and distracted, has poor sleep marked by difficulty falling asleep, and sometimes wakes up early out of fear of oversleeping her alarm. She also reports that in the past she was so anxious her heart was beating out of her chest that she went to the emergency department for fear that she might die.

▶ INCIDENCE AND PREVALENCE

The most common psychiatric disorder; lifetime prevalence 33% among the U.S. population (Bandelow & Michaelis, 2015)

- More prevalent in females than males except for obsessive-compulsive disorder (OCD) and social phobias (social anxiety disorder)
- **Age of onset:** Early adolescence
- Prevalence is highly variable across cultures
- **Etiology:** Various theories regarding underlying cause; no one theory accounts completely for manifestations of anxiety, and numerous factors must be considered in making a diagnosis of exclusion; a meta-theoretically informed approach offers the best chance at developing a therapeutic alliance leading to a good outcome. The neurobiological explanation for anxiety disorder is theoretical and dependent on metaphor for conceptualization.
  - **Neurobiological theories (E. Kraepelin 1856–1926):** Premised on the bio-amine theory of mental illness (neurotransmitter deficits). This theory implicates neuroendocrine, neurotransmitter, and neuroanatomical disruptions as the predisposing factors of anxiety disorder (Martin, Ressler, Binder, & Nemeroff, 2009). Dysfunctions may arise congenitally or as a response to epigenetic stressors during a time of rapid growth and development (in utero, first few years of life, adolescence). A chemical imbalance may be genetically mediated due to structural abnormalities in the limbic system, midbrain, and cerebral cortex.
    - Gamma-aminobutyric acid (GABA), an inhibitory neurotransmitter, is insufficient to contain the effects of norepinephrine (excitatory neurotransmitter).
    - Serotonin deficit leads to insufficient inhibition of the hypothalamic–pituitary axis (HPA) to mitigate the intensity of a stress response.
  - Structural dysfunctions may predispose an individual to an abnormal stress response, which correlates with autonomic excitability, triggering symptoms of elevated heart rate and blood pressure, diaphoresis ease, tremor, and increased respiratory rate.
  - **HPA:** Dysfunctions may predispose the individual to perceiving imagined threats, triggering a hormonal cascade of corticotropin-releasing hormone.
    - The amygdala activates the sympathetic nervous system to trigger the fight, flight, or freeze response more readily than a brain without HPA dysfunction.
    - Adrenocorticotropic hormone (ACTH) is released from the pituitary.
      – Adrenal glands are stimulated to release cortisol to restore homeostasis.

- Inhibitory mechanisms of the amygdala may be ineffective in turning off the fight or flight response, disposing the individual to panic attacks.
- **Psychodynamic theories (S. Freud 1856–1939):** Based on the assumption of long-lasting psychic scars during psychosexual development (Goldstein & Harden, 2000). The psychic injury keeps the individual from mastering their psychological milestones.
  - Anxiety stems from a repression of the sexual drive as the individual is unable to resolve the conflict between the Id and the Superego.
  - Anxiety is manifested as a result of unconscious fear of punishment for indulging the Id.
  - The individual may use immature and neurotic defense mechanisms to relieve stress, leading to pathological behaviors and causing distress to the individual.
- **Interpersonal theory (H. Sullivan 1892–1949):** This theory asserts that anxiety arises out of unmet needs and can first arise in infancy. Persistence of anxiety beyond adolescence is a result of the person perceiving their needs will not be met because of rejection, feelings of inferiority, or an inability to engage socially. The individual forms their identity based on how they perceive others will view them, and if they are worthy of having their needs met.
- **Cognitive behavioral theory:** Premised on the interplay of cognitions, emotions, and behaviors driving treatment and is aimed at altering cognitions and thereby affecting emotions and behaviors. Anxiety is thought to be a learned response in which an individual may utilize avoidance to alleviate distress.

- **Risk factors**
  - Genetic predisposition, history of a first-degree relative with an anxiety disorder
  - Immature defense mechanisms
  - High levels of parental distress
  - Substance use disorder (including tobacco, caffeine, and prescription stimulants, in addition to illicit drugs and herbal supplements)
  - History of psychological trauma

▶ SCREENING TOOLS AND EARLY INTERVENTION

- **History**
  - Rule out an underlying medical condition, substance-induced disorder, malingering, and factitious disorder prior to diagnosing anxiety. Assess the patient for the following factors:
    - Onset of symptoms (specified) including aggravating and alleviating factors, and co-occurring symptoms and situations
    - Answer the question "What does this symptom prevent from happening?"
    - Social history including the present living situation, occupation, educational level, relationship status, legal status
    - Nonrelated multiple somatic complaints without organic etiology
    - Identified current and upcoming stressors
    - Distinguish normative from pathological anxiety (e.g., "How does the anxiety keep you from functioning?")

- How does anxiety interfere with social, occupational, and recreational activities of daily living?
- Range for previous diagnosis of anxiety and misuse of medication

ASSESSMENT AND DIAGNOSIS

- **Physical and mental status exam:** Patient may appear to be in obvious distress; observe for the following signs:
  - Pressured speech
  - Flight of ideas
  - Increased heart rate
  - Increased respirations
  - Increased blood pressure
  - Diaphoresis
  - Compensatory posture for musculoskeletal complaints (e.g., headache, neckache, backache, chest tightness)
- **Muscle spasms, tremors**
- **Dilated pupils**
- **Gastrointestinal complaints:** Cramps, nausea, vomiting, diarrhea, weight loss
- **Appearance:** Psychomotor agitation, restlessness, tremor, pacing, hand-wringing, fidgeting
- **Speech:** Impoverished, pressured, distractible, whispered, increasing in volume, babbling nonsensically, inconsolable
- **Mood:** Worried, nervous, stressed, irritable, dysphoric
- **Affect:** Apprehensive, tearful, fearful, trepidatious
- **Thought process:** Linear, disorganized, goal-directed, distractible, redirectable
- **Thought content:** Thematic, perseverative, no perceptual disturbances
- **Orientation:** Oriented to person, time, place, and purpose; may be disoriented
- **Memory:** Short-term impairment, difficulty learning new information, forgetful, may require frequent reminding and reassurance
- **Concentration:** Inattentive, difficulty concentrating
- **Abstraction:** May be limited by concentration, able to abstract on proverbs and similarities
- **Judgment:** Fair to excellent
- **Insight:** Limited to insightful
- **Diagnostic lab findings:** Many medical conditions share signs and symptoms of generalized anxiety disorder and panic disorder. These conditions can also develop as a result of a panic disorder in a patient with limited physiologic reserve. The typical presentations of certain medical conditions require key findings that can be easily excluded. Anxiety and panic symptoms usually resolve in 15 minutes or less.
- No specific diagnostic tests are indicated for panic disorder but should be guided by index of suspicion and clinical reasoning.
- **Cardiovascular**
  - **Ischemic heart disease:** Chest pressure or pain should not be reproducible and should be consistent for 10 to 15 minutes and relieved by rest; accompanied by diaphoresis, nausea, radiating nature of pain or pressure, numbness, and tingling.

- **Pulmonary embolism:** Pain worse with inspiration, tachypnea, tachycardia, relative hypoxia, adventitious lung sounds including rails, and wheezing

PLANNING

- Help the client distinguish signs and symptoms of anxiety versus panic attack
- Establish hemodynamic stability and prioritize clinical findings
- Identify useful coping strategies and safety planning in the event of a panic attack

INTERVENTION

- **Pharmacological management:** The goal is to reduce the cardiovascular manifestations triggered by chronic or acute anxiety often caused by the associated catecholamine surge accompanying the presentation of symptoms. Most medications act directly or indirectly on the GABA system.
- **Selective serotonin reuptake inhibitors (SSRIs)**
  - First-line treatment for anxiety disorders
  - Steady state requires 4 to 6 weeks
  - Low risk of dependency, however, depending on half-life dose, must be tapered gradually
  - Generally, well-tolerated, low drug–drug interactions
  - Cannot be used on an as-needed basis
  - Black-box warning for children and adolescents regarding increased suicidality
- **Benzodiazepines:** High potential for abuse, addiction, diversion, acute withdrawal can be fatal
  - Rapid onset of action
  - Used on an as-needed basis
  - Commonly prescribed to reduce the activating effects of SSRIs during titration
  - Limit use to the lowest possible dose for the shortest duration
    - Long-term use leads to tolerance, dependence, cognitive impairment, and depressed mood
    - Avoid in patients with a history of substance use disorder or alcohol use disorder, or in those currently on medication-assisted treatment for addiction (MATA)
  - Should not be used with buprenorphine
  - Benzodiazepines with longer half-lives require less frequent dosing and have less severe withdrawal and rebound anxiety effects
    - Clonazepam
    - Diazepam
    - Chlordiazepoxide
  - The shorter the half-life, the more severe the withdrawal and rebound anxiety. These medications should be used for premedication for procedures (MRI, etc.) or very short-term use (e.g., preflight). Highest risk for diversion, abuse, and addiction
    - Alprazolam

- Tricyclics (TCA)
  - Many drug–drug interactions
  - Anticholinergic adverse effects
  - Overdose potential
  - Monitor EKG, avoid in patients with cardiac disease
- Miscellaneous pharmacological agents for anxiety
  - Beta-blockers: Can be taken as needed. If consistently taken, requires taper and follow-up EKG, monitor for angina symptoms during taper
  - Gabapentin: Can be taken as needed, wide therapeutic range
  - Buspirone: Must be taken consistently for 8 weeks for anxiolytic effects
  - Alpha-blockers: Used in children off label, based on weight
- **Nonpharmacological management:** Preferred treatment for anxiety offering the longest-lasting relief from symptoms
  - Cognitive behavioral therapy
    - Systematic desensitization
    - Exposure therapy
    - Relaxation and mindfulness
      - Meditation
      - Biofeedback
      - Hypnosis
      - Distraction
  - Bibliotherapy
  - Support groups
  - Complementary and alternative treatments:
    - Aroma therapy
    - Massage
    - Acupuncture/acupressure
    - Exercise (aerobic) and weightlifting (anaerobic)
    - Animal-assisted therapy (emotional support animals)

EVALUATION

- Determine frequency and intensity of anxiety symptoms at various stages of treatment
- Identify effective coping mechanisms deployed at times of stress
- Identify the incidence and frequency of avoidance behaviors
- Identify the development of new maladaptive coping mechanisms

▶ CULTURAL IMPLICATIONS

- Many cultures do not allow for mental health as traditionally defined in the Western world, and such symptoms of anxiety will often manifest in the form of physical complaints.

- Subcultures can also have different manifestations of what is known as anxiety, depending on the social context.
- Manifestations of anxiety are influenced by how the culture understands bodily functions; for example, Asians have notions influenced by the construct of qi (chi), some cultures may relate to a spiritual aspect as the reason for symptoms and distress.

AGORAPHOBIA

Characterized by a fear of avoidance of multiple situations due to thoughts that it may be difficult to escape the situation if panic symptoms occur. Commonly develops in patients with comorbid panic disorder. The anxiety leads to avoidance behaviors and impairs the individual's ability to work, socialize, travel, and carry out activities of daily living (Wittmann et al., 2018). Usually, agoraphobia is a progression of generalized anxiety disorder. It is like the following disorders but is distinguished in the following manner:

- **Social anxiety disorder:** Characterized by an avoidance of social situations in which the person perceives they will be critiqued by others
- **Specific phobia:** Characterized by avoidance of situations specifically related to the likelihood of encountering the object related to the fear (e.g., trapped in an elevator, trapped in a crowd, encountering a dog)
- **Posttraumatic stress disorder (PTSD) or acute stress disorder:** Characterized by avoidance of situations that arouse upsetting memories, thoughts, or feelings about a specific traumatic event
- **Major depressive disorder:** Avoids going outside due to apathy, fatigue, fear of crying in public, or being unable to experience pleasure
- **Delusional disorder/psychotic features:** Characterized by the avoidance resulting from a delusional concern (e.g., will not go outside because they believe they are being followed)
- **Obsessive compulsive disorder:** Characterized by an avoidance behavior that is intended to prevent triggering an obsession or compulsion (avoids going outside because of becoming contaminated and unable to wash hands)
- **Separation anxiety disorder:** Characterized by avoidance of situations that require being away from the major attachment figure, which can lead to avoidance of going out of one's house (e.g., child does not want to go to school because they will be away from mother)

▶ CLINICAL VIGNETTE OF THE PROTOTYPICAL PATIENT

A 36-year-old male with a history of anhedonia and apathy has become increasingly isolative and narrowing the focus of interest increasingly more each day and reports increased distress to the point of panic at the thought of leaving the safety of his home because he thinks he will be followed due to his unusual appearance.

▶ INCIDENCE AND PREVALENCE

- Varies greatly as symptoms can be episodic and hard to quantify and is often comorbid with generalized anxiety disorder or panic disorder

▶ SCREENING TOOLS AND EARLY INTERVENTION

- Hamilton Anxiety Rating Scale
- Overall Anxiety Severity and Impairment Scale
- Help the client elicit antecedents to the feelings of distress and note the time to resolution of acute symptoms
- Listen for cognitive distortions, including catastrophic thinking and fortune-telling

ASSESSMENT AND DIAGNOSIS

- Patients may be ashamed or embarrassed when they realize their symptoms are not physical but psychological in nature. Using a normalizing approach that assumes everything and assumes nothing is often most helpful
  - "Some people have problems with crowds, busses, subways, restaurants, bridges, or driving places. Do you have problems like this too?"
  - "Some people get anxious when they leave their home, do you feel this way too?"

PLANNING

- Help the client distinguish signs and symptoms of anxiety versus panic attack
- Establish hemodynamic stability and prioritize clinical findings
- Identify useful coping strategies and safety planning in the event of a panic attack

INTERVENTION

- **Nonpharmacological management:** Preferred treatment for anxiety offering the longest lasting relief from symptoms
  - Cognitive behavioral therapy
    - Systematic desensitization
    - Exposure therapy
    - Relaxation and mindfulness
      - Meditation
      - Biofeedback
      - Hypnosis
      - Distraction
  - Bibliotherapy
  - Support groups

- Complementary and alternative treatments:
    - Aroma therapy
    - Massage
    - Acupuncture/acupressure
    - Exercise (aerobic) and weightlifting (anaerobic)
    - Animal-assisted therapy (emotional support animals)

EVALUATION

- Determine frequency and intensity of anxiety symptoms at various stages of treatment
- Identify effective coping mechanisms deployed at times of stress
- Identify the incidence and frequency of avoidance behaviors
- Identify the development of new maladaptive coping mechanisms

▶ CULTURAL IMPLICATIONS

- Many cultures do not allow for mental health as traditionally defined in the Western world, and such symptoms of anxiety will often manifest in the form of physical complaints.
- Subcultures can also have different manifestations of what is known as anxiety, depending on the social context.
- Manifestations of anxiety are influenced by how the culture understands bodily functions; for example, Asians have notions influenced by the construct of qi (aka chi), some cultures may relate to a spiritual aspect as the reason for symptoms and distress.

OBSESSIVE COMPULSIVE DISORDER

Characterized by recurrent thoughts, urges, or images experienced as intrusive and unwanted that the patient attempts to ignore or suppress, and/or repetitive behaviors or mental acts that the person is compelled to perform in response to the thoughts according to rules that must rigidly be applied for the purpose of reducing the individual's subjective anxiety level (Apergis-Schoute et al., 2018).

- **Obsessions:** Recurrent and persistent thoughts, impulses, or images that cause distress
    - Thoughts of contamination, dirt, or germs
    - Persistent doubts such as having hit somebody or hurt somebody
    - The drive to have things organized in a very specific order followed by great distress when that order is not maintained
    - Aggressive or horrific thoughts
    - Persistent sexual imagery

- Obsessions are not usually grounded in reality
  - Patients recognize that thoughts and impulses are a product of their own minds
  - Person spends a considerable amount of time trying to suppress the thoughts and impulses to override them with other thoughts and behaviors
  - Patients may exhibit avoidance behavior in which the content of the session may be encountered such as public transportation with respect to contamination with germs
- **Compulsions:** Repetitive behaviors or mental actions that the person is driven to perform in response to the obsession in order to relieve the distress.
  - Handwashing
  - Excessive cleaning
  - Persistent checking of lights, the burner, locks
  - Persistent organizing and reorganizing
  - Counting
  - Silently repeating words
  - Praying
  - Patients may attach superstitious meanings or magical thinking to behaviors and thoughts
- Pediatric autoimmune neuropsychiatric disorders associated with streptococcal infections (PANDAS) should be considered when acute onset signs and symptoms arise in children.

▶ CLINICAL VIGNETTE OF THE PROTOTYPICAL PATIENT

A 26-year-old man spends much of his day ruminating about all the germs he may possibly come into contact with and is fearful of contaminating surfaces and himself that he washes his hands frequently with a new bar of soap each time.

▶ INCIDENCE AND PREVALENCE

- Lifetime prevalence is approximately 2% in the United States
- 76% have a lifetime history of another anxiety disorder
- 64% have a lifetime history of mood disorder
- 25% may also have obsessive-compulsive personality disorder
- 29% have a lifetime history of tic disorder comorbidly

▶ SCREENING TOOLS AND EARLY INTERVENTION

- Hamilton Anxiety Rating Scale
- Overall Anxiety Severity and Impairment Scale
- Help the client elicit antecedents to the feelings of distress and note the time to resolution of acute symptoms
- Listen for cognitive distortions, including catastrophic thinking and fortune-telling

ASSESSMENT AND DIAGNOSIS

- Patients rarely volunteer these embarrassing symptoms without being expressly asked. Asking in a normalizing fashion, assuming nothing, and assuming everything can put the patient at ease to disclose their symptoms.
- Some people are comforted when they wash their hands frequently, check and double-check things, or have annoying thoughts pop up in their heads frequently. "Do you sometimes feel driven to wash or straighten things, or have recurrent thoughts, or mental rituals around certain words or numbers, or find yourself holding on to a lot of things for fear of needing them one day or being caught off guard?"
- "Often people may feel if they do not do certain actions something bad will happen. Do you feel that way too?"

PLANNING

- Help the client distinguish signs and symptoms of anxiety versus panic attack
- Establish hemodynamic stability and prioritize clinical findings
- Identify useful coping strategies and safety planning in the event of a panic attack

INTERVENTION

- **Nonpharmacological management:** Preferred treatment for anxiety offering the longest-lasting relief from symptoms.
  - Cognitive behavioral therapy
    - Systematic desensitization
    - Exposure therapy
    - Relaxation and mindfulness
      - Meditation
      - Biofeedback
      - Hypnosis
      - Distraction
  - Bibliotherapy
  - Support groups

EVALUATION

- Determine frequency and intensity of anxiety symptoms at various stages of treatment
- Identify effective coping mechanisms deployed at times of stress
- Identify the incidence and frequency of avoidance or checking behaviors
- Identify the development of new maladaptive coping mechanisms; the client may experience stress at the lack of things to do as the OCD behavior had previously occupied so much time that they may take on other maladaptive behaviors.

CULTURAL IMPLICATIONS

- Ruminations and hyper-vigilance may be survival skills learned and passed down through the generations as being conscientious and rewarded.
- Certain cultures may encourage what the secular world calls a religious preoccupation, but the patient and the culture from which they hail may see this as a virtue. They may be distressed that they are not doing it enough.

PANIC DISORDER

A discrete episode of heightened arousal characterized by intense apprehension, fearfulness, terror; often associated with an impending sense of doom.

- Signs and symptoms are consistent with that of generalized anxiety disorder, which also include the following:
  - Chest pressure, tightness, discomfort
  - Shortness of breath
  - Palpitations associated with increased heart rate
  - Fear of death
  - Fear of losing control
  - Diaphoresis, paresthesia, chills, hot flashes
  - Nausea, vomiting, diarrhea
  - Tremulousness
- After the first attack, the patient may continue to live in fear of having another panic attack, which can lead to meeting criteria for agoraphobia, generalized anxiety disorder, or major depressive disorder.
- Patients are often intolerant or overly concerned with common side effects of medication.

CLINICAL VIGNETTE OF THE PROTOTYPICAL PATIENT

A 36-year-old man presents to the emergency department for the second time in a month with chest palpitations and an impending sense of doom, difficulty breathing, sweating, and nausea. The symptoms seem to have come out of the blue and lasted approximately 10 to 15 minutes.

INCIDENCE AND PREVALENCE

- Lifetime prevalence in the United States is approximately 3%
- 35% of people have reported panic attack in the previous year but do not meet criteria for panic disorder
- Panic attacks are more common than panic disorder
- Panic attacks can occur in patients without generalized anxiety disorder or underlying panic disorder

SCREENING TOOLS AND EARLY INTERVENTION

- There are no specific early interventions for panic attacks as they occur without known precipitant; however, encouraging effective coping, adequate rest, food, hydration, and consistent exercise and meditation practices can reduce the likelihood of recurrence.

ASSESSMENT AND DIAGNOSIS

- Direct questions can help identify patients who have had panic attacks or who may go on to develop panic disorder.
  - "Have you ever had a panic or anxiety attack?"
  - "A panic attack is a sudden rush of fear and nervousness in which your heart is pounding, and you are short of breath, and you have a fear of losing control or dying. Has this ever happened to you?"
  - Asking them to describe what they felt, what they were doing at the time when it happened, how long did it last are both instructive and therapeutic

PLANNING

- Help the client distinguish signs and symptoms of anxiety versus panic attack
- Establish hemodynamic stability and prioritize clinical findings
- Identify useful coping strategies and safety planning in the event of panic attack

INTERVENTION

- **Nonpharmacological management:** Preferred treatment for anxiety offering the longest lasting relief from symptoms
  - Cognitive behavioral therapy
    - Meditation
    - Biofeedback
    - Hypnosis
    - Distraction
  - Bibliotherapy
  - Support groups

EVALUATION

- Determine frequency and intensity of anxiety symptoms at various stages of treatment
- Identify effective coping mechanisms deployed at times of stress
- Identify the incidence and frequency of avoidance or checking behaviors

- Identify the development of new maladaptive coping mechanisms; the client may experience stress at the lack of things to do as the OCD behavior had previously occupied so much time that they may take on other maladaptive behaviors

▶ CULTURAL IMPLICATIONS

- While commonly occurring around the world, the interpretation of the phenomenon varies greatly.

PHOBIAS

Patients will experience a clinically significant level of distress when presented with the object of their phobia. The stress can occur simply by thinking about the object or situation in anticipation of having to confront the object or situation (e.g., heights, spiders, dogs, snakes).

- Patient may be aware that the fear is unreasonable and excessive.
- Risk factors for phobias include past traumatic exposure (e.g., near-drowning event), vicarious trauma (e.g., peer drowns or nearly drowns), excessively transmitted information (frequent parental warnings; e.g., you will drown if you go in the pool).
- Family history of phobia causing a learned response.

▶ CLINICAL VIGNETTE OF THE PROTOTYPICAL PATIENT

A 36-year-old man sees a spider on the edge of the bathtub where he was taking a shower; out of terror, he runs screaming naked out of the house.

▶ INCIDENCE AND PREVALENCE

- An estimated 2% to 7% of adults in the United States have a lifetime phobia

▶ SCREENING TOOLS AND EARLY INTERVENTION

- Inquiring directly: Do you have any special fears, such as of insects, flying, or clowns? Have you ever had a panic attack around the specific thing you are afraid of?

ASSESSMENT AND DIAGNOSIS

- Key criteria include excessive and unreasonable fear of a specific object or situation
- Exposure to the phobic stimulus causes intense anxiety

PLANNING

- Help the client distinguish signs and symptoms of anxiety versus panic attack
- Establish hemodynamic stability and prioritize clinical findings
- Identify useful coping strategies and safety planning in the event of a panic attack

INTERVENTION

- **Nonpharmacological management:** Preferred treatment for anxiety offering the longest lasting relief from symptoms.
  - Cognitive behavioral therapy
    - Systematic desensitization
    - Exposure therapy
    - Relaxation and mindfulness

EVALUATION

- Quantify the level of fear and anxious reaction after therapeutic interventions

▶ CULTURAL IMPLICATIONS

- Taijin kyofusho appears almost exclusively among those of Japanese and Korean descent and much less often among other Asian cultures. It is the fear of one's appearance, physical body, or actions offending others.
- Koro is a phobia specific to Asian males. It is the fear of the genitals retracting into the body, eventually leading to death.
- Daht is the fear of losing semen, which is based on a misperception in Indian culture that semen is a precious and scarce bodily fluid and should be saved for procreation.

POSTTRAUMATIC STRESS DISORDER (PTSD)

Characterized by reexperiencing an extremely traumatic event after the direct exposure to, witnessing of, or hearing about an actual or threatened death, serious injury, or sexual violence. Symptoms may also arise in first responders collecting human remains or those exposed to or dealing with victims of abuse or assault (American Psychiatric Association Task Force on *DSM-5*, 2013). The person's response must have involved intense fear, helplessness, or horror.

- Characterized by symptoms of increased arousal and avoidance of stimuli associated with the trauma persisting for 1 month or longer

- **Reexperiencing symptoms** (one or more of the following):
  - Recurrent and intrusive thoughts recollecting the event
  - Flashbacks
  - Dissociative state lasting hours to days
  - Nightmares regarding the event
  - Intense distress at exposure to cues symbolizing the event
  - Physiologic reactivity upon exposure to cues symbolizing the event
- **Avoidance symptoms** (three or more of the following):
  - Persistent avoidance of stimuli associated with the traumatic event
  - Effort expended to avoid talking about the traumatic event
  - Inability to recall important aspects about the event
  - Significant anhedonia
  - Persistent feelings of detachment and estrangement from others
  - Restricted range of affect
  - Impending sense of foreboding or shortened future, premature death
- **Persistent hyperarousal symptoms** (two or more of the following):
  - Difficulty falling asleep
  - Irritability or outbursts of anger
  - Difficulty concentrating
  - Hypervigilance
  - Exaggerated startle response
- Symptoms are considered acute if they last less than 3 months, chronic if they last more than 3 months, delayed onset if the symptoms occur at least 6 months after the event
  - Adjustment disorder can be diagnosed if the patient does not meet specific criteria for PTSD

▶ CLINICAL VIGNETTE OF THE PROTOTYPICAL PATIENT

A 50-year-old man who reports hyper-vigilant arousal, avoidant behavior, insomnia due to nightmares, irritability, and dysthymia had a history of past sexual assault.

▶ INCIDENCE AND PREVALENCE

- Prevalence in the United States is 9% in the general adult population

▶ SCREENING TOOLS AND EARLY INTERVENTION

- Pre-trauma risk factors include age at trauma, race, education level, separated, divorced, or widowed
- Adverse Childhood Events screening tool
- Initial severity of reaction to a traumatic event

ASSESSMENT AND DIAGNOSIS

- Do you have memories or dreams of a terrible experience that you thought your life was endangered or you felt very powerless as in a physical or sexual attack, accident, war, or natural disaster?
- Does the experience come back to haunt you, or do you find yourself thinking about it all the time?
- Do you have nightmares related to the incident?
- Do you find yourself avoiding certain activities or people related to your incident?

PLANNING

- Help the client distinguish signs and symptoms of anxiety versus panic attack
- Establish hemodynamic stability and prioritize clinical findings
- Identify useful coping strategies and safety planning in the event of a panic attack

INTERVENTION

- **Nonpharmacological management:** Preferred treatment for anxiety offering the longest lasting relief from symptoms
  - Cognitive behavioral therapy
    - Systematic desensitization
    - Exposure therapy via virtual reality
    - Relaxation and mindfulness
      - Meditation
      - Biofeedback
      - Hypnosis
      - Distraction
  - Bibliotherapy
  - Support groups

EVALUATION

- Determine frequency and intensity of anxiety symptoms at various stages of treatment
- Identify effective coping mechanisms deployed at times of stress
- Identify the incidence and frequency of avoidance or checking behaviors
- Identify the development of new maladaptive coping mechanisms; the client may experience stress at the loss of identity as a victim. Retelling of trauma can create a dopamine feedback system in which remain stuck in the familiar is easier than overcoming

▶ CULTURAL IMPLICATIONS

- Symptoms of PTSD exist in every culture; the distinction lies in how the symptoms are interpreted.
- Some subcultures prize rising above and overcoming and growing from trauma, while others may acknowledge the trauma as a scar that one must learn to live with. These subcultures are found in all ethnicities.
- Black, Hispanic, and Asian people are more likely to delay seeking professional help in comparison to Caucasians.

KNOWLEDGE CHECK: CHAPTER 10

1. A 25-year-old female presents to the emergency department, having just witnessed an accident. Her speech is pressured. She states, "There were a lot of people in need of care at the scene, and I should know because I have traveled to many Third World countries. I know how bad needs can get. The people were injured, and she was hit by a car before but did not suffer any injuries. There were a lot of police cars and ambulances." The patient was triaged to Psychiatry. Which of the following best describes the patient's thought process?

   A. Circumstantial
   B. Tangential
   C. Flight of ideas
   D. Loose associations

2. A 45-year-old man is reporting chest pressure, difficulty breathing, numbness, and tingling in his hands and lips. He has been seen in the emergency department, where he underwent a negative cardiac workup. He was subsequently triaged to Psychiatry for evaluation. The psychiatric-mental health nurse asks how he came to the hospital. He states, "I felt awful, my heart was pounding, I was sweating so much, I thought I was going to die. My father had a similar problem, but he died 10 years ago." Which of the following best describes the patient's thought process?

   A. Circumstantial
   B. Tangential
   C. Flight of ideas
   D. Loose associations

3. A 29-year-old man presents to the emergency department stating he is very anxious and feels his heart is going to beat out of his chest. He is diaphoretic, with pressured speech and unable to be calmed. A psychiatric consult was called because the patient seems uncooperative, and a proper history cannot be obtained. Which of the following conditions must be excluded first?

   A. Hypochondriasis
   B. Phobia
   C. Cocaine-induced mood disorder
   D. Panic attack

(See answers next page.)

1. A) Circumstantial

Circumstantial describes a speech pattern that is overly inclusive and includes a lot of unnecessary details and digressions but eventually reaches the point. Tangential describes a thought pattern that uses a lot of unnecessary details and digressions but never returns to the main point. Flight of ideas describes a thought pattern with erratic direction changes with an identifiable connection between thoughts. Loosening of association is characterized by an illogical connection between thoughts digressing in multiple directions, but sentence structure remains intact.

2. B) Tangential

Tangential describes a thought pattern that uses a lot of unnecessary details and digressions but never returns to the main point. Circumstantial describes a speech pattern that is overly inclusive and includes a lot of unnecessary details and digressions but eventually reaches the point. Flight of ideas describes a thought pattern with erratic direction changes with an identifiable connection between thoughts. Loosening of association is characterized by an illogical connection between thoughts digressing in multiple directions, but sentence structure remains intact.

3. C) Cocaine-induced mood disorder

Cocaine-induced mood disorder must be ruled out first as it can trigger myocardial infraction and would prohibit the use of beta-blockers in the management of vasospasm and anxiety due to the unopposed effects of the alpha blockade on the heart worsening ischemia. Phobia and hypochondriasis are not life-threatening conditions, and panic attacks spontaneously resolve within 20 minutes.

4. A 22-year-old medical student has had several episodes of impending doom over the last 4 months. The events last 10 to 20 minutes and are associated with tremors, sweating, dizziness, and being unable to concentrate. He is now perpetually worried that these attacks will happen when doing his clerkship. The psychiatrist in the student health center diagnoses him with panic disorder without agoraphobia. Which medications should the psychiatric-mental health nurse reinforce through psychopharmacology teaching?

   A. Klonopin
   B. Fluoxetine
   C. Chlordiazepoxide
   D. Lithium

5. An 18-year-old girl was visiting colleges with her family and was involved in a fatal car accident 2 weeks ago. Since that time, she continually has flashbacks, difficulty sleeping, persistent ruminations, and is afraid to drive. She has become apprehensive about her family members driving as well. Which of the following conditions most likely explains her symptoms?

   A. Posttraumatic stress disorder
   B. Generalized anxiety disorder
   C. Adjustment disorder
   D. Acute stress disorder

6. A 34-year-old woman comes to an appointment because she is bothered by disturbing and recurrent thoughts of harming her 7-month-old infant. She reports that her thoughts are distressing enough that she has removed all sharp objects from the kitchen so that she cannot stab her baby with a knife. She has not shared these thoughts with her husband for fear of how he may react to her. For which of the following conditions should the psychiatric-mental health nurse provide education?

   A. Obsessive compulsive disorder
   B. Generalized anxiety disorder
   C. Bipolar disorder with peripartum onset
   D. Acute stress disorder

(See answers next page.)

4. B) Fluoxetine

Fluoxetine, a selective serotonin reuptake inhibitor (SSRI), is the first-line psychopharmacological agent for panic disorders and anxiety disorders. Benzodiazepines like Klonopin, while useful in the short term, are highly addictive and lead to tolerance. Lithium is not indicated for panic or anxiety disorders.

5. D) Acute stress disorder

Acute stress disorder best describes her symptoms of intrusive memory, rumination, hypervigilance, apprehensiveness, and avoidance because the incident was less than 4 weeks ago. Posttraumatic stress disorder would have the same symptoms, but they must persist longer than 4 weeks. Generalized anxiety disorder is not associated with a specific traumatic event, and the symptoms must persist a majority of the time and include irritability lasting at least 6 months. Adjustment disorder is characterized by the development of mood and anxiety symptoms, not precipitated by a traumatic event.

6. A) Obsessive compulsive disorder

The client's recurrent thoughts are ego dystonic, and she is attempting to ignore and suppress them and does not discuss them with her husband. She tries to mitigate the risk by getting rid of all the knives. Bipolar disorder with peripartum onset usually occurs within 2 weeks of childbirth and has accompanying mood disorders, hallucinations, and delusions. It is often associated with severe insomnia, rapid mood changes, anxiety, irritability, and psychomotor agitation. Generalized anxiety disorder is not associated with a specific traumatic event, and the symptoms must persist a majority of the time and include irritability lasting at least 6 months. Acute stress disorder best describes her symptoms of intrusive memory, rumination, hypervigilance, apprehensiveness, and avoidance because the incident happened less than 4 weeks ago.

7. A 38-year-old Middle Eastern male veteran of Operation Iraqi Freedom is evaluated at the mental health clinic. He reports that he saw many of his battle buddies get killed in action. He has been stateside for 2 years, but since that time he has had trouble sleeping and as such he is very irritable to be around. He reports ongoing nightmares and flashbacks to an explosion, and he feels on edge most of the time. He avoids large crowds and loud noises. He finds that having a few beers helps calm him and makes him more pleasant to be around and allows him to socialize rather than isolate himself. For which of the following medications should the psychiatric-mental health nurse provide education?

   A. Risperdal
   B. Lorazepam
   C. Sertraline
   D. Imipramine

8. A 32-year-old man presents on referral from his primary care provider. He reports a 6-month history of recurrent bouts of anxiety associated with chest pain, tachycardia, tremors, nausea, diaphoresis, and an impending sense of doom. The episodes last approximately 20 minutes, and he is unable to identify a precipitating event. The patient has become increasingly isolated for fear of not wanting to have this sort of episode in public. The primary care provider started him on a selective serotonin reuptake inhibitor (SSRI) 6 months ago, but he continues to have the symptoms. Which adjunctive psychotherapy would be most appropriate for this patient?

   A. Eye movement desensitization and reprocessing (EMDR) therapy
   B. Interpersonal therapy
   C. Supportive psychotherapy
   D. Cognitive behavioral therapy

9. A 32-year-old male was referred from the urologist for erectile dysfunction. He has been prescribed a phosphodiesterase-5 inhibitor (PD5-I) with variable success despite a negative physiological workup. Which form of therapy is indicated for this sexual dysfunction?

   A. Cognitive behavioral therapy
   B. Interpersonal therapy
   C. Supportive psychotherapy
   D. Eye movement desensitization reprocessing (EMDR) therapy

(See answers next page.)

7. C) Sertraline
Sertraline and other selective serotonin reuptake inhibitors (SSRIs) are indicated for symptoms of posttraumatic stress disorder (PTSD) as indicated by his symptoms. The patient does not demonstrate any psychotic symptoms, so there is no need for antipsychotic medication given the risk of metabolic syndrome and limited efficacy for monotherapy and PTSD. Benzodiazepines are highly addictive and should be avoided in this population. Tricyclic antidepressants have a host of anticholinergic adverse effects and should be reserved for chronic pain conditions and failure of first and second-line therapies.

8. D) Cognitive behavioral therapy
Cognitive behavioral therapy is an evidence-based psychotherapeutic approach indicated for anxiety disorders and mood disorders. EMDR is specifically developed for the treatment of posttraumatic stress disorder (PTSD). Interpersonal therapy looks at the relationships contributing to depression. Supportive psychotherapy aims to strengthen the patient's defense mechanisms to restore function and is typically reserved for patients with more primitive coping mechanisms.

9. A) Cognitive behavioral therapy
Cognitive behavioral therapy is an evidence-based psychotherapeutic approach indicated for anxiety disorders and the primary treatment for sexual dysfunction. EMDR is specially developed for the treatment of posttraumatic stress disorder (PTSD). Interpersonal therapy looks at the relationships contributing to depression. Supportive psychotherapy aims to strengthen the patient's defense mechanisms to restore function and is typically reserved for patients with more primitive coping mechanisms.

10. A 29-year-old woman has been diagnosed with panic disorder and is requesting a psychiatric home visit because she continues to experience feelings that her environment is not real despite the fluoxetine she had been prescribed. She states that this is very unsettling and, as a result, has stopped going out of her home. Which of the following best describes the symptoms reported?

    A. Depersonalization
    B. Derealization
    C. Psychosis
    D. Depressive symptoms

11. A 34-year-old Korean male pediatric dentist is referred to Psychiatry for persistent anxiety. Upon further assessment, he reveals that his penis is shrinking into his abdomen. Despite the reassurance he has received from numerous health care providers in the past he remains convinced of this belief. This culture-bound delusion is known as:

    A. Zar
    B. Taijin kyofusho
    C. Koro
    D. Kuru

12. A 32-year-old White male was formerly employed as a corporate lawyer and has recently started his own business. He has started experiencing symptoms of intense anxiety when taking the subway to work. The symptoms include feeling short of breath, chest pressure, sweaty, irritability, and an impending sense of doom. Which of the following therapeutic modalities would be most helpful?

    A. Electroconvulsive therapy
    B. Ketamine infusion therapy
    C. Cognitive behavioral therapy
    D Dialectical behavioral therapy

13. A 30-year-old female is referred by her women's health nurse practitioner for vaginismus. The woman is distraught and embarrassed because she has not been able to consummate her marriage. Which therapeutic technique would be most helpful?

    A. Systematic desensitization
    B. Exposure therapy
    C. Distraction
    D. Group therapy

(See answers next page.)

10. B) Derealization
Derealization is common in anxiety disorders, and it is characterized by the sense of one's surroundings being strange or unfamiliar and not real. Depersonalization is the feeling that one's identity has been lost as if they are outside their own body. Psychosis is characterized by disordered thought patterns and gross disorganization accompanied by hallucinations or delusions. Depressive symptoms commonly include sleep disruption, anhedonia, apathy, guilt, fatigue, and hopelessness.

11. C) Koro
Koro is the delusion that the penis is shrinking into the abdomen, found in South and East Asian cultures. Zar is a culture-bound syndrome delusion of being spirit possessed, found in North and East African cultures and Middle Eastern cultures. Taijin kyofusho is a Japanese culture-bound syndrome in which one perceives their body to be offensive to others. Kuru is a neurodegenerative prion disease that leads to death, found in New Guinea and transmitted through the cannibalistic funeral ritual of eating the brains of the dead.

12. C) Cognitive behavioral therapy
Cognitive behavioral therapy is most effective in treating agoraphobia, specifically systematic desensitization. Electroconvulsive therapy is best for major depression with psychotic features. Ketamine is indicated for refractory depression. Dialectical behavioral therapy is used in borderline personality disorder to help reduce self-injurious behaviors.

13. A) Systemic desensitization
Systematic desensitization is a modality of cognitive behavioral therapy in which the patient controls the stressful impetus until a more muted response is produced. Exposure therapy prematurely provided may worsen and entrench the anxiety-provoking occurrence. Distraction can be included in systematic desensitization but is not a first-line treatment. Group therapy may be helpful eventually, but it is essential to build a therapeutic alliance before making a referral.

14. A 15-year-old boy has refused to go to school for the past month. Every morning he has a new symptom that necessitates his having to be picked up from school. When he is home, the symptoms disappear. On weekends the symptoms never present. Which of the following best explains the condition?

    A. Separation anxiety
    B. Social anxiety
    C. Agoraphobia
    D. Panic disorder

15. A patient tells the psychiatric-mental health nurse that her anxiety is quite high, and her mood is low. The patient states she is thinking about suicide. Which of the following is the best response?

    A. Let me review some relaxation techniques with you
    B. Call the physician to obtain as-needed anxiolytic medication
    C. Ask about the client's plan to commit suicide
    D. Encourage the client to attend group activities

(*See answers next page.*)

14. A) Separation anxiety

Separation anxiety is characterized by developmentally inappropriate, excessive apprehensiveness and worry related to separating from significant attachment figures or a source of comfort. Social anxiety is characterized by marked fear or anxiety about social situations in which the individual is exposed to possible scrutiny by others. There is not sufficient information in the presentation to suggest social anxiety to be this patient's diagnosis. Agoraphobia is characterized by the fear and avoidance of multiple situations due to thoughts that it may be difficult to escape should a panic attack occur. Panic disorder is a discrete episode of heightened arousal characterized by intense apprehension, fear, terror, or the impending sense of doom.

15. C) Ask about the client's plan to commit suicide

When a client endorses a suicidal ideation, the psychiatric-mental health nurse must assess the lethality of the situation by asking about intent, means, and protective factors. The other response does not take priority over the suicide assessment.

REFERENCES

American Psychiatric Association. Task Force on *DSM-5*. (2013). *Diagnostic and statistical manual of mental disorders* (5th ed.). Washington, DC: American Psychiatric Publishing.

Apergis-Schoute, A. M., Bijleveld, B., Gillan, C. M., Fineberg, N. A., Sahakian, B. J., & Robbins, T. W. (2018). Hyperconnectivity of the ventromedial prefrontal cortex in obsessive-compulsive disorder. *Brain and Neuroscience Advances, 2*, 239821281880871. doi:10.1177/2398212818808710

Bandelow, B., & Michaelis, S. (2015). Epidemiology of anxiety disorders in the 21st century. *Dialogues in Clinical Neuroscience, 17*(3), 327–335. Retrieved from http://www.ncbi.nlm.nih.gov/pubmed/26487813

Goldstein, M. A., & Harden, C. L. (2000). Epilepsy and anxiety. *Epilepsy & Behavior, 1*(4), 228–234. doi:10.1006/ EBEH.2000.0080

Grant, J. E., Chamberlain, S. R., Redden, S. A., Leppink, E. W., Odlaug, B. L., & Kim, S. W. (2016). *N* -Acetylcysteine in the treatment of excoriation disorder. *JAMA Psychiatry, 73*(5), 490. doi:10.1001/jamapsychiatry.2016.0060

Lavallee, K. L., & Schneider, S. (2019). Separation anxiety disorder. *Pediatric Anxiety Disorders, 1*, 151–176. doi:10.1016/ B978-0-12-813004-9.00008-6

Martin, E. I., Ressler, K. J., Binder, E., & Nemeroff, C. B. (2009).The neurobiology of anxiety disorders: Brain imaging, genetics, and psychoneuroendocrinology. *The Psychiatric Clinics of North America, 32*(3), 549–575. doi:10.1016/j. psc.2009.05.004

Phillips, K. A., & Castle, D. J. (2001). Body dysmorphic disorder in men. *BMJ (Clinical Research Ed.), 323*(7320), 1015–1016. doi:10.1136/bmj.323.7320.1015

Swart, S., Wildschut, M., Draijer, N., Langeland, W., & Smit, J. H. (2019). Dissociative subtype of posttraumatic stress disorder or PTSD with comorbid dissociative disorders: Comparative evaluation of clinical profiles. *Psychological Trauma: Theory, Research, Practice and Policy, 12*(1), 38–45. doi:10.1037/tra0000474

Wittmann, A., Schlagenhauf, F., Guhn, A., Lueken, U., Elle, M., Stoy, M., … Ströhle, A. (2018). Effects of cognitive behavioral therapy on neural processing of agoraphobia-specific stimuli in panic disorder and agoraphobia. *Psychotherapy and Psychosomatics, 87*(6), 350–365. doi:10.1159/000493146

Child/Adolescent and Developmental Disorders

> **OBJECTIVES**
> - Identify the ages and stages of normal growth and development
> - Identify red flags that prompt a focused assessment and signs of maltreatment
> - Review the common child and adolescent psychiatric disorders

FAST FACTS

- **Ages and stages:** It is important to consider antepartum and peripartum factors when evaluating the child for the achievement of normal growth and developmental milestones, particularly in the first 2 years of life (Table 11.1). Children who are born prematurely may demonstrate developmental incongruence with their chronological age in the course of their normal trajectory of growth and development. The neurodevelopment must be assessed according to the corrected or adjusted age rather than the chronological age (American Academy of Pediatrics, 2004).
- Adjusted age is used until the age of 24 months (another acceptable method is to multiply the number of weeks premature by a factor of 10 to provide the number of weeks necessary to correct for normal growth and development).

ATTENTION-DEFICIT HYPERACTIVITY DISORDER (ADHD)

Characterized by consistent symptoms of inattention in at least two domains (academic, social, occupational), and may or may not have hyperactivity and impulsivity that is inconsistent with the developmental age, and negatively impacts function, causing distress (Gelenberg et al., 2010; Kroenke et al., 2001; Polanczyk, Salum, Sugaya, Caye, & Rohde, 2015; Royal College of Psychiatrists, 2017; Strawn, Dobson, & Giles, 2017). It is sometimes comorbid with the following conditions, sharing symptoms but distinguished with characteristics discussed here:

- **Oppositional defiant disorder (ODD):** Characterized by resistance to work and school tasks because of resistance to authority, accompanied by hostility and defiance. In ADHD, the aversion to school or work is due to the difficulty in sustaining attention, forgetting instructions, and impulsivity.

Table 11.1 Growth and Development Milestones (0 to 12 Months)

Age	Child		Parent	
	Developmentally Appropriate	Cause for concern	Anticipatory Guidance	Cause for Concern
0–3 months	■ Reacts and turns toward sounds ■ Watches faces, follows objects ■ Coos and babbles ■ Develops social smile ■ Develops sleep–wake routine	■ Unable to move each limb independently ■ Difficulty tracking light or faces ■ Inconsolable crying for hours at a time	■ Do not be afraid to spoil your child (hold, cuddle, comfort) ■ Respond promptly to cries (comfort, feed, change, rocking) ■ Converse with baby as if there is mutual understanding	■ Parent is unsure when to feed or change or how to comfort baby ■ Becomes upset whenever baby cries ■ Allows for prolonged crying ■ Does not enjoy time with the baby or feels the baby does not fit in with the family
4–7 months	■ Babbles chains of sounds ■ Responds to other's emotions ■ Recognizes own hand, hand to mouth exploration ■ Sits with support initially, progresses to sitting without support	■ Unable to hold head up or rollover ■ Does not respond to other sounds or attention ■ Resists all efforts for comforting ■ Shows no interest in exploration ■ Strongly resists all routines of sleep and wake times	■ Give baby much attention, attune to baby's cues for hunger, fatigue, diaper change ■ Allow exploration through touch and taste with safe limits ■ Provide supervised time for crawling, sitting, and rolling	
8–12 months	■ Increased tonal variability in babbling ■ 2–3-word vocabulary ■ Dadda, Mamma with exclamation ■ Imitates sounds and gestures ■ Sensory exploration ■ Pulls self up to standing	■ No babbling or sounds of communication ■ Unable to self soothe ■ Does not respond to names or verbal requests ■ No interest in exploring ■ No reaction when caregiver leaves the room or returns		

Source: From Zakhari, R. (2015). Pregnancy and fetal development. *Sound Cloud.* Retrieved from https://soundcloud.com/raymond-zakhari/pregnancy-fetal-development.

- **Intermittent explosive disorder:** Characterized by high levels of impulsive behavior with episodes of serious aggression toward others (not commonly found in ADHD alone).
- **Conduct disorder:** Characterized by high levels of impulsivity with an associated pattern of antisocial behavior.
- **Disruptive mood dysregulation disorder (DMDD):** Characterized by persistently pervasive irritability and low frustration tolerance.
- **Medication-induced hyperactivity and inattention:** Bronchodilators, antipsychotics, steroids, and caffeine can cause symptoms of hyperactivity, impulsivity, and restlessness, which, when stopped, symptoms resolve.
  - **Etiology:** Unknown, but many theories regarding biopsychosocial factors are implicated, including structural brain abnormalities, neurotransmitter dysfunction, and abnormalities in the reticular activating system. Other factors may include learned behaviors and unrealistic, developmentally inappropriate expectations.

▶ CLINICAL VIGNETTE OF THE PROTOTYPICAL PATIENT

A 10-year-old boy is reported to spend much of his time in school daydreaming, often forgets his pencil, notebooks, and other school supplies; he also frequently loses gloves and jacket, makes careless errors in writing, easily gets distracted from the task at hand, has many unfinished projects and chores. There is increasing tension in the home as the father yells because the boy seems not to be listening to him. The child reports he finds it very difficult to get started on tasks, especially things he dislikes. The mother reports he can be very focused on something he is fascinated with and can give prolonged and sustained attention. The teacher reports a constant need to remind him to stop talking to his neighbor, stop fidgeting, staying in his seat, and stop calling out answers.

▶ INCIDENCE AND PREVALENCE

- **Demographics:**
  - 5% of U.S. children diagnosed with ADHD
  - More common in males than females
  - 60% of patients will persist with inattention symptoms into adulthood
- **History findings:**
  - Consistent inattentiveness
  - Carelessness
  - Seems not to be listening
  - Difficulty completing tasks
  - Disorganized schoolwork
  - Task avoidance
  - Distractibility
  - Blurting and interrupting
  - Fidgeting
  - General restlessness
  - Difficulty with leisure activities

▶ SCREENING TOOLS AND EARLY INTERVENTION

- Standardized assessments from multiple domains and self-report
  - Conner's Parent-Teacher Rating Scale
  - Barkley Home Situations Questionnaire
  - Wender Utah Rating Scale
  - Rule out adjustment disorder, primary mood disorder, anxiety disorder, posttraumatic stress disorder first
- Model appropriate behavior
- Teach language skills and identification of feelings
- Label objects
- Identify precipitants to common behavior problems: attention-seeking, feeling lonely, fearful, boredom, anger, dislike of a task and preempt the behavior
- Help the child learn distress tolerance and appropriate self-soothing behaviors

ASSESSMENT AND DIAGNOSIS

- Predominant inattentive type
- Predominant hyperactive-impulsive type
- Combined type

PLANNING

- Distinguish age-appropriate behavior from problem behavior
- Identify priority outcomes based on the maladaptive behavior giving priority to physiological and safety needs
- Help the child express their thoughts and feelings in a constructive manner
- Identify motivating factors to behavior change
- Encourage healthy habit formation
- Help children identify consequences of behaviors (both positive and negative)
- Help parents identify teachable moments and attune to the child's emotional state to intervene before behavioral escalations
- Teach parents and children to distract from impulses that violate their values

INTERVENTION

- **Pharmacological:** Primarily stimulants followed by selective norepinephrine reuptake inhibitors and alpha agonists.
  - **Methylphenidate (Ritalin, Metadate, Concerta):** Mixed inattention/hyperactivity
    - Dextromethamphetamine (Dexedrine)
    - Amphetamine (Adderall)
    - Dexmethylphenidate (Focalin)
    - Lisdexamfetamine (Vyvanse)

- **Serotonin–norepinephrine reuptake inhibitor (SNRI)/dopamine reuptake inhibitor:** Attention
  - Atomoxetine (Strattera)
  - Bupropion (Wellbutrin)
- **Alpha-blockers:** Hyperactivity and impulsivity
  - Guanfacine (Intuniv)
  - Clonidine (Catapres)
- **Monitor for adverse effects and side effects**
  - Anorexia
  - Weight loss
  - Gastrointestinal (GI) upset
  - Headache
  - Irritability
  - Psychosis
  - Hypertension/hypotension
  - Electrocardiogram (EKG)
  - Growth suppression
- **Nonpharmacological:** Environmental restructuring (including behavioral classroom management), and behavioral therapy including behavioral parent training (BPT), and social skills training.
  - Psychoeducation
  - Treatment of learning disorders
  - Family therapy
  - Supportive care and anticipatory guidance for parents regarding:
    - Stress management
    - Self-blame
    - Social isolation
    - Embarrassment
    - Depressive reaction
    - Marital discord
    - Substance use disorders
    - Risk-taking behaviors

EVALUATION

- Identify outcomes that show behavior modifications have been adopted
- Identify mastery of psychosocial task development
- Family and teacher reports of improved school behavior and reduced symptoms on objective screening tests

CULTURAL IMPLICATIONS

- Norms vary and can be inappropriately pathologized
- Hispanic cultures may organize activities in a circular fashion where many things are worked on at the same time

- European cultures organize in a linear fashion, applying a stepwise approach and working on one thing at a time
- Families of different cultures will react in disparate ways to a diagnosis or treatment for a condition and may prefer more culturally familiar solutions to their pressing problems
- Distinguishing a lack of cultural assimilation from a pathology is crucial in order to provide appropriate care

AUTISM SPECTRUM DISORDER (ASD)

Primarily characterized by persistent social interaction deficits across multiple contexts with associated restricted range of interests, repetitive patterns of behavior (Hagberg, Aicardi, Dias, & Ramos, 1983; Neul et al., 2010; Percy, 2011; Stahmer & Aarons, 2009).

▶ CLINICAL VIGNETTE OF THE PROTOTYPICAL PATIENT

A 7-year-old boy who had delayed speech, very low distress tolerance, avoids eye contact, with repetitive self-soothing behaviors rocking, hyper-focused on a few things, does not engage with his peers, becomes explosive when there is a deviation from the daily routine.

▶ INCIDENCE AND PREVALENCE

- **Demographics**
  - Male to female ratio 4:1, with concordant rate for identical twins (60%), affecting 1 in 59 children, onset of symptoms by age 3

▶ SCREENING TOOLS AND EARLY INTERVENTION

- **Key indicators**
  - Impaired social interactions, communication, peer relationships
  - Impaired emotional reciprocity or spontaneous pleasure seeking
  - Delayed communication with impaired ability to initiate and sustain conversations, repetitive stereotyped use of language, inability for interactive play
  - No cooing by age 1, no single words by 16 months, no two-word phrases by 24 months
  - No imaginary play
  - Little interest in other children
  - Extremely short attention span
  - No response when called by name
  - Poor eye contact
  - Intense tantrums

- Single object fixations
- Unusually strong resistance to change routines
- Overly sensitive to certain sounds, textures, smells
- Nonsuicidal self-injurious behavior

ASSESSMENT AND DIAGNOSIS

- ASD is like the following conditions but distinguished in the following manner:
  - **Rett syndrome:** Includes disruptions beyond social interactions during the regressive phases and is characterized by impaired physical growth, loss of hand movements, and poor coordination
  - **Childhood-onset schizophrenia:** Develops after a period of normal growth and development with the prodromal phase, including social impairment, atypical interests, and delusional beliefs that often have accompanying perceptual disturbance (auditory hallucinations), which are not characteristic of ASD
  - **Selective mutism:** Characterized by normal early developmental behavior and generally appropriate social communication and function in contexts perceived as safe (at home, with family members)
  - **Intellectual disability:** Characterized by a general impairment in intellectual function and social adaptability, but incongruent with developmental stage

PLANNING

- Distinguish age-appropriate behavior from problem behavior, and allow for skill acquisition on a more expansive timeline
- Identify priority outcomes based on the maladaptive behavior giving priority to physiological and safety needs
- Help the child express their thoughts and feelings in a constructive manner
- Identify motivating factors to behavior change that are developmentally appropriate
- Encourage healthy habit formation in both parents and child
- Help children identify consequences of behaviors (both positive and negative)
- Help parents identify teachable moments and attune to the child's emotional state to intervene before behavioral escalations
- Teach parents and children to distract from impulses that violate their values

INTERVENTION

- Environmental restructuring (including behavioral classroom management) and behavioral therapy, including behavioral parent training (BPT), social skills training, and ABA therapy
  - Psychoeducation
  - Treatment of learning disorders
  - Family therapy
  - Supportive care and anticipatory guidance for parents and children regarding:

- Stress management
- Self-blame
- Child blaming
- Social isolation
- Embarrassment
- Depressive reaction
- Marital discord
- Substance use disorders
- Risk-taking behaviors

EVALUATION

- Identify outcomes that show behavior modifications have been adopted
- Identify mastery of psychosocial task development, and lower frustration levels in the child and family
- Family and teacher reports of improved school behavior and reduced symptoms on objective screening tests

▶ CULTURAL IMPLICATIONS

- The word "autism" does not exist in many cultures and is difficult to classify, and some cultures have long descriptions that do not fit exactly with standardized assessments.
- Cultural factors include myths about disabilities that may deter help-seeking behavior.
- Societal gender roles may also delay diagnosis, as girls may be expected to be more reserved, shy, and withdrawn, and boys may be expected to be energetic and outgoing.
- Many myths may abound in various subcultures or may develop within the family as a means of understanding their circumstances.
  - A 3-year-old girl who does not relate well to her peers but is considered mature because she relates better with adults.
  - A 4-year-old boy who has not yet spoken and the family is not concerned because Indian boys tend to have speech delays.
  - A 5-year-old who keeps to herself and is quiet much of the time is thought to be an angel because she is no trouble at all.
- Symptom descriptions, interpretations, and acceptance can vary widely among cultures.
- Direct eye contact in some Asian cultures, from children to authority figures, may be a sign of disrespect, yet this is a key diagnostic criterion in autism.

CONDUCT DISORDERS

Characterized by a repetitive and persistent pattern of disregard for social norms, rules, and the basic rights of others (Connolly & Beaver, 2016). In adults, this is called antisocial personality disorder.

- **Etiology:** More common in children of parents with antisocial personality disorder and families with dysfunctional interpersonal patterns of relating.

▶ CLINICAL VIGNETTE OF THE PROTOTYPICAL PATIENT

Johnny is a 12-year-old boy who has been increasingly irritable in the past year, with explosive rage episodes, antagonistic and argumentative behavior with most authority figures, and spiteful and unforgiving behavior toward peers whom he has perceived have wronged him. The mother is at her wit's end because she feels alone in her plight as her husband has increasingly spent more and more time at work.

▶ INCIDENCE AND PREVALENCE

- **Demographics**
  - More common in boys than girls, affects up to 10% of the general U.S. population. Onset of symptoms:
    - Boys age 10 to 12
    - Girls age 16

▶ SCREENING TOOLS AND EARLY INTERVENTION

- Most common in families in which a primary relative has a substance use disorder or primary mood disorder
- More common in families with interpersonal chaos and single-parent homes
- Homes lacking parental supervision
- Blended families due to inconsistent discipline practices and insecurity regarding future abandonment
- Exposure to domestic and community violence

ASSESSMENT AND DIAGNOSIS

- **Assessment/diagnostic indicators:** Requires three or more signs in the past year, with one sign in the previous 6 months, and one criterion met before age 10 and associated with significant impairment in social or academic function:
  - Aggression toward people and animals
  - Destruction of property
  - Deceitfulness or theft
  - Serious violation of rules

- Conduct disorder is like the following conditions but distinguished in the following manner:
  - **ODD:** Characterized by less-severe disruptive behaviors and does not include aggression toward people or animals, no willful destruction of property, and no pattern of deceit or theft. ODD is also associated with emotional dysregulation
  - **ADHD:** Behavioral problems do not violate social norms or the rights of others
  - **Mood disorder:** Bipolar and major depression behavioral disruptions are caused by the presence of mood symptoms (irritability, aggression) in concert with the behavioral dysregulation. In the absence of mood symptoms, behavior does not violate social norms or the rights of others
  - **Intermittent explosive disorder:** Symptoms are limited to impulsive aggression rather than premeditated, and the intent was not to achieve a tangible objective
  - **Antisocial behavior in psychosis:** Aggressive behaviors are only in response to perceptual disturbances and delusions
  - **Adjustment disorder with disturbed conduct:** Characterized by a time-limited conduct problem that is in response to a psychosocial stressor rather than a long-standing problem. Careful history is needed to distinguish from children with long-standing and numerous psychosocial stressors leading to habituation
- **Mental status exam**
  - Affect
    - Irritability, anger, uncooperative
  - Mood
    - Anger, anxious, impervious
  - Thought content
    - Without empathy or regard for social norms, and rights of others
    - Tangential and circumstantial
  - Cognition
    - Distractible
  - Insight and judgment
    - Poor
- May be diagnosed in patients over age 18 if not meeting full criteria for antisocial personality disorder

PLANNING

- Distinguish age-appropriate behavior from problem behavior and allow for skill acquisition on a more expansive timeline
- Identify priority outcomes based on the maladaptive behavior giving priority to physiological and safety needs
- Help the child express their thoughts and feelings in a constructive manner
- Identify motivating factors to behavior change that are developmentally appropriate
- Encourage healthy habit formation in both parents and child
- Help children identify consequences of behaviors (both positive and negative)
- Help parents identify teachable moments and attune to the child's emotional state to intervene before behavioral escalations
- Teach parents and children to distract from impulses that violate their values

INTERVENTION

- **Treatment**
  - Primarily behavioral modification, cognitive restructuring, and pharmacology to treat comorbid mood disorder
  - Anticipate and address underlying triggers for expressed behaviors
    - Anxiety, fear, loss of control, physical or emotional pain leading to rage, escapism, noncompliance, nagging, school refusal, yelling, aggression, and bullying

EVALUATION

- Identify outcomes that show behavior modifications have been adopted
- Identify mastery of psychosocial task development
- Family and teacher reports of improved school behavior and reduced symptoms on objective screening tests

CULTURAL IMPLICATIONS

- Asian cultures have far less tolerance for behavioral dysregulation that does not conform to societal norms, specifically suppression of aggression.
- Latino cultures in which close familial attachments strict familial monitoring of children tend to have fewer reports of oppositional behavior.
- Cultures in which family honor and unity are prized over individuality as a means of survival have report fewer conduct disorders and oppositional behavior.

EATING DISORDERS

Characterized by a disordered eating pattern combined with a persistent preoccupation of a distorted self-perception relating to body shape and size (Chen et al., 2010). Patients may fluctuate between types of eating disorders and engage in many weight gain prevention and weight loss promotion behaviors, including:

- Self-induced vomiting
- Laxatives
- Diuretics
- Stimulants
- Fasting
- Excessive exercise

▶ CLINICAL VIGNETTE OF THE PROTOTYPICAL PATIENT

A 16-year-old girl is described as anxiously disposed and melancholic with persistent irritability and severe food rituals that include restricting behaviors, very focused on specific nutrients to the exclusion of others. She takes 2 hours to finish eating a very small amount of food. She wears oversized clothing, with sleeves pulled over her hands.

▶ INCIDENCE AND PREVALENCE

- Epidemiology:
  - Most prevalent in industrialized societies
  - 1% of the U.S. population has some form of an eating disorder
  - More common in females than males (10:1)
    - Males may suffer from body dysmorphia (bigorexia) in which they do not perceive their muscles big enough or may engage in avoidant/restrictive eating behaviors for specific athletic endeavors.
  - Age of onset is early to late adolescence (14–18 years)
  - 50% to 70% improve in the second decade of life
  - More common in dancers, gymnasts, male wrestlers, models, and so on

▶ SCREENING TOOLS AND EARLY INTERVENTION

- **Anorexia nervosa:** Manifests as a restriction of caloric intake relative to requirements, leading to a significantly lower than expected body mass index (BMI); associated with an intense fear of gaining weight, and a delusion in the way in which one's body weight or shape is experienced. Diagnostic criteria include (FADE):
  - Fear of gaining weight or becoming fat
  - Amenorrhea
  - Delusion related to body weight
  - Expected body weight (failure to maintain at least 85%)
- **Bulimia nervosa:** Characterized by recurrent episodes of binge eating accompanied by inappropriate compensatory behaviors of elimination (emesis and enemas) to prevent weight gain. Diagnostic criteria include (BASTE):
  - Binge eating
  - Anorexia nervosa excluded
  - Self-worth based on weight
  - Twice weekly for 3 months purging
  - Excessive exercise, emesis, enemas
- **Binge eating disorder:** Characterized by recurrent episodes of binge eating associated with significant distress without compensatory measures to prevent weight gain or enhance weight loss despite overvaluation of body weight and shape (Gelenberg et al., 2010; Kroenke, Spitzer, & Williams, 2001; Royal College of Psychiatrists, 2017). Sufferers often have comorbid obesity

ASSESSMENT AND DIAGNOSIS

- **Physical exam and diagnostic findings**
  - Anorexia
    - Low body weight (<85% of expected)
    - Autonomic instability (e.g., tachycardia, bradycardia, hypotension, hypothermia)
    - Prolonged QTc

- Xerosis, brittle hair, and nails
- Lanugo
- Elevated amylase
- Pancytopenia
- Metabolic acidosis
- Anion gap
- Bulimia
  - Weighing in 90% of expected body weight
  - Eroded dental enamel
  - Russell's sign (scarred calluses on the dorsum of fingers due to induced vomiting)
  - Hypertrophic salivary glands (chipmunk cheeks)
  - Rectal prolapse
  - Autonomic instability (tachycardia, bradycardia, hypotension, hypothermia)
  - Prolonged QTc
  - Pancytopenia
  - Metabolic acidosis
  - Anion gap
  - Hypokalemia, hyponatremia/hypernatremia if dehydration is paramount
- Binge eating disorder
  - BMI >30
  - Elevated liver enzymes
  - Dyslipidemia
  - Impaired glucose tolerance
- **Mental status exam:** Varies depending on severity of symptoms
  - Affect
    - Constricted, fixed to labile
  - Mood
    - Dysphoric
  - Thought content
    - Low self-worth
    - Weight and size
    - Food rituals and avoidance
    - Suicidal ideations
  - Concentration
    - Impaired and inattentive
  - Insight and judgment
    - Poor

PLANNING

- Depending on the severity of the physiological symptoms with respect to hemodynamic stability, the patient may need acute hospitalization
- Assessing readiness for discharge from acute care
- **Identifying physiological criteria**: weight gain, electrolyte stability, fluid volume balance, normal elimination, resting heart rate, and orthostatic vital signs

INTERVENTION

- **Treatment**
  - Pharmacology is only adjunctive to psychotherapy with the primary goal of hemodynamic stability and weight restoration in the short term, and cognitive restructuring in the long term
    - Fluoxetine is approved by the U.S. Food and Drug Administration (FDA) for bulimia nervosa
    - Psychopharmacology is targeted at symptoms associated with comorbid mood disorder, anxiety disorder, or psychotic disorder
    - Nutritional counseling, be mindful of refeeding syndrome when starting consistent nutritional support
    - Vitamin supplementation
    - Correct electrolyte abnormalities
    - Dental care
    - Individual psychotherapy, cognitive behavioral therapy
    - Family therapy
    - **Group therapy:** If decline in physiological parameters is noted, consider stopping group therapy and other eating disorder support groups, as patients may be listening for ways to be more subtle in their maladaptive behavior

EVALUATION

- Assess if physiologic stability has been achieved
- Identify anxiety reduction strategies
- Identify outcomes that show behavior modifications have been adopted
- Identify mastery of psychosocial task development

CULTURAL IMPLICATIONS

- Primarily a phenomenon in industrialized countries that prize high achievement, which is often linked to the thin body image
- Often patients with anorexia or bulimia may seek social support outside the home identifying with the pro-ana (pro-anorexia) or pro-mia (pro-bulimia) subculture connected online through websites, discussion boards, and chat rooms

KNOWLEDGE CHECK: CHAPTER 11

1. A 16-year-old male is being evaluated in a partial hospital program for adolescents for major depressive disorder. In addressing safety planning with the boy and his parents, they raised the question of possible suicidality with the use of selective serotonin reuptake inhibitors (SSRIs). What question should the psychiatric-mental health nurse ask regarding the most common means of suicide and adolescence?

   A. Does the home contain ligature risks?
   B. Is the medicine cabinet locked?
   C. Are there firearms in the home?
   D. Can all the knives be secured?

2. A 16-year-old girl with no past medical history was referred by her primary care provider, who saw her for a sports physical, because she said she was depressed. During the interview, the girl revealed that she has been feeling tired, sad, is crying easily, and has difficulty falling asleep. She reports that she has also been eating a lot more, and to keep from gaining weight she has been taking laxatives and on occasions makes herself vomit. She has dropped out of the yearbook committee, and she is not sure she wants to go to college anymore. Which nonpharmacological intervention is most appropriate?

   A. Group therapy
   B. Psychoanalysis
   C. Family therapy
   D. Cognitive behavioral therapy

3. A 17-year-old girl with major depressive disorder (single episode) and bulimia nervosa is unable to actively participate in psychotherapy because she says she feels too sleepy during the day as she is unable to sleep at night. In addition, she is inattentive, irritable, finds it difficult to concentrate, and has no desire to do anything. She wants to know if there is any medication that can help her. Which pharmacological agent is preferred for monotherapy?

   A. Atypical antipsychotic
   B. Selective serotonin reuptake inhibitor
   C. Tricyclic antidepressant
   D. Mood stabilizer

(See answers next page.)

1. C) Are there firearms in the home?

The most common means of committing suicide are by firearms. Drug overdose is the most common method of attempted suicide. Hanging, cutting, and stabbing are not as common methods of suicide.

2. D) Cognitive behavioral therapy

Cognitive behavioral therapy is the preferred psychotherapeutic intervention for major depressive disorder and bulimia nervosa. Group therapy, psychoanalysis, and family therapy may also be effective long term, but the evidence supports cognitive behavioral therapy above these other modalities.

3. B) Selective serotonin reuptake inhibitor

Selective serotonin reuptake inhibitors (SSRIs) are the first-line agent for major depressive disorder in children and adolescents and are very difficult to overdose. Tricyclic antidepressants (TCAs) are associated with numerous adverse effects and are much easier to overdose. Stabilizers are primarily used for bipolar disorder and only as augmentation for major depression. Antipsychotics are associated with weight gain and are not indicated for major depression in children or adolescents.

4. A mother 4 months' postpartum is referred to infant psychiatry as the baby has failed to gain weight over the last 2 months. He has dropped from the 75th percentile to the 50th percentile. The mother states that up until 8 weeks of age he was gaining weight and growing just fine. The baby is generally happy and continues to meet his developmental milestones. Of note, the mother has returned to work after her postpartum leave 2 months ago, and the baby is in daycare 5 days a week. The mother notes that he has been increasingly spitting up for the last month soon after receiving breast milk via the bottle. She has also started to supplement with formula out of concern for his poor weight gain. Which of the following disorders is this clinical description most consistent?

   A. Bulimia nervosa
   B. Pica
   C. Rumination disorder
   D. Anorexia

5. A 10-year-old boy is referred by the school nurse because of persistent stomachache every morning in school. On evaluating the boy, it is learned that he does not like to go to school and insists on coming home immediately and sleeps in his parent's bed at night. His clinical description is most characteristic of which of the following conditions?

   A. Social phobia
   B. Separation anxiety
   C. Reactive attachment disorder
   D. Posttraumatic stress disorder (PTSD)

6. A 4-year-old boy is brought to the pediatric emergency department kicking and screaming while trying to run away from the sharks he fears are going to eat him. Which of the following diagnostic tests would be most appropriate?

   A. Complete blood count
   B. Comprehensive metabolic profile
   C. Urine toxicology
   D. Electrocardiogram (EKG)

7. The psychiatric-mental health nurse is offering primary prevention services in the area high schools regarding mental illness. The most common psychiatric emergency in children and adolescents is:

   A. Sexually inappropriate behavior
   B. Homicidal behavior
   C. Suicidal behavior
   D. Psychotic behavior

(See answers next page.)

4. C) Rumination disorder

Rumination disorder is a feeding disorder of infancy and early childhood characterized by regurgitation shortly after eating without swallowing the spit-up food, lasting at least 1 month following a period of normal function. Rumination disorder is common in infants who have a variety of caretakers or are maintained in an unstable environment. There is no indication of deliberate food avoidance consistent with anorexia nervosa; the infant does not have episodes of binge eating followed by purging and is not self-inducing vomiting or afraid of becoming fat. There is no report of eating nonnutritive substances, elevated lead level, or anemia.

5. B) Separation anxiety

Separation anxiety best describes this clinical presentation characterized by developmentally inappropriate and excessively anxious disposition regarding separation from the home or other sources of comfort. Social phobia would require persistent fear of social or performance situations in which exposure triggers near-panic attacks or temper tantrums. PTSD would require hypervigilance and avoidance behaviors at least 4 weeks after a trauma. Reactive attachment disorder requires severely disturbed social relationships, in most contexts beginning before 5 years of age.

6. C) Urine toxicology

Urine toxicology is the most appropriate diagnostic test; it is a substance-induced psychotic disorder and is the most common etiology for florid visual hallucinations in children. It is essential to rule out potential ingestion of prescription drugs, illicit drugs, over-the-counter medications, or other household agents. A complete blood count, a comprehensive metabolic profile, and an EKG may be helpful in providing supportive care.

7. C) Suicidal behavior

Suicidal behavior is the most common psychiatric emergency in the child adolescent population. Psychotic behavior, homicidal behavior, and sexually inappropriate behavior are far less common.

8. A 10-year-old boy who had been prescribed fluoxetine for major depressive disorder presents to the psychiatric emergency department (ED) for running into the street in front of a car on the way home from school. In the ED, he has been selectively mute, but the nurse practitioner student was able to elicit his desire to be dead. He has been medically cleared pending a psychiatric evaluation. What is the most common sign of major depressive disorder in children?

   A. Weight change
   B. Hypersomnia
   C. Psychomotor agitation
   D. Hopelessness

9. A 16-year-old boy with a history of substance use disorder reports fatigue, apathy, and anhedonia almost every day, and his mother reports increasing irritability and raging behavior. The boy says he smokes marijuana daily just to feel good and is unwilling to give it up. The mother wants some sort of medication to help him feel better so that he stops smoking marijuana. The psychiatric-mental health advanced practice nurse (PMH-NP) agrees to prescribe fluoxetine 20 mg daily. What psychoeducation should the psychiatric-mental health nurse reinforce as the most common side effect associated with this medication?

   A. Hypotension
   B. Nausea
   C. Weight gain
   D. Sedation

10. Child Protective Services is requested for an evaluation of a 9-month-old girl in foster care whose mother was on a methadone maintenance program and using cocaine while pregnant. The child is HIV negative and during the assessment the psychiatric-mental health nurse learns of a 3-year-old brother who is HIV positive. The psychiatric-mental health nurse is asked to recommend placement for both of these children. Which of the following is the best recommendation?

    A. A hospital
    B. A group home
    C. A nursing home
    D. A foster home

11. An 8-year-old boy is referred to you for evaluation for disruptive behavior in school. The teachers report that without warning the boy will make disruptive sounds or shout out in class. Other than these instances, the boy is described as polite and well kempt but restless. Which of the following interventions should be recommended?

    A. Referral to behavior management classroom for oppositional defiant disorder
    B. Parental education regarding conduct disorder
    C. Referral to pediatrician for suspicion of Tourette's syndrome
    D. Psychoeducation for the teacher regarding separation anxiety disorder

(See answers next page.)

8. C) Psychomotor agitation
Psychomotor agitation is more commonly observed in children than adolescents with major depressive disorder. They may also appear more anxious, irritable, dysphoric, and selectively mute, with a flat affect. Hypersomnia, changes in weight, and hopelessness are more common in adolescents with major depressive disorder.

9. B) Nausea
The most common adverse effect associated with selective serotonin reuptake inhibitors (SSRIs) is nausea. Other adverse effects include insomnia, agitation, and headache. Weight gain and sedation are not associated with SSRIs in children.

10. D) A foster home
A foster home is the optimal place for young children, especially those with HIV, so that they may benefit from psychological belonging and adequate individual emotional support rather than in a group setting. The risk of opportunistic and nosocomial infection is greater in group homes, nursing homes, and hospitals.

11. C) Referral to pediatrician for suspicion of Tourette's syndrome
Referral to pediatrician for suspicion of Tourette's syndrome is the most likely diagnosis as the outbursts are consistent with vocal tics and motor tics are often incorrectly identified as restless behavior. He does not meet the criteria for oppositional defiant disorder or conduct disorder, as he is described as polite and well kempt without hostility, destructive tendencies, or angry behaviors. There are no signs or symptoms consistent with anxious behaviors in the setting of separation from a comforting figure or object.

12. An 8-year-old boy diagnosed with leukemia is referred to child psychiatry because he is consistently displaying a flat affect, irritability, angry acting out, and occasional physical aggression toward his 6-year-old brother. What approach should the psychiatric-mental health nurse take when interviewing this child?

    A. Ask the child direct questions about how he feels about his disease
    B. Provide toys and allow the child to play
    C. Encourage the child to talk about whatever is on his mind
    D. Sit quietly and allow the child to talk

13. The psychiatric-mental health nurse is evaluating a 22-month-old girl whose mother is concerned about aggressive behavior toward her 4-month-old brother. The mother states that her daughter is often angry and irritable with directed hostility toward the baby. Which of the following responses is best?

    A. You should ignore your daughter's behavior, and it will pass
    B. Your daughter's behavior is normal for her age
    C. Each day, schedule some time for you and your daughter to spend together without the baby
    D. Explain to your daughter that the baby needs more attention than she does right now

14. Which of the following developmental milestones should a 2-year-old child be able to accomplish?

    A. Ride a tricycle
    B. Copy a circle
    C. Identify age and gender
    D. Copy a square

15. A 12-year-old child is seen for follow up after starting on a stimulant for attention-deficit hyperactivity disorder. Which of the following parameters should the psychiatric-mental health nurse assess?

    A. Fingerstick glucose
    B. Height and weight
    C. Waist circumference
    D. Attentiveness

(See answers next page.)

12. B) Provide toys and allow the child to play
A play interview in which the child is provided with toys and allowed to play is an effective and efficient way to interview children. Even with encouragement and direct questions, children are unlikely to produce sufficient spontaneous dialogue in an uncomfortable setting with a stranger. It is unlikely that the child will spontaneously express his thoughts and feelings to a stranger who sits by quietly.

13. C) Each day, schedule some time for you and your daughter to spend together without the baby
Each day schedule alone time with the daughter without the baby as she may be feeling rejected, jealous, or angry. She needs to know that she is still loved and wanted. Ignoring the behavior may cause it to escalate or entrench the message that her needs are not important. Although it is normal behavior, it must be addressed.

14. B) Copy a circle
Copying a circle is developmentally appropriate for a 24-month-old child. At 3 years, they can identify age and gender, and ride a tricycle. At 5 years, they can draw a square.

15. B) Height and weight
Height and weight should be tracked, as stimulants are known to be appetite suppressing; improper nutrition can impair growth and proper physiological function. Stimulants are not known to cause diabetes or metabolic syndrome or weight gain. Attentiveness would indicate how effective the medication is helping with symptoms, but the physiological needs take priority over psychological needs.

REFERENCES

American Academy of Pediatrics. (2004). Policy statement: Age terminology during the perinatal period. *Pediatrics, 11*, 1362–1364. doi:10.1542/peds.2004–1915

Chen, L. P., Murad, M. H., Paras, M. L., Colbenson, K. M., Sattler, A. L., Goranson, E. N., ... Zirakzadeh, A. (2010). Sexual abuse and lifetime diagnosis of psychiatric disorders: Systematic review and meta-analysis. *Mayo Clinic Proceedings, 85*(7), 618–629. doi:10.4065/mcp.2009.0583

Connolly, E. J., & Beaver, K. M. (2016). Considering the genetic and environmental overlap between bullying victimization, delinquency, and symptoms of depression/anxiety. *Journal of Interpersonal Violence, 31*(7), 1230–1256. doi:10.1177/0886260514564158

Correll, C. U., Kratochvil, C. J., & March, J. S. (2011). Developments in pediatric psychopharmacology. *The Journal of Clinical Psychiatry, 72*(05), 655–670. doi:10.4088/JCP.11r07064

Costello, E. J., He, J., Sampson, N. A., Kessler, R. C., & Merikangas, K. R. (2014). Services for adolescents with psychiatric disorders: 12-month data from the national comorbidity survey–adolescent. *Psychiatric Services, 65*(3), 359–366. doi:10.1176/appi.ps.201100518

Gelenberg, A. J., Marlene Freeman, C. P., Markowitz, J. C., Rosenbaum, J. F., Thase, M. E., Trivedi, M. H., ... Silbersweig, D. A. (2010). *Practice guideline for the treatment of patients with major depressive disorder, third edition: Work group on major depressive disorder*. Retrieved from https://psychiatryonline.org/pb/assets/raw/sitewide/practice_guidelines/guidelines/mdd.pdf

Hagberg, B., Aicardi, J., Dias, K., & Ramos, O. (1983). A progressive syndrome of autism, dementia, ataxia, and loss of purposeful hand use in girls: Rett's syndrome: Report of 35 cases. *Annals of Neurology, 14*, 471–479. doi:10.1002/ana.410140412

Kroenke, K., Spitzer, R. L., & Williams, J. B. (2001). The PHQ-9: Validity of a brief depression severity measure. *Journal of General Internal Medicine, 16*(9), 606–613. doi:10.1046/J.1525-1497.2001.016009606.X

Lempp, T., de Lange, D., Radeloff, D., & Bachmann, C. (2012). The clinical examination of children, adolescents and their families. In J. M. Rey (Ed.), *IACAPAP e-textbook of child and adolescent mental health*. Geneva, Switzerland: International Association for Child and Adolescent Psychiatry and Allied Professions. Retrieved from https://pdfs.semanticscholar.org/5cf3/c42fff0caec7a8b88fdb57f867f8ea590cec.pdf

Neul, J. L., Kaufmann, W. E., Glaze, D. G., Christodoulou, J., Clarke, A. J., Bahi-Buisson, N., ... Percy, A. K. (2010). Rett syndrome: Revised diagnostic criteria and nomenclature. *Annals of Neurology, 68*, 944–950. doi:10.1002/ana.22124

Percy, A. K. (2011). Rett syndrome: Exploring the autism link. *Archives of Neurology, 68*, 985–989. doi:10.1001/archneurol.2011.149

Polanczyk, G. V., Salum, G. A., Sugaya, L. S., Caye, A., & Rohde, L. A. (2015). Annual research review: A meta-analysis of the worldwide prevalence of mental disorders in children and adolescents. *Journal of Child Psychology and Psychiatry, 56*(3), 345–365. doi:10.1111/jcpp.12381

Royal College of Psychiatrists. (2017). *The management of diabetes in adults and children with psychiatric disorders in inpatient settings* (May). Retrieved from https://www.diabetes.org.uk/resources-s3/2017-10/Management%20of%20 diabetes%20 in%20adults%20and%20children%20with%20psychiatric%20disorders%20in%20 inpatient%20settingsAugust-2017.pdf

Stahmer, A., & Aarons, G. (2009). Attitudes toward adoption of evidence-based practices: A comparison of autism early intervention providers and children's mental health providers. *Psychological Services, 6*(3), 223–234. Retrieved from http://psycnet.apa.org/journals/ser/6/3/223/

Strawn, J. R., Dobson, E. T., & Giles, L. L. (2017). Primary pediatric care psychopharmacology: Focus on medications for ADHD, depression, and anxiety. *Current Problems in Pediatric and Adolescent Health Care, 47*(1), 3–14. doi:10.1016/j.cppeds.2016.11.008

Zakhari, R. (2015). Pregnancy and fetal development. *Sound Cloud*. Retrieved from https://soundcloud.com/raymond-zakhari/pregnancy-fetal-development

Personality Disorders

OBJECTIVES
- Identify personality disorders associated with the three clusters of categories
- Describe the etiology of personality disorders
- Compare and contrast the key features of personality clusters
- Identify nonpharmacological evidence-based treatments for personality disorders

FAST FACTS

- Diagnosis of personality disorder is rarely made in a single visit regardless of how obvious the symptomatology and should be reserved in children <18 years old.
  - The exception to diagnosing a personality disorder is in patients suspected of having antisocial personality disorder, in which case the criteria for oppositional defiant disorder should be considered until the age of majority.
  - Early indicators of dependent personality disorder include physical illness (chronic or episodic) associated with separation anxiety.
  - Personality disorders are chronic in nature, difficult to change, and require a high degree of consistency in approach, preferably from the same therapist over the course of 5 to 10 years.
    - Borderline personality disorder is among the most treatable.
    - Narcissistic personality disorder is among the most difficult to treat, and some sources would say it is untreatable.
    - Often, treatment goals should focus on day-to-day coping, harm reduction, and symptom management if the patient is unwilling or unable to develop insight.
    - Prognosis is most improved earlier in life (late teens to late 20s).
    - Prognosis is poor without treatment.
- **Cluster categories:** Patients often overlap classification systems and do not fit the precise characterization of a personality disorder. Personality disorders are grouped into category clusters in which the diagnostic process focuses on traits and symptom clusters.

CLUSTER A PERSONALITY DISORDERS

Traits in this category show patterns of consistent and persistent distrust and suspiciousness, and the patient demonstrates unusual behaviors in a variety of contexts. The level of distrust does not rise to the level of psychosis, although the patient may manifest a brief psychotic disorder under times of stress (Barnhill, 2013; First, 2013; Parker, 2014).

- Consistent findings include:
  - Limited social networks, poor interpersonal relationships
  - Guarded and evasive
  - Difficulty reading social cues
  - Pathological jealousy
  - Seemingly indifferent
  - Rigidity in cognitive distortions, prone to stereotypes, negative perception of others
  - Highly litigious
- **Paranoid personality disorder:** Characterized by a pervasive, persistent, and consistent distrust and suspiciousness of others such that motives are interpreted as malevolent. It is distinguishable from the following disorders in the following manner:
  - **Delusional disorder:** The personality disorder must have occurred before the onset of psychotic symptoms and must persist when the psychotic symptoms are treated
  - **Schizotypal personality disorder:** Does not include magical thinking, unusual perceptual disturbance, or odd speech or behavior pattern
  - **Schizoid personality disorder:** Paranoid ideations are not pervasive.
- **Schizoid personality disorder:** Characterized by a pervasive pattern of detachment from social relationships and a restricted range of expression of emotions in interpersonal settings (Barnhill, 2013; First, 2013; Parker, 2014). It is distinguishable from the following disorders in the following manner:
  - **Schizophrenia:** Characterized by a period of persistent psychosis, diminished emotional expression, social withdrawal, disorganized speech, and perceptual disturbance (hallucinations). The personality disorder must have been present before the psychosis and persist when psychotic symptoms are treated into remission
  - **Autism spectrum disorder:** More severely impaired social interaction with stereotyped behaviors and interests
  - **Schizotypal personality disorder:** Characterized by cognitive and perceptual disturbance in addition to social isolation
  - Paranoid personality disorder: Characterized by paranoia and suspiciousness.
- **Schizotypal personality disorder:** Characterized by a consistent and persistent pattern of social deficits associated with acute discomfort and reduced capacity for close relationships, complicated by cognitive and perceptual distortions and eccentric behaviors. It is distinguishable from the following disorders in the following manner:
  - **Delusional disorders, psychotic disorders, and mood disorders with psychotic features**: The personality disorder must have been present before and persist after the psychotic symptoms are treated into remission

- **Autism spectrum disorder:** More severe social impairment with stereotyped behaviors and interests
- **Language disorders:** A severe disturbance in expressive ability with compensatory efforts to communicate by other means
- **Paranoid and schizoid personality disorders:** These do not have the cognitive and perceptional distortions and lack the eccentric behaviors
- **Avoidant personality disorder:** Active desire for relationships but limited by fear of embarrassment or rejection
- **Transient schizotypal traits in adolescents:** Transient emotional distress that does not persist beyond the developmental stage

▶ CLINICAL VIGNETTE OF THE PROTOTYPICAL PATIENT

Professor Constantine is a 58-year-old underemployed adjunct professor with a blunted affect, mildly disheveled, oddly related, with paranoid ideations that all police are out to get her, and fixed bizarre delusions that people can unhinge their jaws and swallow others whole. She had been married twice but has remained emotionally unavailable in the relationship yet very possessive and would not let either spouse have a key to their home. She remains busy with many side art projects, which do produce some financial gain; however, she is fairly disorganized in her personal effects (mail piles up, bills go unpaid, food is forgotten in the refrigerator, she showers a couple of times per week, but has a standing appointment with a hairdresser).

▶ INCIDENCE AND PREVALENCE

- **Incidence:** Exact statistics are difficult to estimate due to the subjective nature of the diagnostic process, the low frequency of hospitalization, and the frequency by which individuals seek treatment. It is commonly assumed to range from 1% to 5% of the general U.S. population.
  - Risk factors include learned behavior patterns in the family of origin, early life traumas, genetic predispositions, verbal abuse, highly reactive home life during developmental years in which maladaptive coping strategies were inadvertently rewarded.

▶ SCREENING TOOLS AND EARLY INTERVENTION

- **Prevention and screening:** There are no agreed-upon prevention strategies for personality disorders, but many epigenetic theories abound. Providing a stable home life through the developmental years with good role modeling is believed to reduce the incidence of a full-blown personality disorder, but traits can develop through the completion of adolescents. Screening is done to distinguish between a mood, psychotic, developmental, or neurological disorder, and interventions are aimed at facilitating coping skills and mastering developmental tasks.

- Anticipatory guidance for expectant and new parents
- Community education regarding early signs and symptoms
- Encourage personal accountability and moral reasoning

ASSESSMENT AND DIAGNOSIS

- Symptoms must be persistent and consistent with maladaptive coping, causing dysfunction to interpersonal relationships and distress in multiple domains
- Often requires several interviews with collateral information to clarify a diagnosis
- Detailed developmental history to include onset, duration, and severity of symptoms, and aggravating and alleviating factors as well as helpful and harmful coping strategies to date
  - School history
  - Legal history
  - Social and intimate relationships over time
  - Vocational history
  - Factors related to cultural assimilation
  - Religious influences on behavior and identity

PLANNING

- **Career planning:** activities that capitalize on the traits of the disorder
- Prioritize and anticipate defense mechanisms associated with high-stress situations
- Express empathy toward the patient's perceived need to utilize maladaptive coping strategies
- Avoid power struggles
- Always maintain professional boundaries

INTERVENTION

- Limit setting for inappropriate and unsafe behaviors
- Express empathy and validate feelings without agreeing or disagreeing
- Remain consistent in the team's approach to minimize splitting behaviors
- Remain vigilant for physical safety of the milieu
- Validate feelings and encourage alternative coping strategies that reduce harm and promote well-being
- Role model appropriate behavior and positive interactions
- Help the client identify cognitive distortions
- Praise the use of mature defense mechanisms
- **Nonpharmacological treatment options:** There are no medications approved for the diagnosis of a personality disorder, but medications are sometimes used to treat the perceived anxiety in order to enhance daily function (Sadock, Sadock, & Ruiz, 2015)
  - Various therapeutic approaches are used; primarily cognitive behavioral therapy and dialectical behavioral therapy for patients using more immature defense mechanisms

- The aim of therapy is to reduce cognitive distortions and to enhance a sense of control and accountability for individual actions
- Group therapy is often used alone or in conjunction with individual therapy to allow for structured peer feedback and to capitalize on the domains of group dynamics
- Helping the client develop realistic expectations of themselves and others

EVALUATION

- Distinguish characteristic behaviors exhibited between various personality disorders
- Distinguish isolated maladaptive coping in an acute stress response from pervasive behavior pattern
- Identify personality traits and the triggers for acting out

▶ CULTURAL IMPLICATIONS

- Clients may manifest certain behaviors and interpersonal expressions only in certain contexts in which the client's behavior may not be viewed as disordered but rather an assimilation and survival strategy.
- Culture can include ethnographic or local context (e.g., frat house, group of socialites, prison population, hostage situation, professional group).
- Personality traits should be present across multiple domains and increasingly maladaptive, particularly at times of high stress or perceived stress.

CLUSTER B PERSONALITY DISORDERS

Traits are consistent and persistent regarding interpersonal relationship disruptions in a variety of contexts and do not rise to the level of psychosis; however, brief psychotic episodes can occur in times of acute stress, and symptoms may require acute hospitalization. Signs and symptoms include dramatic expressions of a fluctuating emotional state, and the severity of the disorder is determined by the varying degrees of affective instability, the type of interpersonal disruption, and the behaviors manifested (Barnhill, 2013; First, 2013; Parker, 2014).

- **Antisocial personality disorder:** Characterized by a consistent and persistent pervasive disregard for the rights of others since the age of 15 and often has a previous diagnosis of a conduct disorder. This cannot be diagnosed until the individual is 18 years of age and is distinguished from the following disorders in the following manner:
  - **Isolated antisocial behavior due to substance use:** This is exclusively related to substance use and is not part of a pattern that began in childhood
  - **Conduct disorder:** Consistent and persistent pattern of violating the rights of others and can be diagnosed at any age

- **Narcissistic personality disorder:** The glibness, exploitation, and lack of empathy are not characterized by impulsivity, aggressiveness, or previous pattern consistent with conduct disorder
- **Histrionic personality disorder:** The superficial emotionality is not characterized by impulsivity, aggressiveness, or previous conduct disorder
- **Borderline personality disorder:** The manipulative behavior is not characterized by impulsivity, aggressiveness, or previous conduct disorder
- **Paranoid personality disorder:** The antisocial behavior is motivated by revenge rather than personal gain

■ **Borderline personality disorder:** Characterized by an unstable sense of self and unstable interpersonal relationships, the individual is distressed by an unstable internal psychic state and chronic feelings of emptiness, exacerbated by intense separation anxiety, and an inability to be alone without persistent concern for the availability of other people to help reduce the internal distress. It is distinguished from the following disorders in the following manner:
- **Histrionic personality disorder:** Does not contain the self-injurious behaviors, the anger with disruption to relationships, or the chronic feelings of emptiness and loneliness
- **Schizotypal personality disorder:** The paranoid ideations are not related to interpersonal conflicts and may be further exacerbated with psychosocial support
- **Paranoid personality disorder and narcissistic personality disorder:** The paranoid ideations and angry reactions to minor stimuli are characterized by relative stability in the self-image and decreased propensity to self-destructive tendencies and impulsive actions to a real or imagined sense of abandonment
- **Antisocial personality disorder:** Manipulation in this disorder is motivated by a desire for power, profit, or personal gain rather than a desire for nurturance
- **Dependent personality disorder:** Abandonment concerns in this disorder are characterized by reacting to the threat of abandonment with increased appeasement and submission with attempts to seek a replacement relationship to provide caregiving support

■ **Histrionic personality disorder:** Characterized by a consistent and persistent pervasive pattern of excessive emotionality and other attention-seeking (negative, positive, pity, sympathy) behaviors. This is distinguished from the following disorders in the following manner:
- **Borderline personality disorder:** Characterized by self-destructive reactions and angry disruptions in close relationships due to an unstable identity and fear of abandonment
- **Antisocial personality disorder:** The manipulative aspect is for a desire for personal gain, profit, or power rather than for attention or approval
- **Narcissistic personality disorder:** Attention-seeking behavior is for the purpose of praise or being perceived as superior
- **Dependent personality disorder:** Characterized by excessive dependence on others for praise and guidance without the dramatic emotions

■ **Narcissistic personality disorder:** Characterized by a persistent inferiority complex in which they attempt to overcompensate with an overinflated sense of importance and being perceived as special. The grandiosity serves as a defense against not feeling valued while defensively putting off their need for others, despite craving constant admiration and reassurance from others. Individuals with narcissistic personality disorder feel entitled yet dependent on others with whom they often demonstrate a lack of empathy and concern, culminating in their disappointment and leading to rage. It is distinguished from the following disorders in the following manner:

- **Histrionic personality disorder:** The need for attention is related to the need for approval rather than admiration
- **Antisocial personality disorder:** The lack of empathy is characterized by impulsivity and aggression rather than a need for admiration by others
- **Borderline personality disorder:** The need for attention is triggered by the instability in the self-image and is accompanied by self-destructive, impulsive behaviors as a reaction to a sense of real or imagined abandonment
- **Obsessive compulsive personality disorder:** The perfectionism is characterized by a striving to attain perfection and a belief that others cannot do things as well rather than the belief that the perfection has already been attained
- **Schizotypal personality disorder and paranoid personality disorder:** The suspiciousness and social withdrawal are related to paranoid ideations as opposed to fears that imperfections will be revealed
- **Mania:** The grandiosity only occurs during manic phases and is absent when in remission or in the depression phase

▶ CLINICAL VIGNETTE OF THE PROTOTYPICAL PATIENT

A 25-year-old female with a history of nonsuicidal self-injurious behavior who often sees the world in all or nothing, black and white terms. She easily falls in "love" idolizing the object of her affection only to become emotionally dysregulated at the perception of any perceived loss, manifesting help-seeking and help-rejecting tendencies, mood fluctuates are rapid within the span of minutes to hours. She may drastically alter her physical appearance from day to day out of desperate attempts to form an identity.

▶ INCIDENCE AND PREVALENCE

- **Incidence:** Exact statistics are difficult to estimate due to the subjective nature of the diagnostic process, the low frequency of hospitalization, and the frequency by which individuals seek treatment. It is commonly assumed to range from 1% to 5% of the general U.S. population.
    - Risk factors include learned behavior patterns in the family of origin, early life traumas, genetic predispositions, verbal abuse, highly reactive home life during developmental years in which maladaptive coping strategies were inadvertently rewarded.

▶ SCREENING TOOLS AND EARLY INTERVENTION

- **Prevention and screening:** There are no agreed-upon prevention strategies for personality disorders, but many epigenetic theories abound. Providing a stable home life through the developmental years with good role modeling is believed to reduce the incidence of a full-blown personality disorder, but traits can develop through the completion of adolescents. Screening is done to distinguish between a mood, psychotic, developmental, or neurological disorder, and interventions are aimed at facilitating coping skills and mastering developmental tasks.
  - Anticipatory guidance for expectant and new parents
  - Community education regarding early signs and symptoms
  - Encourage personal accountability and moral reasoning

ASSESSMENT AND DIAGNOSIS

- Symptoms must be persistent and consistent with maladaptive coping, causing dysfunction to interpersonal relationships and distress in multiple domains
- Often requires several interviews with collateral information to clarify a diagnosis
- Detailed developmental history to include onset, duration, and severity of symptoms, and aggravating and alleviating factors, as well as helpful and harmful coping strategies to date
  - School history
  - Legal history
  - Social and intimate relationships over time
  - Vocational history
  - Factors related to cultural assimilation
  - Religious influences on behavior and identity

PLANNING

- **Career planning:** Activities that capitalize on the traits of the disorder
- Prioritize and anticipate defense mechanisms associated with high-stress situations
- Expression empathy towards the patient's perceived need to utilize maladaptive coping strategies
- Avoid power struggles
- Always maintain professional boundaries

INTERVENTION

- Limit setting for inappropriate and unsafe behaviors
- Expressing empathy and validate feelings without agreeing or disagreeing
- Remain consistent in the team's approach to minimize splitting behaviors
- Remain vigilant for physical safety of the milieu
- Validate feelings and encourage alternative coping strategies that reduce harm and promote well-being

- Role model appropriate behavior and positive interactions
- Help the client identify cognitive distortions
- Praise the use of mature defense mechanisms
- **Nonpharmacological treatment options:** There are no medications approved for the diagnosis of a personality disorder, but medications are sometimes used to treat the perceived anxiety in order to enhance daily function (Sadock, Sadock, & Ruiz, 2015)
    - Various therapeutic approaches are used, primarily cognitive behavioral therapy and dialectical behavioral therapy for patients using more immature defense mechanisms
    - The aim of therapy is to reduce cognitive distortions and to enhance a sense of control and accountability for individual actions
    - Group therapy is often used alone or in conjunction with individual therapy to allow for structured peer feedback and to capitalize on the domains of group dynamics
    - Helping the client develop realistic expectations of themselves and others

EVALUATION

- Distinguish characteristic behaviors exhibited between various personality disorders
- Distinguish isolated maladaptive coping in an acute stress response from pervasive behavior pattern
- Identify personality traits and the triggers for acting out

▶ CULTURAL IMPLICATIONS

- Clients may manifest certain behaviors and interpersonal expressions only in certain contexts in which the client's behavior may not be viewed as disordered but rather an assimilation and survival strategy.
- Culture can include ethnographic or local context (e.g., frat house, group of socialites, prison population, hostage situation, professional group).
- Personality traits should be present across multiple domains and increasingly maladaptive, particularly at times of high stress or perceived stress.

CLUSTER C PERSONALITY DISORDERS

Characterized by a consistent and persistent pattern of fear and anxiety in a variety of contexts across multiple domains of functioning in which the individual demonstrates maladaptive coping mechanisms (avoidance behaviors, procrastination, difficulty in following through on tasks, difficulty unwinding), motivated by fear of rejection or criticism, not rising to the level of psychosis although brief psychotic episodes can occur in times of acute stress (Barnhill, 2013; First, 2013; Parker, 2014).

- **Avoidant personality disorder:** Characterized by a consistent and persistent pervasive pattern of social inhibition, feelings of inadequacy, and a hypersensitivity to real or perceived critiques. It is distinguished from the following disorders in the following manner:
  - **Agoraphobia:** The avoidance aspect of this disorder starts after the onset of a panic attack and varies based on the intensity and frequency of the panic attack
  - **Dependent personality disorder:** The feelings of inadequacy and sensitivity to criticism and need for reassurance arise from concerns of being cared for rather than the avoidance of humiliation or rejection
  - **Schizoid and schizotypal personality disorders:** The social isolation is preferred as it brings a sense of contentment
  - **Paranoid personality disorder:** The reluctance to confide in others is motivated by fear that the personal information will be used for malevolent intent rather than by fear of embarrassment
- **Dependent personality disorder:** Characterized by a consistent and persistent pervasive pattern of maladaptive behaviors arising from an excessive need to be cared for and leading to submissive, clinging behavior with the goal of reducing the chance of separation. It is distinguished from the following disorders in the following manner:
  - **Separation anxiety disorder:** This is characterized by an excessive and persistent fear of being physically separated from a specific attachment figure and not the fear of being uncared for or having unmet needs
  - **Borderline personality disorder:** The fear of abandonment stems from real, perceived, or anticipated abandonment, resulting in feelings of emptiness, rage, and the use of immature defense mechanisms
  - **Histrionic personality disorder:** The need for reassurance and approval are made known through dramatic expressions with the intent of drawing any attention
  - **Avoidant personality disorder:** The social withdrawal stems from a fear of rejection or humiliation until the individual is assured of social acceptance
- **Obsessive compulsive personality disorder:** Characterized by a consistent and persistent pervasive pattern of obsession with perfectionism, order, and inter-/intrapersonal control at the expense of openness, flexibility, and efficiency coupled with an excessive devotion to work. It is distinguished from the following disorders in the following manner:
  - **Obsessive compulsive disorder:** Characterized by the presence of a true obsession (recurrent thoughts, urges, images) that are intrusive and unwanted, which the individual attempts to control or suppress, leading to compulsive acts that the individual must engage in to relieve the distress caused by the obsession. The individual is not attempting to get others to behave in a similarly compulsive manner
  - **Hoarding disorder:** Characterized by a consistent and persistent pervasive pattern of difficulty in discarding any possession regardless of value leading to an unlivable cluttered dwelling
  - **Narcissistic personality disorder:** Perfectionist tendencies are thought to already have been achieved rather than being goals
  - **Antisocial personality disorder:** The lack of generosity is done for the purpose of self-indulgence rather than a miserly spending style toward self and others

- **Schizoid personality disorder:** The social detachment occurs in the context of an inability to be intimate and of discomfort with emotion

▶ CLINICAL VIGNETTE OF THE PROTOTYPICAL PATIENT

A 68-year-old writer who lives alone and insists on certain rituals of daily life, which include washing his hands with a new bar of soap under extremely hot running water, checking if the door is locked exactly four times, avoiding walking on any cracks in the sidewalk, he must sit at the same table in the same restaurant and insists on the same waitress every day. He is a prolific writer completing a new novel each year. He does not see his behaviors as odd and believes others should adopt his regimented lifestyle and are delinquents if they do not.

▶ INCIDENCE AND PREVALENCE

- **Incidence:** Exact statistics are difficult to estimate due to the subjective nature of the diagnostic process, the low frequency of hospitalization, and the frequency by which individuals seek treatment. It is commonly assumed to range from 1% to 5% of the general U.S. population.
  - Risk factors include learned behavior patterns in the family of origin, early life traumas, genetic predispositions, verbal abuse, highly reactive home life during developmental years in which maladaptive coping strategies were inadvertently rewarded.

▶ SCREENING TOOLS AND EARLY INTERVENTION

- **Prevention and screening:** There are no agreed-upon prevention strategies for personality disorders, but many epigenetic theories abound. Providing a stable home life through the developmental years with good role modeling is believed to reduce the incidence of a full-blown personality disorder, but traits can develop through the completion of adolescents. Screening is done to distinguish between a mood, psychotic, developmental, or neurological disorder, and interventions are aimed at facilitating coping skills and mastering developmental tasks.
  - Anticipatory guidance for expectant and new parents
  - Community education regarding early signs and symptoms
  - Encourage personal accountability and moral reasoning

ASSESSMENT AND DIAGNOSIS

- Symptoms must be persistent and consistent with maladaptive coping, causing dysfunction to interpersonal relationships and distress in multiple domains
- Often requires several interviews with collateral information to clarify a diagnosis

- Detailed developmental history to include onset, duration, and severity of symptoms, and aggravating and alleviating factors as well as helpful and harmful coping strategies to date
  - School history
  - Legal history
  - Social and intimate relationships over time
  - Vocational history
  - Factors related to cultural assimilation
  - Religious influences on behavior and identity

PLANNING

- **Career planning:** Activities that capitalize on the traits of the disorder
- Prioritize and anticipate defense mechanisms associated with high-stress situations
- Expression empathy toward the patient's perceived need to utilize maladaptive coping strategies
- Avoid power struggles
- Always maintain professional boundaries

INTERVENTION

- Limit setting for inappropriate and unsafe behaviors
- Expressing empathy and validate feelings without agreeing or disagreeing
- Remain consistent in the team's approach to minimize splitting behaviors
- Remain vigilant for physical safety of the milieu
- Validate feelings and encourage alternative coping strategies that reduce harm and promote well-being
- Role-model appropriate behavior and positive interactions
- Help the client identify cognitive distortions
- Praise the use of mature defense mechanisms
- **Nonpharmacological treatment options:** There are no medications approved for the diagnosis of a personality disorder, but medications are sometimes used to treat the perceived anxiety in order to enhance daily function (Sadock, Sadock, & Ruiz, 2015)
  - Various therapeutic approaches are used; primarily cognitive behavioral therapy and dialectical behavioral therapy for patients using more immature defense mechanisms
  - The aim of therapy is to reduce cognitive distortions and to enhance a sense of control and accountability for individual actions
  - Group therapy is often used alone or in conjunction with individual therapy to allow for structured peer feedback and to capitalize on the domains of group dynamics
  - Helping the client develop realistic expectations of themselves and others

EVALUATION

- Distinguish characteristic behaviors exhibited between various personality disorders
- Distinguish isolated maladaptive coping in an acute stress response from pervasive behavior pattern
- Identify personality traits and the triggers for acting out

▶ CULTURAL IMPLICATIONS

- Clients may manifest certain behaviors and interpersonal expressions only in certain contexts in which the client's behavior may not be viewed as disordered but rather an assimilation and survival strategy.
- Culture can include ethnographic or local context (e.g., frat house, group of socialites, prison population, hostage situation, professional group).
- Personality traits should be present across multiple domains and increasingly maladaptive, particularly at times of high stress or perceived stress.

KNOWLEDGE CHECK: CHAPTER 12

1. A 56-year-old widow has deeply held beliefs about various conspiracy theories where the government is spying on her, and her sister is trying to control her money. She attends writing classes, sings in the choir, and works as a mailroom clerk in a law firm. Which of the following is the most likely diagnosis of this patient?

   A. Paranoid personality disorder
   B. Schizotypal personality disorder
   C. Schizoid personality disorder
   D. Schizophrenia

2. A 35-year-old man is found to have a flat affect, very few current social contacts, and prefers to be alone. He was referred by the employee assistance program for evaluation after someone reported him for odd behavior. His boss reports that in 20 years he has never called out sick, does not attend company outings, and has never spoken of a significant other. Which of the following is the most likely diagnosis?

   A. Paranoid personality disorder
   B. Schizotypal personality disorder
   C. Schizoid personality disorder
   D. Schizophrenia

3. A 68-year-old woman who has been self-employed as a copyeditor avoids social gatherings and would rather stay home and read. She has a few distant friends who check in on her occasionally and who report her entire home is covered in bedsheets. She attends church weekly but quickly leaves after the service. She is known to never be without her feather boa. Which of the following best describes this patient?

   A. Paranoid personality disorder
   B. Schizotypal personality disorder
   C. Schizoid personality disorder
   D. Schizophrenia

(See answers next page.)

1. A) Paranoid personality disorder

The most likely diagnosis for this patient is paranoid personality disorder due to the pervasive paranoia and delusional thinking. Schizotypal personality disorder includes magical thinking, unusual perceptual disturbance, and odd speech or behavior. Schizoid personality is not characterized by paranoid ideations. Schizophrenia requires a period of persistent psychotic symptoms for at least 6 months with impaired functioning, including hallucinations congruent with delusions, disorganized speech, impaired cognition, and agitation.

2. C) Schizoid personality disorder

Schizoid personality disorder is characterized by a pervasive pattern of detachment from social relationships and restricted range of expressions. Paranoid personality disorder is characterized by a consistent and persistent thought pattern without perceptual disturbance. Schizotypal personality disorder is characterized by a consistent and persistent pattern of social deficits associated with acute discomfort in social settings with associated cognitive and perceptual distortions and eccentric behaviors. Schizophrenia requires a period of persistent psychotic symptoms for at least 6 months with impaired functioning, including hallucinations congruent with delusions, disorganized speech, impaired cognition, and agitation.

3. B) Schizotypal personality disorder

Schizotypal personality disorder is characterized by a consistent and persistent pattern of social deficits associated with acute discomfort in social settings with associated cognitive and perceptual distortions and eccentric behaviors. Paranoid personality disorder is characterized by a consistent and persistent thought pattern without perceptual disturbance. Schizoid personality disorder is characterized by a pervasive pattern of detachment from social relationships and restricted range of expressions. Schizophrenia requires a period of persistent psychotic symptoms for at least 6 months with impaired functioning, including hallucinations congruent with delusions, disorganized speech, impaired cognition, and agitation.

4. A 40-year-old man with a history of oppositional defiant behavior as a child has recently been released on parole for possession of marijuana and theft. He tells the probation officer to send him to the psychiatrist so he can get some disability. The psychiatric-mental health nurse should plan care according to which of the following personality traits?

   A. Cluster C personality
   B. Cluster B personality
   C. Cluster A personality
   D. Malingering

5. An 18-year-old high school senior with a history of substance use disorder and school refusal brags to her peers about her shoplifting exploits. To which personality disorder group should the psychiatric-mental health nurse assign the patient when admitting her to the partial hospital program?

   A. Antisocial personality disorder
   B. Borderline personality disorder
   C. Histrionic personality disorder
   D. Narcissistic personality disorder

6. A 30-year-old female is admitted to the emergency department after slashing her arms when her boyfriend left for a weeklong business trip. She states she did not want to kill herself but rather wanted him to come back home. Which intervention would be most helpful for this patient's emotional distress?

   A. Set firm limits that she is not act out
   B. Allow for a stuffed animal reminding her of the boyfriend
   C. Speak in soft tones with simple commands
   D. Reply in a matter of fact tone and validate her underlying fear

(See answers next page.)

4. D) Malingering
Malingering is the faking of symptoms for financial or material gain, commonly comorbid in people with antisocial personality disorder. Cluster B traits are characterized by persistent and consistent relationship disruptions in a variety of contexts with transient episodes of psychosis in acute stress states; symptoms include dramatic expressions of emotion and fluctuating emotional state with low frustration tolerance. Cluster A personality disorders are characterized by a pattern of consistent and persistent distrust and suspiciousness with odd behaviors in various contexts. Cluster C disorders are characterized by a consistent and persistent pattern of fear and anxiety in a variety of contexts across multiple domains in which the person expresses avoidance coping behaviors.

5. A) Antisocial personality disorder
Antisocial personality disorder is characterized by a pervasive lack of empathy, impulsivity, aggression, and manipulation of others for personal gain. Borderline personality disorder is characterized by an unstable sense of self, intense interpersonal relationships, and emotional volatility. Histrionic personality disorder is characterized by a consistent and pervasive pattern of excessive emotionality and other attention-seeking behaviors. Narcissistic personality disorder is characterized by a persistent and consistent inferiority complex overcompensated by an inflated sense of self-importance and need to be admired and perceived as special.

6. B) Allow for a stuffed animal reminding her of the boyfriend
Provide a stuffed animal as a transitional object; borderline personality disorder is characterized by an unstable sense of self, intense interpersonal relationships, and emotional volatility. Speaking in soft tones with simple commands is appropriate for histrionic personality disorder characterized by a consistent and pervasive pattern of excessive emotionality and other attention-seeking behaviors. Replying in a matter-of-fact tone while validating underlying fears helps the patient with narcissistic personality disorder, which is characterized by a persistent and consistent inferiority complex overcompensated by an inflated sense of self-importance and need to be admired and perceived as special. Setting firm limits clearly communicates the rules for the group or any engagement for the person with antisocial personality disorder. It is characterized by a pervasive lack of empathy, impulsivity, aggression, and manipulation of others for personal gain.

7. A 28-year-old female enters the room with wide gestures and declares, "I have arrived; let the fun begin." She struts her way through the room, bumping her way through the crowd and stepping on a few toes. How should the psychiatric-mental health nurse approach this patient?

    A. Set firm limits
    B. Provide a stuffed animal
    C. Speak to her in a soft tone explaining the limits of the environment
    D. Reply in a matter of fact tone and validate his underlying fear

8. A 24-year-old man who has been diagnosed with substance-induced mood disorder is doing well, maintaining his sobriety for the past 5 years. He complains of being lonely but is afraid of going to any social events lest he encounter alcohol. He requires much reassurance that he is okay, he will be fine, and that he is good enough to be around others whom he perceives to be better adjusted to life. These characteristics are most consistent with which of the following disorders?

    A. Avoidant personality disorder
    B. Dependent personality disorder
    C. Obsessive compulsive personality disorder
    D. Paranoid personality disorder

9. Mr. Smith is complaining about another failed romantic relationship. He says his girlfriend described him as needy all the time, avoidant of confrontation at all costs, agreeable to all her requests, and never disagreeable with her. She told him she was done with his passive ways and was going to find a real man. These traits are most consistent with which of the following disorders?

    A. Avoidant personality disorder
    B. Dependent personality disorder
    C. Obsessive compulsive personality disorder
    D. Paranoid personality disorder

(See answers next page.)

7. C) Speak to her in a soft tone explaining the limits of the environment

Speaking to her in a soft tone explaining the limits of the environment can help model appropriate behavior for the patient with histrionic personality disorder is characterized by a consistent and pervasive pattern of excessive emotionality and other attention-seeking behaviors. Replying in a matter-of-fact tone while validating underlying fears is more useful in speaking to someone with narcissistic personality disorder, which is characterized by a persistent and consistent inferiority complex overcompensated by an inflated sense of self-importance and need to be admired and perceived as special. Setting firm limits is preferred for someone with antisocial personality disorder, which is characterized by a pervasive lack of empathy, impulsivity, aggression, and manipulation of others for personal gain. A stuffed animal is preferred for someone with borderline personality disorder, which is characterized by an unstable sense of self, intense interpersonal relationships, and emotional volatility.

8. A) Avoidant personality disorder

Avoidant personality disorder is characterized by a consistent and persistent pervasive pattern of social inhibition, feelings of inadequacy, and a hypersensitivity to real or perceived critique. Dependent personality disorder is characterized by a consistent and persistent pervasive pattern of maladaptive behaviors arising from an excessive need to be cared for, leading to submissive, clingy behaviors with the goal of reducing the chance of separation. Obsessive compulsive personality disorder is characterized by a consistent and persistent pervasive pattern of obsessions of perfectionism, order, and inter- and intra-personal control at the expense of openness, flexibility, and efficiency coupled with an excessive devotion to work. Paranoid personality disorder manifests as the reluctance to confide in others and is motivated by fear that the personal information will be used for malevolent intent rather than for fear of embarrassment.

9. B) Dependent personality disorder

Dependent personality disorder is characterized by a consistent and persistent pervasive pattern of maladaptive behaviors arising from an excessive need to be cared for, leading to submissive, clingy behaviors with the goal of reducing the chance of separation. Avoidant personality disorder is characterized by a consistent and persistent pervasive pattern of social inhibition, feelings of inadequacy, and a hypersensitivity to real or perceived critique. Obsessive compulsive personality disorder is characterized by a consistent and persistent pervasive pattern of obsessions of perfectionism, order, and inter- and intra-personal control at the expense of openness, flexibility, and efficiency coupled with an excessive devotion to work. Paranoid personality disorder manifests as the reluctance to confide in others and is motivated by fear that the personal information will be used for malevolent intent rather than for fear of embarrassment.

10. In a movie, Jack Nicholson played a meticulous writer who was highly productive, very concerned about germ contamination, and very ritualistic about walking on sidewalk cracks. In addition, he would turn the lights on and off repeatedly and use a brand-new bar of soap to wash his hands with exceedingly hot water. These traits are characteristic of which personality disorder?

    A. Avoidant personality disorder
    B. Dependent personality disorder
    C. Obsessive compulsive personality disorder
    D. Paranoid personality disorder

11. In treating personality disorders, the role of psychopharmacology is to:

    A. Alleviate comorbid mood symptoms
    B. Undo the antecedents leading to the disorder
    C. Modify behaviors
    D. Prevent comorbid conditions from developing

12. Which of the following personality disorders can be diagnosed in a single visit?

    A. Narcissistic personality disorder
    B. Borderline personality disorder
    C. Antisocial personality disorder
    D. Histrionic personality disorder

13. Which of the following characteristics distinguishes schizotypal personality disorder from autism spectrum disorder?

    A. Severity of social impairment and stereotyped behaviors and interests
    B. Severe disturbance in expressive ability with compensatory efforts to communicate in another way
    C. Cognitive perceptual disturbances
    D. Active desire for relationships but fear of rejection

(See answers next page.)

10. C) Obsessive compulsive personality disorder
Obsessive compulsive personality disorder is characterized by a consistent and persistent pervasive pattern of obsessions of perfectionism, order, and inter- and intra-personal control at the expense of openness, flexibility, and efficiency coupled with an excessive devotion to work. Dependent personality disorder is characterized by a consistent and persistent pervasive pattern of maladaptive behaviors arising from an excessive need to be cared for, leading to submissive, clingy behaviors with the goal of reducing the chance of separation. Avoidant personality disorder is characterized by a consistent and persistent pervasive pattern of social inhibition, feelings of inadequacy, and a hypersensitivity to real or perceived critique. Paranoid personality disorder manifests as the reluctance to confide in others and is motivated by fear that the personal information will be used for malevolent intent rather than for fear of embarrassment.

11. A) Alleviate comorbid mood symptoms
Primary treatment for personality disorders is psychotherapy. Medication is only used to alleviate comorbid symptoms associated with the distress caused by the personality disorder. Medications cannot undo past events or prevent disorders from developing or modifying behavior.

12. C) Antisocial personality disorder
Antisocial personality disorder can be diagnosed in a single visit if there is a past history of conduct disorder before age 15 and current signs and symptoms of the pervasive disregard for the rights of others. Narcissistic personality disorder, borderline personality disorder, and histrionic personality disorder require several visits as the novelty of a new situation and situational anxiety can trigger compensatory behaviors that are not consistent or persistent. No diagnosis should ever be made of someone who has not been personally evaluated.

13. A) Severity of social impairment and stereotyped behaviors and interests
Autism spectrum behaviors are associated with more severe social impairment and stereotyped behaviors and interests. A severe disturbance in expressive ability with compensatory efforts is associated with language disorders. Cognitive and perceptual disturbances are associated with paranoid and schizoid personality disturbances. A desire for relationships limited by fear of rejection is associated with avoidant personality disorder.

14. A psychiatric-mental health nurse is teaching a seminar on personality disorders. Which of the following characteristics distinguishes narcissistic personality disorder from antisocial personality disorder?

    A. The need for attention is related to the need for approval rather than admiration
    B. The lack of empathy manifested in impulsivity and aggression rather than the need for admiration
    C. The need for attention is triggered by instability of the self-image and fear of abandonment
    D. The grandiosity only occurs during times of elevated mood

15. A 40-year-old male nurse who works the night shift reports an uneventful childhood and college experience. He spends most of the time alone when he is not at work, does not venture out of the house, and limits his social contacts to work colleagues during his shift. He is an avid cook and spends much of his free time indoors attending to very complicated recipes with esoteric ingredients. He reports that he is quite content with his life. This patient meets the criteria for which of the following conditions?

    A. Agoraphobia
    B. Avoidant personality disorder
    C. Schizoid personality disorder
    D. Schizotypal personality disorder

(See answers next page.)

14. B) The lack of empathy manifested in impulsivity and aggression rather than the need for admiration

Narcissistic personality disorder is driven by a need for admiration rather than a lack of empathy, as in antisocial personality disorder. When the need for attention is driven by a desire for approval rather than admiration, this is consistent with histrionic personality disorder. If the need for attention is triggered by unstable self-image and fear of abandonment, this is consistent with borderline personality disorder. If the grandiosity is only in the context of elevated mood, this is consistent with mania.

15. C) Schizoid personality disorder

People with schizoid personality disorder are not distressed by the lack of social interaction and rather prefer it that way. Agoraphobia is characterized by a fear of panic symptoms in public. People with schizotypal disorder may have similar features to schizoid personality disorder but also have bizarre thought patterns. People with avoidant personality disorder are distressed by the lack of social interaction but fear rejection.

REFERENCES

Barnhill, J. W. (2013). DSM-5® *clinical cases*. Arlington, VA: American Psychiatric Publishing. doi:10.1176/appi. books.9781585624836

Baumert, A., Schmitt, M., Perugini, M., Johnson, W., Blum, G., Borkenau, P., ... Wrzus, C. (2017). Integrating person ality structure, personality process, and personality development. *European Journal of Personality, 31*(5), 503–528. doi:10.1002/per.2115

First, M. B. (2013). *DSM-5® handbook of differential diagnosis*. Arlington, VA: American Psychiatric Publishing. doi:10.1176/ appi.books.9781585629992

Kernberg, O. (1995). *Object relations theory and clinical psychoanalysis*. Retrieved from https://books.google.com/ books?hl=en&lr=&id=X-USb93ZGy 4C&oi=fnd&pg=PP2&dq=object+relations+theory+personality+disor ders&ots=vHwD7hjtaU&sig=OEjF4sFv-hNZKpmT0534081G4iM

Mahler, M., Pine, F., & Bergman, A. (1975). *The psychological birth of the human infant. Symbiosis and individuation*. New York, NY: Basic Books, Inc.

Parker, G. F. (2014). *DSM-5 psychotic and mood disorders. Journal of the American Academy of Psychiatry and the Law, 43*(1), 165–172. Retrieved from http://jaapl.org/content/42/2/182#sec-1

Pine, F. (2004). Mahler's concepts of "symbiosis" and separation-individuation: Revisited, reevaluated, refined. *Journal of the American Psychoanalytic Association, 52*(2), 511–533. doi:10.1177/00030651040520021001

Sadock, B., Sadock, V., & Ruiz, P. (2015). *Synopsis of psychiatry* (11th ed.). New York, NY: Wolters Kluwer.

Twenge, J. M., & Campbell, S. M. (2008). Generational differences in psychological traits and their impact on the work place. *Journal of Managerial Psychology, 23*(8), 862–877. doi:10.1108/02683940810904367

Part III

Practice Test

Practice Test Questions

1. Which of the following elements is reflective of a professional relationship rather than a social relationship?

    A. In a professional relationship, there is no place for social interactions
    B. In a professional relationship, the psychiatric-mental health nurse is solely responsible for making the relationship work
    C. In a professional relationship, the primary focus is on the client and their needs
    D. In a professional relationship, goals are left vague so that the client feels any issue can be discussed

2. The psychiatric-mental health nurse recognizes the essential nature of primary prevention strategies for a community. Which of the following is an example of a primary prevention strategy?

    A. A skills class for at-risk adolescents
    B. A suicide hotline
    C. Mandated treatment
    D. A psychosocial clubhouse for the mentally ill

3. A 45-year-old White female agreed to hospitalization after presenting to the emergency department with passive suicidal ideations. After 24 hours, she states that she wishes to leave because "this place cannot help me." Which of the following actions should the psychiatric-mental health nurse take first?

    A. Prepare the patient to be discharged immediately
    B. The patient must sign forms indicating her actions and acknowledging her actions are against medical advice
    C. Contact the physician and request conversion to an involuntary status
    D. Explain that the patient cannot leave until further assessments are completed, and collateral information is obtained

4. The purpose of a professional organization's scope and standards of practice is to:

    A. Define the roles and actions for that particular profession
    B. Define the differences between professions
    C. Establish the legal authority to practice for a profession
    D. Define the legal statutes that are governing a profession

5. A patient who has been voluntarily admitted is experiencing symptoms of psychosis; he declares he has the right to refuse his medications despite the court order because God told him he would be healed by his faith alone. Based on the psychiatric-mental health nurse's knowledge of court-ordered treatment, which of the following statements is true?

   A. Psychiatric clients cannot refuse treatment
   B. Psychiatric clients can refuse treatment unless it is court-ordered
   C. Psychiatric clients cannot act in their own best judgment
   D. The professional judgment of the psychiatric-mental health nurse supersedes the client's right to refuse medication

6. A 50-year-old physician presents with complaints of fatigue, headache, abdominal distress, and weight loss. His husband reports increasing irritability, inattentiveness, and low libido over the last month. He was seen by his primary care provider, who just notified him he had pre-diabetes, hypercholesterolemia, and hypertension despite weight loss. For which condition will the psychiatric-mental health nurse provide psychoeducation and anticipatory guidance?

   A. Dysthymia
   B. Major depression
   C. Generalized anxiety disorder
   D. Seasonal affective disorder

7. In light of the recent school shootings, the local high schools have noticed an unusually high incidence of depressive symptoms and illicit drug use among their students. The psychiatric-mental health nurse formulates a plan to address the problem. The goal of the program is to enhance the capabilities of families and teachers to identify antecedents of depression and drug use and to prevent new cases from developing. What level of prevention is this strategy?

   A. Tertiary prevention
   B. Secondary prevention
   C. Solution-focused prevention
   D. Primary prevention

8. Which of the following statements made by a client is the best indicator of a therapeutic alliance?

   A. "You have no idea what you are doing"
   B. "You are the only person who has been helpful to me"
   C. "You are not even a doctor"
   D. "I have nothing to say to you"

9. Which Freudian psychodynamic principle assumes all behavior conveys purpose?

    A. The Ego development principle
    B. Psychic determinism principle
    C. The Id principle
    D. The Superego mediation principle

10. A Black man in the fifth decade of life has been seen for several weeks of psychotherapy to discuss his current stressors. He proceeds to curl up in the fetal position and lie on the floor. Which defense mechanism is he manifesting?

    A. Repression
    B. Projection
    C. Denial
    D. Regression

11. A 39-year-old woman has been in therapy for the last 3 months. She has shown much improvement in her functioning and has developed much insight into her illness. This week during her session, the psychiatric-mental health nurse discusses termination, and the client suddenly begins to demonstrate the first symptoms that brought her into therapy initially. What is the best explanation for her symptom return?

    A. Acute stress reaction
    B. Reaction formation
    C. A normal resistance seen in the termination time of therapy
    D. A sign of undiagnosed pathological attachment

12. Which of the following statements gives an example of a mature defense mechanism?

    A. "I am being held against my will because I am being punished"
    B. "I have no idea why I get so nervous around authority figures"
    C. "I have started baking scones for my irritating coworkers"
    D. "When I get nervous, I can't help putting things in my mouth"

13. A 30-year-old man reports low self-esteem, demonstrates poor self-control, exhibits much self-doubt, and requires a high degree of reassurance. What developmental task has he failed to master?

    A. Trust versus mistrust
    B. Industry versus inferiority
    C. Generativity versus stagnation
    D. Integrity versus despair

14. An ambulance brings a 26-year-old female to the emergency department after a suicide attempt by self-mutilation. Which of the following is the most critical factor for the psychiatric-mental health nurse to consider when conducting an assessment?

    A. Past medical and psychiatric history
    B. Hemodynamic stability
    C. The current level of suicidality
    D. Effective coping mechanisms

15. A married couple of 7 years presents for therapy because the wife perceives her husband to be a constant nag. He believes that he is correct and only trying to help. The psychiatric-mental health nurse assigns him a paradoxical directive to schedule 1 hour per day in which he nags her, and once that hour is over, to keep a list and save it until the next day. The therapeutic intervention is a type of which therapy?

    A. Experiential therapy
    B. Strategic therapy
    C. Structural therapy
    D. Solution-focused therapy

16. A patient is prescribed a selective serotonin reuptake inhibitor (SSRI) for depression. When providing psychoeducation, the psychiatric-mental health nurse explains this class is often the first-line drug of choice for depression because of which of the following safety profile?

    A. Ease of dosing for stepwise titration
    B. Promote sleep
    C. Difficulty in overdosing for suicidal patients
    D. Drug-level monitoring capabilities

17. According to family systems theory, which of the following is reflective of homeostasis?

    A. Family members placate each other to keep the peace
    B. Family members behave erratically to reduce predictability
    C. Stability in the interpersonal relationships despite dysfunctions
    D. A crisis restores peace

18. A man diagnosed with major depressive disorder is started on a selective serotonin reuptake inhibitor (SSRI). Which of the following ways is most effective for the psychiatric-mental health nurse to monitor the client's therapeutic response to medication?

    A. An EKG for QTc prolongation
    B. Basic metabolic profile
    C. Urine toxicology screen
    D. A standardized rating scale for depression

19. In helping a client overcome a maladaptive coping mechanism, the psychiatric-mental health nurse would utilize which of the following elements of cognitive behavioral therapy?

    A. Recognizing and accepting automatic thoughts
    B. Recognizing and changing automatic thoughts
    C. Seeing reality as the private provider sees it
    D. Changing reality through environmental restructuring

20. The following statement is reflective of which type of therapy: "If a miracle were to happen the problem that brought you into therapy no longer existed, what would be different?"

    A. Cognitive behavioral therapy
    B. Dialectical behavioral therapy
    C. Solution-focused therapy
    D. Psychoanalysis

21. A patient is referred by his primary care physician for the treatment of panic disorder with agoraphobia. He had been titrated on paroxetine CR 37.5 mg daily and clonazepam 0.5 mg daily as needed. He has been on this regimen for the last year, but he admits that he sometimes requires as many as five clonazepam tablets to get the same effect. Which pharmacokinetic property is influencing this phenomenon?

    A. Potency
    B. Tolerance
    C. Kindling
    D. Addiction

22. The psychiatric-mental health nurse is providing psychoeducation regarding medications for mood disorders. Which of the following neuroleptic mood-stabilizing medications commonly used to treat bipolar disorder is associated with which teratogenic effects?

    A. Divalproex (shortened limbs); lithium (seizure disorder)
    B. Lithium (Ebstein's anomaly); divalproex (neural tube defects)
    C. Divalproex (Ebstein's anomaly); lithium (cleft lip and palate)
    D. Lithium (spina bifida); divalproex (neural tube defects)

23. A 60-year-old male survived heart attack and found himself depressed 6 months after the event. Which class of medication might be contributing to the patient's symptoms?

    A. Proton pump inhibitors
    B. Beta blockers
    C. Antihistamines
    D. PD 5 inhibitors

24. The psychiatric-mental health nurse is facilitating a group for spouses of patient with dementia. Which of the following principles of group dynamics enhances therapeutic efficacy?

   A. Shared decision-making
   B. Acquiring curative factors
   C. Cost efficiency
   D. Enhancing social skills

25. An elderly woman is inquiring as to why she needs her lithium dose reduced since she has been stable on it for the past 30 years. Which of the following conditions occurs with the normal aging process that affects drug metabolism?

   A. Increased muscle mass
   B. Reduced protein binding
   C. Increased liver metabolization pathways leading to toxicity
   D. Decreased body fat

26. A 90-year-old Black woman tells the psychiatric-mental health nurse, "Some days life is just not worth living. I would be less of a burden if I were not here anymore." Which of the following is the most therapeutic response the psychiatric-mental health nurse can make?

   A. "Everybody loves you and likes being around you"
   B. "Tell me what you mean when you say 'life is not worth living'"
   C. Therapeutic use of silence
   D. "Are you thinking suicide might be an option for you?"

27. While performing a mental status exam on a patient, the psychiatric-mental health nurse asks them to interpret this proverb: "A stitch in time saves nine." The patient replies, "The garment would be more likely to rip." How would the psychiatric-mental health nurse interpret these findings?

   A. The patient is psychotic
   B. The patient is anxious
   C. The patient is intellectually disabled
   D. There is not enough information to interpret the statement without knowing the client's age

28. A 36-year-old pharmacist has a history of depression and a suicide attempt 1 month ago by hanging. She had been started on a tricyclic antidepressant but abruptly stopped taking the medication a week after she started, saying it was "ineffective." The psychiatric-mental health nurse meets with this patient to plan care. Which of the following is the most appropriate initial action?

    A. Ask the patient how to help her
    B. Provide teaching about the long timeframe it takes for tricyclic antidepressants (TCAs) to work
    C. Contract with the patient for six sessions of therapy
    D. Tell the patient how suicide might affect her family

29. During the first session of group therapy, the patient makes the following statement: "All my other kids got through their drug use phase and were able to get on with their lives. I have grounded him, taken away his privileges, and I even tried to cut out his allowance, but I'm just not sure what I should do now?" Which of the following is the most therapeutic response the psychiatric-mental health nurse can make?

    A. Therapeutic use of silence
    B. "I wonder if locking him in his room was abusive"
    C. "Maybe that depends on what you're trying to accomplish"
    D. "Perhaps talking to his friends, coaches, and teachers would be helpful"

30. In conducting a psychoeducation group for patients newly prescribed psychotropic medications, the psychiatric-mental health nurse should emphasize that these types of medication treat:

    A. Psychiatric disorders
    B. Psychiatric symptoms
    C. Neurological conditions
    D. Endocrine disorders

31. A client states that he "did not realize the time" and apologized for running late. The psychiatric-mental health nurse replies, "This is the fourth time in a row that you've been late to our sessions; I'm just wondering how committed you are to this therapy." What communication technique was used by the psychiatric-mental health nurse?

    A. Reflecting
    B. Restating
    C. Presenting reality
    D. Validating

32. The psychiatric-mental health nurse completes a comprehensive psychiatric evaluation in order to:

    A. To complete the necessary forms for a maximum reimbursement
    B. To develop a correct diagnosis
    C. To communicate with others about the patient's healthcare needs
    D. To identify the mental health needs of the patient

33. The psychiatric-mental health nurse is providing psychoeducation on the relationship between neurophysiology and mental illness. What purpose does a neurotransmitter serve in the nervous system?

    A. Enzyme breakdown
    B. Amino-acid scaffolding
    C. Communication medium
    D. Enzyme production

34. The psychiatric-mental health nurse will evaluate a recently admitted 22-year-old male and gather data to help formulate the initial treatment plan. The patient asks to go to his room because "people make me nervous." The psychiatric-mental health nurse's action should be based on the awareness that the best location to do an initial evaluation is:

    A. In the patient's room because it's the least noisy and most comfortable for him
    B. In a public area to observe his interactions with others
    C. In a treatment room with the door closed in a neutral location
    D. In a quiet but public place to get assistance should it be required during the evaluation

35. The psychiatric-mental health nurse is providing psychoeducation on the relationship between neurophysiology and mental illness. Which area of the brain regulates appetite, the sleep–wake cycle, and libido?

    A. Hippocampus
    B. Amygdala
    C. Hypothalamus
    D. Limbic system

36. A patient is experiencing memory deficits, difficulty in prioritizing and planning, no insight into problems, and poor impulse control. A dysfunction in which lobe of the brain is most likely responsible for the symptoms?

    A. Parietal lobe
    B. Frontal lobe
    C. Temporal lobe
    D. Occipital lobe

37. A patient who was able to escape the World Trade Center on 9/11 is dysphoric several months after the event and tells the psychiatric-mental health nurse that she does not want to talk about her coworkers who were lost because it hurts so much. Which defense mechanism is being utilized?

    A. Denial
    B. Suppression
    C. Undoing
    D. Projection

38. In completing a magnetic resonance imaging (MRI) safety screening form, which of the following conditions, if noted in the patient's history, is a contraindication for brain MRI?

    A. Automated internal cardiac defibrillator (AICD)/pacemaker
    B. History of traumatic brain injury
    C. Hip replacement
    D. Pregnancy

39. A patient's mother is concerned about the attention-deficit hyperactivity disorder (ADHD) diagnosis given to her son and suspects something else might be wrong. He has a family history of bipolar disorder. Which of the following ADHD symptoms overlap with bipolar disorder in children and adolescents?

    A. Talkativeness, hyperactivity, and distractibility
    B. Insomnia, mood lability, and distractibility
    C. Irritability, talkativeness, and insomnia
    D. Sleep problems, irritability, and mood swings

40. A patient who is not willing to discuss his involvement in a psychological trauma is using which of the following defense mechanisms?

    A. Denial
    B. Suppression
    C. Projection
    D. Undoing

41. Which of the following is a defense mechanism purpose?

    A. Alert to danger
    B. Protect the Id
    C. Resolve conflicts
    D. Suppress intuition

42. A sole survivor from a house fire tells the psychiatric-mental health nurse that she does not remember anything about how she got out. Which defense mechanism is being used?

    A. Suppression
    B. Denial
    C. Repression
    D. Sublimation

43. A man finds his coworkers exceptionally difficult to work with, and he finds them generally incompetent. He does not share his thoughts with his coworkers or his boss out of fear of hurting their feelings. He suddenly has the urge to bring baked goods several times a week. Which defense mechanism best explains this behavior?

    A. Denial
    B. Suppression
    C. Repression
    D. Undoing

44. A 17-year-old male, high school senior who is on the wrestling team is being treated for an eating disorder. He is of average weight, socially engaged, attention seeking at times among his peers. Which of the following eating disorders is most consistent with these symptoms?

    A. Anxiety-induced eating disorder
    B. Binge eating disorder
    C. Bulimia nervosa
    D. Anorexia nervosa

45. Which of the following is the best intervention for a client experiencing ataque de nervios?

    A. Benzodiazepines
    B. Using a family member to interpret
    C. Involuntary admission
    D. Referral to supportive psychotherapy by a therapist who speaks the language

46. A psychiatric-mental health nurse is providing psychoeducation regarding psychotropic medications; they come with a black-box warning, particularly for use in children and young adults. What specific education must the psychiatric-mental health nurse provide to a 22-year-old male?

    A. Risk of increased impulsive behavior
    B. Risk of increased suicidal thoughts
    C. Risk of sexual side effects
    D. Risk of teratogenic sperm production

47. Which of the following is consistent with isolation as may be exhibited by someone with a Cluster C personality disorder?

    A. Not leaving the house for many days, declining social events
    B. Grandiose declarations of one's greatness
    C. Increased goal-directed behaviors
    D. Guarded and reluctant information sharing with flat affect

48. The psychiatric-mental health nurse is conducting a community teaching program to reduce the stigma of mental illness. Which of the following is considered a genetic and social risk factor for a person to develop antisocial personality disorder?

    A. Psychotic disorders
    B. Oppositional defiant disorder
    C. Generalized anxiety disorders
    D. Affective disorders

49. The psychiatric-mental health nurse is reviewing charts for an insurance company. According to the *DSM-5*, personality disorders are categorized according to which of the following?

    A. Axis II
    B. Axis III
    C. Axis IV
    D. In the primary psychiatric disorder

50. A psychiatric-mental health nurse is providing psychoeducation to an 8-year-old girl and her mother regarding stimulants for attention-deficit/hyperactivity disorder (ADHD). What assessments need to be completed before starting stimulant medication?

    A. The ADHD rating scale completed by the grandparents
    B. Rule out a family history of bipolar disorder
    C. Check blood pressure and pulse
    D. Blood pressure, pulse, height, weight, and 12-lead EKG

51. When precepting a new nurse, the psychiatric-mental health nurse explains the classification and traits of personality disorders. Which of the following personality disorders are classified as Cluster C?

    A. Paranoid personality disorder, schizoid personality disorder, schizotypal personality disorder
    B. Antisocial personality disorder, borderline personality disorder, histrionic personality disorder, narcissistic personality disorder
    C. Avoidant personality disorder, dependent personality disorder, obsessive compulsive personality disorder
    D. Paranoid personality disorder, antisocial personality disorder, obsessive compulsive personality disorder, histrionic personality disorder

52. A 35-year-old female with a Cluster A personality disorder states that "I hear people outside the office door during our sessions. Are they listening in on us?" What would be the psychiatric-mental health nurse's best response?

    A. Validate her and ask her to tell of a time in her life when she had a similar experience
    B. Using humor, ask a rhetorical question to stimulate reflection and then reassure her that she is that special
    C. Distract her from the topic and insist that there is no way for someone outside to hear your session
    D. Validate her and inform her that the white noise sound machine muffles the sounds of the session, and it would be hard to hear the conversation outside the office

53. When precepting a new nurse, the psychiatric-mental health nurse explains the classification and traits of personality disorders. Which of the following personality disorders are classified as Cluster A?

    A. Paranoid personality disorder, schizoid personality disorder, schizotypal personality disorder
    B. Antisocial personality disorder, borderline personality disorder, histrionic personality disorder, narcissistic personality disorder
    C. Avoidant personality disorder, dependent personality disorder, obsessive compulsive personality disorder
    D. Paranoid personality disorder, antisocial personality disorder, obsessive compulsive personality disorder, histrionic personality disorder

54. When providing psychotherapy to a 50-year-old man with a Cluster A personality disorder, what would be the best strategy?

    A. Do not challenge his negative views or recollections of past events
    B. Confront misinterpreted thoughts and feelings, especially those that are negative
    C. Make time for a detailed and emotionally engaging dialogue
    D. Deflate any grandiose thoughts he may have

55. What is the primary goal of psychotherapy when treating someone with a personality disorder?

    A. Enhance the client's ego strength and encourage the use of mature defense mechanisms
    B. Review the antecedents to this pathological personality development, paying particular attention to trauma
    C. Help parents and the client to form secure attachments
    D. Make the client change their personality so that they're more adaptable in everyday life

56. When precepting a new nurse, the psychiatric-mental health nurse explains the classification and traits of personality disorders. Which of the following personality disorders are classified as Cluster B?

   A. Paranoid personality disorder, schizoid personality disorder, schizotypal personality disorder
   B. Antisocial personality disorder, borderline personality disorder, histrionic personality disorder, narcissistic personality disorder
   C. Avoidant personality disorder, dependent personality disorder, obsessive compulsive personality disorder
   D. Paranoid personality disorder, antisocial personality disorder, obsessive compulsive personality disorder, histrionic personality disorder

57. During a session with a 17-year-old male with cannabis use disorder, who engages in petty theft and has refused school since 7th grade, the patient makes the following statement: "I don't know why I continue to see you, you just charge my parents so much money, and all I want to do is feel good." The psychiatric-mental health nurse replies, "You feel confused about the process." To which the boy replies, "I never thought I'd have a shrink come to my house." The psychiatric-mental health nurse then replies, "Thank you for allowing me into your home, and I recognize the courage it must have taken to allow this to happen." What motivational interviewing techniques are used in this dialogue?

   A. Affirming and reflecting
   B. Interrupting and reassuring
   C. Open-ended questions and summarizing
   D. Clarification and data collection

58. In working with a 34-year-old man initially seen for substance use disorder who continues in therapy to develop effective coping through the use of mature defense mechanisms, the patient states "I noticed your Rolex watch, is that new? You have exquisite taste." Which of the following is the best response from the psychiatric-mental health nurse?

   A. "You're right, I do."
   B. "I didn't realize you paid such close attention to what I wear."
   C. "I noticed you had a Rolex watch as well. How do you like it?"
   D. "It sounds like you value luxury items. Tell me more about that."

59. An RN from the detox unit reports to the psychiatric-mental health nurse that a 54-year-old man who was admitted 3 days ago for alcohol use disorder has a Clinical Institute Withdrawal Assessment (CIWA)-Alcohol score of 20. What action should the psychiatric-mental health nurse take first?

   A. Assess for hemodynamic stability and call the physician
   B. Administer 1 mg Ativan PO per standing order for withdrawal symptoms
   C. Reassure the patient that all will be well
   D. Review effective coping strategies with the client

60. The psychiatric-mental health nurse sees a 34-year-old male 2 weeks after an opioid detox. The patient states, "I feel like I'm going to die if I don't get something to relieve my symptoms." Which of the following would be the best response?

    A. "This feeling will pass, you just have to tolerate the discomfort for the short term."
    B. "Let me check your vital signs to see if you would be able to tolerate a clonidine patch."
    C. "You have been using OxyContin for a long time, and it will take several months for the withdrawal to end. In the meantime I should see you twice a week."
    D. "You are no longer in withdrawal as it has been 14 days since your last use and your urine tox screen is clean."

61. When asking an adolescent male about his cannabis use disorder, which of the following signs or symptoms would the psychiatric-mental health nurse expect him to report?

    A. Enhanced motor skills
    B. Accelerated time passage
    C. Heightened sensitivity to external stimuli
    D. Lower heart rate

62. The psychiatric-mental health nurse is providing psychotherapy for a patient with a personality disorder. Which of the following defense mechanisms are most commonly used in patients with Cluster C personality disorders?

    A. Displacement and reaction formation
    B. Motivation and disassociation
    C. Projection and distortion
    D. Isolation and intellectualization

63. A 23-year-old male with schizoaffective disorder and a history of four past hospitalizations for manic episodes has been started on clozapine. During the weekly complete blood count with differential, which of the following results would necessitate discontinuing treatment?

    A. Absolute neutrophil count (ANC) less than 2,000
    B. Leukocytes less than 5,000
    C. ANC less than 1,000
    D. Leukocytes less than 2,000 and ANC less than 1,200

64. David is a 43-year-old veteran of Operation Iraqi Freedom. A psychiatric-mental health nurse is currently providing psychotherapy for generalized anxiety disorder and major depressive disorder. During their last visit, the psychiatric-mental health nurse learned that David had a blast injury and sustained head trauma during his tour in Iraq. At the time, he was diagnosed with a traumatic brain injury. His current regimen includes fluoxetine 40 mg daily and clonazepam 1 mg twice daily. In light of this new information, what are some potential adverse effects?

    A. Benzodiazepines cause memory problems and confusion in clients with a history of traumatic brain injury
    B. Benzodiazepines increase the risk of a subsequent traumatic brain injury
    C. Benzodiazepines are addictive, and therefore banned from the Veterans' Affairs (VA) formulary
    D. Benzodiazepines lower the seizure threshold, particularly in clients with traumatic brain injury

65. One of the most common problems encountered by a psychiatric-mental health nurse in geriatric psychiatry is delirium. Why must the psychiatric-mental health nurse maintain a high index of suspicion for this condition?

    A. High risk of a 1-year mortality rate
    B. High risk for depression
    C. High risk for self-harm and harm to others
    D. High risk for persistent psychosis

66. A psychiatric-mental health nurse in private practice is experiencing feelings of resentment toward a patient who missed his last two appointments at the last minute because he forgot. Which of the following is an example of a therapeutic response?

    A. "You seem ambivalent about seeking treatment"
    B. "It's obvious you don't want to come for treatment"
    C. "You knew you would have to be charged for missed appointments"
    D. "Help me understand what's going on so we can figure out how to proceed"

67. When providing care to a patient who has been non-adherent with pharmacologic treatment for human immunodeficiency virus (HIV) or their mood disorder, which of the following is the best treatment for acquired immunodeficiency syndrome (AIDS)-related complex dementia?

    A. Anti-Parkinson agents
    B. Nonpharmacological supportive care
    C. Antiretroviral therapy
    D. Acetylcholinesterase inhibitors

68. A 42-year-old White female presents with concerns about her memory. She states that her grandmother experienced Alzheimer's dementia and that her 63-year-old mother, with obesity, hypertension, and depression, is also increasingly forgetful. The patient wants to do everything possible to prevent or significantly postpone the onset of dementia. She currently works full time, is the mother of two children, is president of the Parent-Teacher Association (PTA), attends church regularly, exercises three to four times a week, volunteers for various organizations, and is sexually active with her husband of 10 years. She occasionally forgets dates and misplaces things. What is the best response to this patient?

   A. "Continue your regular activities but be careful of the exercise, less because of injury to self but because a prolonged hospitalization and loss of independence would increase your risk for dementia."
   B. "We can start you on some fish oils, vitamin E supplements, and medication to enhance your memory."
   C. "While most brain development occurs early in life, we still form new brain cells in various areas of the brain throughout our lives. Continue with your activities because they offer the best protection of cognitive function."
   D. "Researchers know that we do continue to form new brain cells throughout the entire brain during adulthood. Keep up with your activities because you are producing new brain cells in the frontal lobe and this will decrease your risk of dementia."

69. In planning a therapeutic response consistent with the transtheoretical model, which stage of change is the patient in if they acknowledge there is a problem with their current behavior?

   A. Precontemplation
   B. Contemplation
   C. Preparing to take action
   D. Taking action

70. A psychiatric-mental health nurse is contracted to a student health clinic to work with incoming freshman and transfer students for several weeks. The psychiatric-mental health nurse encounters a student who describes himself as shy and uncomfortable in social situations. He reports having few friends in high school and has realized that he needs a few drinks to loosen up before going out to party. Upon further questioning, it is revealed he consistently drinks two to three beers on the weekend to enhance his socialization. According to the *DSM-5*, does this student have a mental illness?

   A. Yes, mild alcohol use disorder
   B. No, the student does not meet the criteria for mental illness
   C. Yes, adjustment disorder with mixed features
   D. Yes, social anxiety disorder

71. The psychiatric-mental health nurse is asked to review a medical malpractice case for merit focusing on the standard of care on an inpatient psychiatric unit in which a patient committed suicide. Which elements must be present to substantiate a claim of negligence?

    A. Deceit, breach of standards of care, and intent to harm
    B. Breach of care, violation of ethics, and patient abandonment
    C. Beneficence, nonmaleficence, veracity, and breach of standards
    D. Duty to care, breach of a standard of care, and injury related to the breach of the standard of care

72. Dialectical behavioral therapy (DBT) therapy involves reconciling the tension to find the truth between:

    A. Experience and avoidance
    B. Radical acceptance and change
    C. Crisis survival and radical acceptance
    D. Confrontation and avoidance

73. A 33-year-old married gay man employed as a corporate attorney wonders aloud to the PMHNP: "Things are going well in our relationship, our 8-year-old boy is about to enter third grade, our 6-year-old girl is entering first grade, my husband is a successful published author, but for some reason I don't feel happy. I think I have been depressed for much of my life." Which of the following demonstrates a core concept in transactional analysis (TA)?

    A. The patient may have experienced long periods of separation from his parents or guardians as a child, which may be affecting his ability to accept love and experience happiness
    B. The patient may have experienced an event that forced him into a parentified role
    C. The patient may have a distorted thought pattern affecting interpersonal relationships
    D. The patient may have had a traumatic event in his childhood in which thoughts and feelings have become locked together and are inaccessible to the conscious mind

74. A psychiatric-mental health nurse has been appointed to a community board tasked with conducting a risk–benefit analysis regarding healthcare resource utilization in the planning of a psychosocial clubhouse for an at-risk population. What are two economic concepts that must be considered in allocating public funds to demonstrate a return on investment and access to care with the greatest number of people?

    A. Affordability and quality
    B. Equity and efficiency
    C. Cost and benefits
    D. Opportunities and risks

75. The psychiatric-mental health nurse will provide psychoeducation regarding antipsychotic medications. Which of the following best summarizes the evidence-based practice guidelines regarding the initiation of antipsychotic medication?

   A. Physical exam to include blood glucose, lipid profile, height and weight, blood pressure, waist circumference, and a review of cardiovascular risk factors and the family history
   B. Physical exam to include a comprehensive metabolic panel, body mass index, complete blood count, and thyroid function
   C. Serum glucose or hemoglobin A1C, lipid profile, weight, body mass index, blood pressure, waist circumference, and review of family cardiovascular disease
   D. Serum glucose, complete blood count, assessment of family history regarding cardiovascular disease, and cancer

76. A 59-year-old man has been seeing the psychiatric-mental health nurse for schizophrenia. He was first diagnosed when he was 21 years old. He remains medication compliant. In getting to know the patient, it is revealed that he has very few social interactions, prefers to be alone, and has never had a romantic interest or desire to pursue one. Which type of symptoms has persisted in this clinical course?

   A. Affective disorder
   B. Positive symptoms
   C. Negative symptoms
   D. Self-care deficit

77. Which of the following hallucinations is more common in patients with an organic etiology such as substance-induced altered mental status or delirium rather than in patients with psychosis such as schizophrenia, schizophreniform disorder, and brief psychotic episode?

   A. Tactile hallucinations
   B. Auditory hallucinations
   C. Visual hallucinations
   D. Combined hallucinations

78. A psychiatric-mental health nurse would like to start a fee-for-service model specifically targeting patients recently discharged from the hospital after their first manic episode or with a diagnosis of bipolar disorder with the goal of reducing recidivism through medication compliance and administering long-acting injectable medications. This service is an example of which kind of prevention strategy?

   A. Primary prevention
   B. Secondary prevention
   C. Tertiary prevention
   D. Acute treatment

79. A middle-aged married man has been attending a psychoeducation group for people with mood disorders. During a session, he reports his symptoms include fatigue throughout the day, leading him to drink five to six cups of coffee daily to stay awake; this leads to him feeling too wired to sleep at night. He drinks one to two drinks every night. He has no trouble falling asleep. However, his wife kicks him due to his snoring and describes him as a restless sleeper, and he also sweats profusely every night. Which of the following suggestions should the psychiatric-mental health nurse offer this client?

   A. Coping strategies for attention deficit disorder which he is medicating with caffeine
   B. Refer him to addiction and detox treatment for alcohol withdrawal syndrome
   C. Coping strategies to reduce caffeine use
   D. Encourage an appointment with a psychiatrist or psychiatric-mental health nurse practitioner for obstructive sleep apnea

80. An 88-year-old female is prescribed fluvoxamine for generalized anxiety disorder. Which of the following must the psychiatric-mental health nurse be cognizant of in elderly patients?

   A. Drugs are metabolized more slowly through the liver
   B. Treatment is shorter in duration
   C. The therapeutic dose is higher than for children
   D. Titration should be faster to delay first-pass effects

81. A 36-year-old female reports increasing fatigue, decreased energy, difficulty concentrating, sleepiness throughout the day, and anhedonia. The most bothersome symptom was the impaired concentration. She was started on venlafaxine 37.5 mg once daily 1 week ago by her primary care provider and referred to the psychiatric-mental health nurse as a bridge until she can see a psychiatrist. During the evaluation, the psychiatric-mental health nurse notes pressured speech, her affect is expansive, she continues to report difficulty sleeping but states her energy is terrific, and she can "get so much done." Which of the following is a plausible explanation for this clinical presentation?

   A. She is psychotic
   B. She has become euthymic
   C. She is hypomanic
   D. These are adverse effects of venlafaxine

82. A board-certified psychiatric-mental health nurse is working in a rural critical access hospital-based clinic and providing psychoeducation regarding medication management for a patient with bipolar 2 disorder, who has comorbid hypertension. When checking his blood pressure, the psychiatric-mental health nurse notes that the client is hypertensive, and upon further questioning, the client states he has not seen his primary care provider for 9 months because he finds the cost of the visit and the medication prohibitive. What is the most appropriate action?

   A. Call the pharmacy to confirm the medication and dosage and ask for a refill for 1 month until the patient can see his primary care provider
   B. Advise the patient to go to the emergency department if any signs and symptoms develop
   C. Send the patient to urgent care for and refill of the antihypertensive medication
   D. Call the patient's primary care provider to explain the situation, coordinate an appointment, and plan for medication refills

83. According to the American Nurses Association position statement, which of the following is aimed at reducing human error and creating an open and fair environment for interprofessional equality and collaboration to promote patient safety?

   A. Just culture
   B. Personnel policies and HIV in the workplace
   C. Standardization of health information technology
   D. Civil disobedience

84. When a patient is treated over objection by court order, which ethical principle has been trumped?

   A. Beneficence
   B. Justice
   C. Nonmaleficence
   D. Autonomy

85. A psychiatric-mental health nurse is opening a private practice and decided to offer free screening for depression in her local church during their annual health fair. Testing for disease is an example of which kind of prevention category?

   A. Primary prevention
   B. Secondary prevention
   C. Tertiary prevention
   D. Preventive care

86. A nonprofit organization would like to develop a vaccination program, but the grant organization requires an integrative care approach, and they have selected a psychiatric-mental health nurse from the visiting nurse service to sit on this task force. Vaccination programs are an example of which kind of prevention category?

    A. Preventive care
    B. Primary prevention
    C. Secondary prevention
    D. Tertiary prevention

87. What is the process by which the psychiatric-mental health nurse identifies signs and symptoms of mental illness and provides essential psychiatric nursing care?

    A. Psychiatric interview
    B. Physical examination
    C. Interdisciplinary treatment planning
    D. Neurological examination

88. The psychiatric-mental health nurse is working in a movement disorders clinic due to the incidence of depression and dementia associated with Parkinson's disease. The patient is unable to shrug his shoulders. Which cranial nerve might be affected?

    A. XII
    B. XI
    C. IX
    D. V

89. The psychiatric-mental health nurse is seeing a 10-year-old boy for supportive psychotherapy and anticipatory guidance for a diagnosis attention-deficit/hyperactivity disorder (ADHD). The boy has been experiencing increasing anxiety leading up to his visit with his pediatric nurse practitioner, who is planning to give him the human papillomavirus (HPV) vaccine. The mother would like to relieve the anxiety by just skipping the vaccine. She asks the psychiatric-mental health nurse during their session "why would a boy even need the shot?" The best response is:

    A. "My son received the vaccine at 10 too, and it was not that bad"
    B. "The Centers for Disease Control and Prevention recommends it, but every parent has the right to choose what is best for their child, so you can refuse it for him"
    C. "The Centers for Disease Control and Prevention recommends the human papillomavirus (HPV) vaccine for all children at age 10 because HPV can cause cancer in both men and women. The vaccine protects against the three most common forms of the virus. What is your concern?"
    D. "There will be many anxiety-causing things in life that he will have to face; he should start now"

90. The psychiatric-mental health nurse is evaluating a man who reveals that his girl-friend screams at him and has repeatedly slapped, kicked, and tripped him down the stairs. He states that she has also thrown things at him, including a plate, a glass of wine, and once even hitting their 3-year-old son inadvertently. What duty does the psychiatric-mental health nurse have concerning reporting this to child protective services?

   A. No duty; the child is not the patient
   B. Yes, the psychiatric-mental health nurse must report
   C. Nothing to report because the assault on the child was inadvertent
   D. Safer not to notify child protective services because the violence may escalate

91. Which cranial nerve is the psychiatric-mental health nurse assessing when the patient is asked to stick out their tongue?

   A. II-optic nerve
   B. III-oculomotor nerve
   C. X-vagus nerve
   D. XII-hypoglossal nerve

92. The psychiatric-mental health nurse is conducting a mental status exam and notes that the patient is speaking loudly but non-pressured. Which cranial nerve may be affected and warrant further investigation?

   A. Optic
   B. Trigeminal
   C. Vestibulocochlear
   D. Facial

93. When reviewing the results of the mini-mental status exam of a 70-year-old woman, the psychiatric-mental health nurse notes that the score is 18. How should this test be interpreted?

   A. Severe dementia
   B. Mild cognitive impairment
   C. Moderate cognitive impairment
   D. Normal exam

94. The psychiatric-mental health nurse observes the newly admitted patient as having ideas of reference. Which of the following statements would lead the psychiatric-mental health nurse to make this assessment?

   A. "The people on television are talking to me."
   B. "The voice in my head is telling me I should die."
   C. "I see little people at the end of my bed."
   D. "You think people are watching us?"

95. A psychiatric-mental health nurse on a disaster response team deployed to a mass casualty. In the immediate aftermath of a school shooting which of the following is the priority crisis intervention assessment?

   A. Current living situation and coping skills
   B. Immediate safety of people involved
   C. Quickly gather collateral information on each victim
   D. Assess for allergies to medications for all victims involved

96. A psychiatric-mental health nurse working in the subspecialty of addictions may often refer clients to Alcoholics Anonymous and Narcotics Anonymous meetings. Which of the following therapeutic factors emerge in peer-led groups, according to Yalom's group dynamics process?

   A. Reflection on existential matters
   B. Psychological relief
   C. Peer support
   D. Hopefulness

97. In a closed therapy group for adults dealing with a family of origin conflict issue, members have begun to model aspects of other group members and the group leader. Which group dynamic has manifested?

   A. Imitative behavior
   B. Confrontational behavior
   C. Avoidant behavior
   D. Mocking behavior

98. In planning for the aftercare of the patient who is treated for schizophrenia, the nurse reads the PPD at 10-mm induration on his tuberculosis skin test. What is the next action for the psychiatric-mental health nurse to take?

   A. Order a STAT chest x-ray to rule out tuberculosis
   B. Cancel the discharge and repeat the test in 2 weeks
   C. Order acid-fast bacilli sputum
   D. Continue with the discharge as the test is negative

99. In cognitive behavioral therapy, it is often helpful to prescribe the symptom that is bothersome as the treatment. This is known as a paradoxical directive. In which type of therapy would a paradoxical directive be utilized?

   A. Psychoanalysis
   B. Narrative therapy
   C. Strategic therapy
   D. Psychodynamic therapy

100. The psychiatric-mental health nurse understands that elements of cognitive behavioral therapy (CBT) inform dialectical behavioral therapy (DBT). Which of the following are characteristic of DBT?

   A. Mindfulness, meditation, and emotional regulation
   B. Systematic desensitization, reintegration, and attachment
   C. Harm reduction, systematic desensitization, and aversion therapy
   D. Aversion therapy, mindfulness, and systematic desensitization

101. The psychiatric-mental health nurse is completing an intake interview on a homeless man with schizophrenia. She notes that the patient is scratching his arms and legs during the interview. When the patient rolls up his sleeves, she notices multiple papules and vesicles with an excoriated maculopapular rash around the webs of his fingers. Which action should the psychiatric-mental health nurse take?

   A. Place the patient on contact isolation for possible scabies
   B. Call the doctor for antibiotics for impetigo
   C. Place the patient on airborne and contact precautions for shingles
   D. Apply moisturizer for dermatitis

102. A patient who has been diagnosed with microcytic hypochromic anemia for 3 years may have which of the following symptoms?

   A. Irritability
   B. Pallor
   C. Fatigue
   D. Pica

103. A patient has been started on valproic acid for the management of his mood disorder. On rounds, the psychiatric-mental health nurse notices altered mental status and asterixis. After notifying the psychiatrist, what tests would the psychiatric-mental health nurse expect to be ordered?

   A. Magnetic resonance imaging (MRI) of the brain with and without contrast
   B. Liver function and ammonia level
   C. Renal function and complete blood count
   D. Heart enzymes

104. Which of the following patients is at the lowest risk for suicide?

   A. A 60-year-old White man who was recently laid off
   B. A 25-year-old male with bipolar disorder and substance use disorder
   C. A 45-year-old woman with a major depressive disorder whose mother committed suicide
   D. A 16-year-old boy with only one close friend with whom he likes to hunt

105. The patient has been on lithium for 6 months and has had a level of 0.8. What test would the psychiatric-mental health nurse expect to be checked in addition to renal function labs?

    A. Thyroid function
    B. Liver function
    C. Cardiac enzymes
    D. 12-lead EKG

106. A 50-year-old female with no past psychiatric history referred by her physician for psychiatric issues reports new gradual onset of cyclical mood swings. She reports that she can sleep through the night, except sometimes she awakens to find herself in a pool of sweat. The symptoms began gradually about 5 months ago. She also reports her periods have been irregular most of her life. What would be the best intervention?

    A. Psychoeducation regarding mood stabilizers
    B. Psychoeducation regarding antidepressants
    C. Anticipatory guidance regarding normal physiological changes with age
    D. Psychoeducation regarding how emotions cause physical symptoms

107. A 40-year-old man who is HIV positive has a 10-mm induration from his Mantoux test. What should the psychiatric-mental health nurse do next?

    A. Notify the nurse practitioner
    B. Do nothing; this test is negative
    C. Put the patient on airborne precautions
    D. Request transfer the patient to the medical service

108. The psychiatric-mental health nurse would expect which of the following tests done at baseline when starting the patient on lithium for bipolar disorder?

    A. Cardiac enzymes
    B. Renal function
    C. Liver function
    D. Complete blood count

109. A 38-year-old man with Down syndrome begins to develop cognitive impairment, particularly in his daily routines. His primary care provider completed a history and physical with unremarkable findings. For which of the following conditions should the psychiatric-mental health nurse provide supportive psychotherapy?

    A. Delirium
    B. Alzheimer's disease
    C. Cerebrovascular accident
    D. Attention-deficit hyperactivity disorder (ADHD)

110. Which of the following is a breach of medical confidentiality?

    A. Releasing records to an insurance company
    B. Releasing records under subpoena
    C. Notifying the public health department of a reportable disease
    D. Disclosing a diagnosis to the spouse

111. The purpose of board certification for the psychiatric-mental health nurse is to:

    A. Convey expertise in the field of psychiatric mental health
    B. To restrict access to care
    C. To preserve the reimbursement structure
    D. To encourage litigation

112. In providing anticipatory guidance to a loved one of an elderly woman who is suspected of having dementia, what is the best initial method for assessing for signs and symptoms consistent with this condition?

    A. Magnetic resonance imaging (MRI) of the brain
    B. Comprehensive psychiatric evaluation with collateral information
    C. Positron emission tomography (PET) scan of the brain
    D. Electroencephalogram (EEG)

113. The practice of a professional registered nurse is regulated by the:

    A. State Nurse Practice Act
    B. Medicare regulations
    C. Collaborating physician
    D. Institution in which they practice

114. Which of the following psychopharmacologic agents should the nurse focus on for patients in a support group for obsessive compulsive disorder in high doses of monotherapy?

    A. Tricyclic antidepressants
    B. Benzodiazepines
    C. Antipsychotics
    D. Selective serotonin reuptake inhibitors

115. The psychiatric-mental health nurse is providing peer education to colleagues regarding geriatric psychopharmacology. Which of the following medications is most likely to cause delirium in the elderly?

    A. Diphenhydramine, digoxin, oxybutynin
    B. Ibuprofen, acetaminophen, omeprazole
    C. Docusate, psyllium, senna
    D. Penicillin, cephalosporins, aminoglycosides

116. A 62-year-old female is recently diagnosed with obsessive compulsive disorder. Which of the following symptoms are characteristic of the obsession?

A. Handwashing
B. Checking the gas
C. Anxiety
D. Rumination

117. A patient with a history of alcohol use disorder tells the psychiatric-mental health nurse during his admission to rehabilitation that the Sinclair method is what he prefers rather than a monthly injection. Which of the following best describes the patient's preferred method?

A. Every day
B. 1 hour before intended alcohol use
C. Monthly
D. Daily Antabuse

118. In conducting a community education intervention, which of the findings in a patient's history would reduce the likelihood of elder abuse?

A. Delayed medical care
B. New-onset sexually transmitted infection
C. Patients over 80 years of age with a high care burden
D. A consistent and attentive caretaker

119. In conducting a community outreach at a local church, the psychiatric-mental health nurse informs attendees that the most common form of dementia in the United States is:

A. Multi-infarct dementia
B. Alzheimer's disease
C. Frontotemporal dementia
D. Parkinson's dementia

120. A patient with post-traumatic stress disorder (PTSD) reports middle insomnia secondary to nightmares. Which pharmacological class is used specifically to treat this symptom?

A. Selective serotonin reuptake inhibitors (SSRIs)
B. Alpha blockers
C. Beta blockers
D. Benzodiazepines

121. A daughter is concerned that her mother may have dementia. Which of the following criteria distinguishes delirium from dementia?

    A. Rate of onset
    B. Confusion
    C. Persistence of symptoms
    D. Cognitive impairment

122. A patient presents to the emergency department with abdominal pain in the epigastric and left upper quadrant. He has history of alcohol use disorder, increasing his risk of pancreatitis. Which of the following would indicate this finding?

    A. Renal function
    B. Blood alcohol level
    C. Serum lipase
    D. Brain natriuretic peptide

123. A 36-year-old investment banker has been experiencing chest tightness, palpitations, and diaphoresis. He has had these symptoms three times in the last 3 months. Each time, he calls 911 and gets admitted. Myocardial infarction is ruled out, and his findings are unremarkable. Which of the following conditions should psychoeducational interventions target?

    A. Generalized anxiety disorder
    B. Panic disorder
    C. Factitious disorder
    D. Malingering

124. The psychiatric-mental health nurse is providing psychoeducation for a newly diagnosed patient with schizophrenia. Which of the following symptoms offers the patient a better prognosis?

    A. Persistent flat or blunted affect
    B. Persistent apathy or anhedonia
    C. High premorbid and social functioning
    D. Delayed onset of psychotic symptoms

125. The psychiatric-mental health nurse is admitting a patient who is homeless and has a diagnosis of schizophrenia. The patient is complaining of insects infesting his arms. Which of the following actions should the psychiatric-mental health nurse take first?

    A. Administer olanzapine 5 mg by mouth for tactile hallucinations
    B. Check the client's body for signs of infestation
    C. Explain to the client that his hallucination is not real
    D. Collect urine for a toxicology screening

126. How should the psychiatric-mental health nurse respond to a patient who exclaims, "I see dead people"?

   A. "A dead person can't walk around"
   B. "Why do you think you see dead people?"
   C. "That must be frightening as it seems so real, but I don't see dead people"
   D. "I don't see the dead people that you're talking about"

127. A psychiatric-mental health nurse is performing psychoeducation to a group of parents with children who have been diagnosed with schizophrenia. Which of the following symptoms experienced by the client would predict a poor prognosis?

   A. Having little or no interest in work or social activities
   B. Continuously repeating words and phrases
   C. Thinking that people on television are talking about them
   D. Hearing command auditory hallucinations

128. A patient who was admitted to the inpatient psychiatric unit appears hypervigilant and scanning the environment. What should the psychiatric-mental health nurse do with regard to the client's behavior?

   A. Place the patient in therapeutic seclusion
   B. Help the patient formulate a discharge plan
   C. Establish a therapeutic relationship with the client
   D. Teach the patient about the importance of medication adherence

129. Which of the following interventions is an example of milieu therapy?

   A. Expressly stating the rules of the group while allowing for peer pressure to govern social interactions
   B. Providing family therapy and facilitating effective coping mechanisms for life stressors
   C. Engaging in individual therapy to explore family dynamics
   D. Engaging in role-play to enhance interpersonal skills

130. The psychiatric-mental health nurse is caring for a patient with paranoid schizophrenia on an inpatient unit. Which of the following actions would help reduce the patient's distress?

   A. Place the patient on 1:1 observation changing the mental health worker every hour, so the patient learns to trust the staff
   B. Place the patient on 1:1 observation with a consistent staff member
   C. Encourage the patient to attend all group activities
   D. Teach the client that his paranoia is causing anxiety

131. A 36-year-old dentist who has never received psychiatric care in the past presents at the prompting of his wife so that the patient can deal with his issues. Which of the following statements regarding psychotherapy should the psychiatric-mental health nurse tell this prospective client?

   A. Rapid improvement can be expected with immediate psychotherapy
   B. Major changes will happen in the brain in the acute phase of psychotherapy
   C. Psychotherapy requires a lot of patience, and his clients often relapse in the process
   D. Psychotherapy is a short-term intervention that is rarely successful

132. Which of the following psychotherapeutic interventions is most appropriate for a patient diagnosed with schizophrenia?

   A. The psychiatric-mental health nurse should establish a relationship that is respectful of the client's dignity
   B. The nurse should convey closeness with the client in order to decrease their suspiciousness
   C. The nurse should befriend the patient to reduce social isolation
   D. The nurse should exhibit paternalism to ensure adherence to medication

133. A patient is expressing their delusions to the psychiatric-mental health nurse. What should be the first intervention to address the problem?

   A. Reorient the patient and help them test reality
   B. Specifically state the delusion is false
   C. Present a logical argument to refute the delusion
   D. Thank the client for trusting you enough to share their delusional thought

134. Which of the following interventions demonstrates a behavioral therapy approach?

   A. Encouraging discussions of feelings
   B. Establishing therapeutic alliance
   C. Attaching consequences to coping mechanisms
   D. Providing psychoeducation about psychotropic medications

135. The psychiatric-mental health nurse is facilitating a group for patients with personality disorder traits. A member of the group asks, "Does being diagnosed with schizoid personality disorder mean that I will develop schizophrenia?" Which response would be the most appropriate?

   A. Tell me more about what you know of schizophrenia
   B. Some clients who developed schizophrenia have had schizoid personality traits early on
   C. Not all people with schizoid personality disorder go on to develop schizophrenia
   D. You seem upset about the possibility of developing schizophrenia

136. A patient was admitted this afternoon to inpatient psychiatry ward on voluntary status. He states that he has been known to sleepwalk, particularly at times of increased stress. Which of the following actions should the psychiatric-mental health nurse take?

   A. Apply a bed alarm
   B. Encourage bedtime exercise routine
   C. Limit caffeine
   D. Encourage sleep hygiene

137. The psychiatric-mental health nurse is facilitating a psychoeducation group. A client who has been admitted to alcohol rehab states that he "used to get lit off of a 6-pack," and now he needs to "down a case" to "feel the same." What would be the best response?

   A. Explain the process of alcohol withdrawal
   B. Explain the effects of tolerance and how it indicates alcohol use disorder
   C. Reframe the client's statement and highlight how he is minimizing the reality of his disorder
   D. Directly confront the client regarding misinformation

138. A client has a diagnosis of mood disorder and expresses low self-worth. Which of the following actions should the psychiatric-mental health nurse take?

   A. Encourage group attendance
   B. Engage in role-play to promote assertiveness
   C. Tell the client to journal daily to analyze her feelings
   D. Refocus on the client's objective accomplishments and past struggles that have been overcome

139. When teaching a client about psychopharmacology principles in general, which of the following is most important to include?

   A. Avoid alcohol while taking medication due to risk of addiction
   B. Take the medication exactly as prescribed as onset of actions can be delayed as much as 3 weeks
   C. Pay close attention to feelings between visits so medication can be increased as needed
   D. It is essential to have monthly labs for antidepressants to avoid toxicity

140. A patient abruptly stopped taking his alprazolam after a year of daily use. Which of the following signs or symptoms would the patient report or the psychiatric-mental health nurse observe?

   A. Increased sedation
   B. Diarrhea
   C. Piloerection
   D. Tremor

141. A 36-year-old man with a history of sexual abuse in childhood while working on the set of a television show becomes triggered whenever he sees reruns of the show come on. He has a diagnosis of post-traumatic stress disorder and reports his current anxiety as a 10 out of 10 because he has learned there will be a marathon airing of his show. Which of the following medications would most likely be prescribed?

   A. Lexapro
   B. Clozapine
   C. Ativan
   D. Lithium

142. A patient reports symptoms to the triage nurse, including not eating very much lately, increasing irritability, lack of interest, depressed mood, and poor sleep. Which of the following actions should the psychiatric-mental health nurse take first?

   A. Triage the patient to psychiatry for evaluation
   B. Complete a focused physical exam of the cardiopulmonary system including vital signs
   C. Triage the patient to 1:1 observation pending psychiatric evaluation
   D. Put the patient in a room alone and remove all harmful objects

143. A patient diagnosed with generalized anxiety disorder has been prescribed escitalopram 10 mg daily and gabapentin 300 mg at bedtime. Which of the following statements, if made by the patient, indicates that the psychoeducation was effective?

   A. The patient states he can have two drinks with the gabapentin if he cannot sleep
   B. The patient states it may take several weeks to achieve the anti-anxiety effect of the Lexapro
   C. The patient states that he can take an extra gabapentin when he feels a panic attack
   D. The patient states the Lexapro should work within a few days

144. A patient reporting headaches, blindness, and palpitations is admitted to psychiatry for anxiety. Which of the following actions should the psychiatric-mental health nurse take first?

   A. Place the patient in therapeutic seclusion
   B. Encourage the patient to express their feelings
   C. Encourage the patient to attend groups
   D. Sit with the patient and engage them with a calm and directive approach

145. The psychiatric-mental health nurse is evaluating a patient with polysubstance use disorder. Which of the following actions would help validate the patient's reporting of the history of present illness?

    A. Instructing the patient on the adverse effects of illicit drug use
    B. After obtaining consent, corroborate the information with others who know the patient
    C. Clearly document the patient's report of history of present illness
    D. Teach the client what he can expect during the detox process

146. A patient reports poor appetite, poor sleep, difficulty concentrating, and anhedonia. The psychiatric-mental health nurse is administering trazodone 100 mg as ordered. The patient states that he is not depressed. What is the best response by the psychiatric-mental health nurse?

    A. "Trazadone is known to exert a sedating effect which can help with your poor sleep"
    B. "Trazadone is an antidepressant that can stimulate your appetite"
    C. "Trazadone is an antipsychotic which can help with your bedtime anxiety"
    D. "Trazadone is an antianxiety medication to reduce your nighttime restlessness"

147. The psychiatric-mental health nurse is providing information regarding alcohol use disorder and recovery. Which of the following statements made by a client indicates that the learning has occurred?

    A. "Al-Anon can be helpful in my recovery process"
    B. "Once I have gone through detox my recovery is complete"
    C. "I realize that recovery is a lifelong process"
    D. "I know that the goal of recovery is to reduce my drinking"

148. Which of the following patients should the psychiatric-mental health nurse attend to first?

    A. A 31-year-old male with rapid, pressured speech and poor personal boundaries
    B. A 62-year-old woman expresses homicidal ideations toward the president of the United States
    C. A 25-year-old man who has only slept for 2 hours for the last three nights
    D. A 40-year-old woman who isolates and refuses to go to groups

149. A Vietnamese woman who has struggled with generalized anxiety disorder has recently moved to a new city in North America. She is surprised and cries when her neighbors sent a bouquet of flowers. Which of the following response by the psychiatric-mental health nurse is best?

   A. "What do flowers mean in your culture?"
   B. "It seems you have very friendly neighbors"
   C. "Do you hate flowers?"
   D. "You seem touched by your neighbor's generosity"

150. A patient reports multiple somatic complaints and feeling hopeless, helpless, and screaming at times. What action should the psychiatric-mental health nurse take?

   A. Help the patient test reality by connecting consequences with impulsive behaviors
   B. Help the patient complete activities of daily living
   C. Have the patient express their feelings
   D. Teach the patient to reframe her thoughts

Practice Test Answers

1. C) In a professional relationship, the primary focus is on the client and their needs
Professional relationships are focused exclusively on the client's needs and outcomes. Professional relationships should not include advice based on personal experience. The responsibility for the client's well-being is shared between the patient and the treatment team. Professionals should not exploit the therapeutic relationship for personal favors.

2. A) A skills class for at-risk adolescents
A skills class for at-risk individuals is an example of primary prevention. The suicide hotline is an example of secondary prevention because a specific condition with specific interventions is aimed at reducing a specific risk outcome. Mandated treatment and a psychosocial clubhouse are tertiary prevention strategies because they are aimed at improving outcomes and reducing symptoms of a condition that has already occurred.

3. D) Explain that the patient cannot leave until further assessments are completed, and collateral information is obtained
Explain that the patient cannot leave until further assessment and collateral information is obtained with the aim of seeing if she will agree to remain on a voluntary basis. Discharging the patient immediately without further assessment information may increase the risk of suicide. Before the patient signs out against medical advice, further assessment is required for capacity to refuse care. Converting the patient to involuntary status requires further assessment.

4. A) Define the roles and actions for that particular profession
The scope and standards dictated by professional organizations define the role and actions of a particular profession. The government appoints professional boards to define the differences between professions, establish criteria for licensure, and define the legal statutes that govern a profession.

5. B) Psychiatric clients can refuse treatment unless it is court-ordered
The court order trumps the patient's right to exercise self-determination, and the patient cannot refuse treatment. Until the court orders treatment over objection, the psychiatric client may refuse treatment unless the condition imminently threatens life or limb. The professional judgment of two physicians does not allow for treatment unless there is an imminent threat, in which case one opinion is sufficient.

6. B) Major depression
Major depressive symptoms include sleep changes, interest loss, guilt, energy deficit, cognitive impairment, appetite change, psychomotor agitation/retardation, and somatic complaints often comorbid with type 2 diabetes. Dysthymia is associated with anhedonia, hopelessness, lack of productivity, and low self-esteem, with feelings of inadequacy lasting for at least 2 years. Generalized anxiety disorder symptoms include persistent worrying, catastrophic thinking, persistent ambivalence, restlessness, persistent fatigue, and muscle tension. Seasonal affective disorder symptoms include a change in sleep, loss of interest, anhedonia, and cognitive impairment occurring in the fall or winter and remitting in the spring and summer.

7. D) Primary prevention
Primary prevention aims to reduce the incidence of a disease or condition. Secondary prevention aims to detect the presence of a condition early and prevent it from getting worse. Tertiary prevention aims to enhance the quality of life after the disease or condition has occurred. Solution-focused therapy is a counseling approach that assumes the individual has the capacity to articulate a problem and offer solutions.

8. B) "You are the only person who has been helpful to me"
The therapeutic alliance requires genuineness, acceptance, and authenticity reflected in the patient's statement. The other responses indicate continued resistance, dismissiveness, and unwillingness to engage in therapy.

9. B) Psychic determinism principle
Psychic determinism is the psychodynamic principle that assumes all behavior has a purpose. The Ego development principle states that one understands that others have needs and that impulsive actions can cause self-harm. The Id principle seeks pleasure and gratification immediately. The Superego imposes a moral framework, and ethical restraint learned from the environment.

10. D) Regression
Regression is a defense mechanism where the person moves back to a previous phase of psychological development and task mastery. Repression is a defense mechanism in which disturbing thoughts are kept from consciousness. Denial is a defense mechanism that involves blocking external events from awareness. Projection is a defense mechanism involving the attribution of one's own unacceptable thoughts, feelings, and motives to another person.

11. C) A normal resistance seen in the termination time of therapy
Regression is a temporary defense mechanism in response to stress in order to avoid circumstances. Projection is a defense mechanism in response to a stressor in which the patient would tell the psychiatric-mental health nurse they are ending therapy because they cannot be helped. It is common for patients to relapse with symptoms during the termination phase.

12. C) "I have started baking scones for my irritating coworkers"

An example of altruism is a client who states the well-being of others is equally important as his own and perhaps even more important in certain situations. Option A is an example of projection; another example would be a husband who has an anger problem attributing his anger to his wife and saying she has an anger problem. Option B is an example of repression; another example would be a client who has suffered abuse and neglect as a child but has no recollection and has trouble forming relationships. Option D is an example of regression; another example is a woman who is chewing on a pen cap while waiting for the results of a pregnancy test.

13. B) Industry versus inferiority

Industry versus inferiority is the stage of development when children learn skills, take pride in their accomplishments, and develop self-esteem from being valued by peers for their competencies. Trust versus mistrust is the first stage of development; if needs are not met in this phase, the person demonstrates suspiciousness and anxiety over their ability to effect change in their life. Generativity versus stagnation is an adult phase of development in which the individual is concerned with leaving a good lasting impression; success in this stage yields a sense of accomplishment and failure leads to a feeling of low self-worth and apathy. Integrity versus despair is the final stage of development in which the individual contemplates accomplishments; a failure in this phase leads to feelings of guilt and hopelessness.

14. B) Hemodynamic stability

Hemodynamic stability is the priority in any patient assessment. The current level of suicidality and effective coping mechanisms is the next priority, followed by past medical and psychiatric history.

15. B) Strategic therapy

Strategic therapy is a short-term problem focused on an interventional approach to treatment. Experiential therapy is a technique that uses expressive tools and activities to recreate emotional situations from the past or present so they can be resolved in a less threatening manner. Structural therapy is a treatment that addresses patterns of interaction that cause conflict within a family system. Solution-focused therapy aims to enhance individual strengths, and past successes are used to build communal self-efficacy within the family system. Tools include the miracle question, scaling questions, and coping questions.

16. C) Difficulty in overdosing for suicidal patients

Selective serotonin reuptake inhibitor (SSRI) medications are difficult to overdose on and are among the safest psychotropic medications. SSRIs may be activating and impair sleep during periods of titration. SSRI dosing and titration are based on the therapeutic response and tolerability of side effects. SSRI drug levels are not correlated with therapeutic efficacy.

17. C) Stability in the interpersonal relationships despite dysfunctions
Homeostasis is characterized by stability within interpersonal relationships despite individual dysfunctions. Placating, appeasing, erratic behavior, emotional manipulation leading to crisis, and then peace are all examples of a volatile family system.

18. D) A standardized rating scale for depression
A standardized rating scale is the best way to quantify treatment efficacy. Diagnostic tests do not indicate the efficacy of SSRIs. Urine toxicology screening indicates the presence of drugs of abuse.

19. B) Recognizing and changing automatic thoughts
Recognizing and changing automatic thoughts are essential elements of cognitive behavioral therapy (CBT) cognitive restructuring. Acknowledging and accepting automatic thoughts is the problem CBT aims to solve. The psychiatric-mental health nurse should invite perspective rather than impose perspective through Socratic questioning. Environmental restructuring is not a CBT principle.

20. C) Solution-focused therapy
Solution-focused therapy is a goal-directed collaborative approach to motivate psychotherapeutic change and is conducted through direct observation to a series of precisely constructed questions. Cognitive behavioral therapy focuses on challenging and changing cognitive distortions, behaviors, and feelings with personal coping strategies targeting a current problem. Dialectical behavioral therapy is a skill-based approach that focuses on four main areas: emotional regulation, improving distress tolerance, mindfulness, and interpersonal effectiveness. Psychoanalysis is a therapeutic approach that focuses on the interaction of the conscious and unconscious mind that is presumed to be motivating present behavior.

21. B) Tolerance
Tolerance is characterized by a diminished response to a drug, which occurs in response to continued presence. Potency refers to the amount of drug needed to produce an effect. Kindling is the metaphorical theory that small neurobiological reactions lead to full-blown disorders. Addiction is the physiological and psychological dependence on a substance leading to persistent use despite adverse consequences.

22. B) Lithium (Ebstein's anomaly); divalproex (neural tube defects)
Tricuspid regurgitation is associated with Ebstein's anomaly, which may occur with the use of lithium in early pregnancy. Shortened limbs is a teratogenic effect associated with thalidomide. Neural tube defects are associated with folic acid deficiency and antiepileptic drugs. Neonatal abstinence syndrome is characterized by withdrawal symptoms in the baby and is associated with the abrupt cessation of medications used during pregnancy due to delivery.

23. B) Beta blockers
Beta blockers, specifically lipophilic beta blockers, are believed to cross the blood-brain barrier and lead to symptoms of depression (hydrophilic beta blockers are less likely to cause symptoms of depression). Proton pump inhibitors are not associated with exacerbating symptoms of depression but rather renal insufficiency over prolonged use. Antihistamines are not related to symptoms of depression and are sometimes used to control anxiety. PD 5 inhibitors are not known to exacerbate depression but rather promote nitric oxide release commonly used for erectile dysfunction or pulmonary hypertension.

24. B) Acquiring curative factors
The eleven curative factors include instillation of hope (encouragement that recovery is possible through sharing), universality (recognizing shared experiences/similarity among the cohort), imparting information (teaching and learning about a problem and treatment options among peers), altruism (helping and supporting each other while building self-efficacy and developing coping skills), simulation of the family of origin (peers learn to identify and change dysfunctional patterns learned in the primary family), development of social skills (peers learn new ways to talk about feelings, observations, and concerns), imitative behavior (functional patterns can be amplified and emulated), interpersonal learning (vicarious learning and self-awareness is cultivated), group cohesiveness (feelings of belonging and valuing affiliation with a supportive group develops), catharsis (the ability to express emotions in a safe environment), and existential factors (learning to take responsibility for personal actions). Neither shared decision-making nor cost efficiency is principle of group dynamics. Enhancing social skills is only one of eleven curative factors that can enhance therapeutic efficacy.

25. B) Reduced protein binding
Reduced protein binding is due to decreased nutritional absorption associated with aging. Increased muscle mass is not associated with the aging process. Increased liver metabolism does not lead to toxicity. Decreased body fat does not affect drug metabolism but rather may affect storage and excretion.

26. B) "Tell me what you mean when you say 'life is not worth living'"
Saying to the patient "Tell me what you mean when you say 'life is not worth living'" encourages further assessment and fosters the therapeutic alliance. Appealing to the patient's environment and loved ones without further assessment or therapeutic alliance is not helpful. The inappropriate use of therapeutic silence in response to an expression of suicidality may limit the evaluation of lethality. Directly inquiring about suicidality without building a therapeutic alliance is less effective.

27. D) There is not enough information to interpret the statement without knowing the client's age
Abstract thinking develops during the formal operations stage of development (11–15 years). There is not enough information to interpret the statement without knowing the client's age or cultural frame of reference. Patients who are anxious, psychotic, or intellectually disabled may have difficulty with abstract thinking.

(See answers next page.)

28. A) Ask the patient how to help her
Asking the patient how to help her can enhance this therapeutic alliance, which is the most significant predictor of a successful outcome in therapy. Psychopharmacology education may be necessary, but it is essential to establish a therapeutic alliance first. Contracting for safety without therapeutic alliance is ineffective. Explaining the consequences of suicide is futile without a therapeutic alliance.

29. C) "Maybe that depends on what you're trying to accomplish"
Helping clarify goals and establishing therapeutic alliances are essential in the early phases of psychotherapy. Prematurely using silence may convey mixed meanings to the client. Wondering out loud if locking him in his room was abusive before establishing a therapeutic alliance may inhibit further disclosure from the client. Offering advice prematurely risks rupturing the therapeutic alliance.

30. B) Psychiatric symptoms
Psychiatric symptoms are treated with psychotropic medications; these medications are not used to treat disorders but rather specific symptoms that are characteristic of a mental illness. Neurological conditions are discretely defined disorders that may present with psychiatric symptoms, which are sometimes managed with psychotropic agents. Endocrine disorders are discretely characterized disorders that may present with psychiatric symptoms that are treated with psychotropic medications.

31. C) Presenting reality
Presenting reality is an expression of the psychiatric-mental health nurse to invite an alternative interpretation of a situation. Reflecting is a strategy that is used to help the client recognize and accept feelings, have opinions, and make decisions independently. Restating is the repetition of the main idea of the words spoken by the client to convey understanding on the part of the psychiatric-mental health nurse. Validation conveys a shared understanding of meaning by the psychiatric-mental health nurse of words spoken by the client.

32. D) To identify the mental health needs of the patient
Identifying the mental health needs of the patient is the primary goal of the comprehensive psychiatric evaluation. Completing the necessary forms, making a correct diagnosis, and communicating with others about the patient's needs are all individual components of the psychiatric assessment.

33. C) Communication medium
Neurotransmitters serve as the medium of communication within the nervous system. Enzymes are used to break down proteins. Peptide bonds link amino acids together. Hormones are believed to produce enzymes in the brain.

34. D) In a quiet but public place to get assistance should it be required during the evaluation

The psychiatric-mental health nurse must ensure that care is provided in an environment that is safe for all parties involved. Evaluating a new patient alone in their room is unsafe. The evaluation requires one-on-one interaction between the patient and the psychiatric-mental health nurse; simply observing in the milieu is insufficient to complete essential elements. Until rapport and therapeutic alliance are established, the psychiatric-mental health nurse should not be alone with the patient in a closed area.

35. C) Hypothalamus

The hypothalamus, located in the inferior portion of the midbrain, regulates appetite, circadian rhythms, and libido. The hippocampus in the temporal lobe governs learning and memory. The amygdala, located in the temporal lobe, regulates emotional response and sensory processing. The medulla oblongata regulates respiration and circulation.

36. B) Frontal lobe

The frontal lobe is responsible for executive function, cognition, and voluntary movement. The parietal lobe is responsible for information processing related to sensory input. The temporal lobe is responsible for memory integration. The occipital lobe is responsible for vision.

37. B) Suppression

Suppression is a mature defense mechanism characterized by a conscious decision to delay paying attention to a thought or emotion to cope with the present reality. Denial is a pathological defense mechanism characterized by a refusal to accept a fact because it is perceived as too threatening. Undoing a neurotic defense mechanism occurs when a person tries to cancel out a threatening thought or emotion by engaging in a contrary behavior. Projection, an immature defense mechanism, occurs when ego-dystonic thoughts and desires are attributed to another person.

38. A) Automated internal cardiac defibrillator (AICD)/pacemaker

An automated internal cardiac defibrillator (AICD)/pacemaker is an absolute contraindication for MRI scanning. Brain injury is not a contraindication for MRI scanning. Hip replacement is not a contraindication for MRI. MRI imaging during pregnancy is preferred due to a lack of radiation exposure.

39. A) Talkativeness, hyperactivity, and distractibility

Talkativeness, hyperactivity, and distractibility are overlapping symptoms of ADHD and bipolar disorder in children and adolescents. Avoidance behaviors, mood lability, irritability, recklessness, hypervigilance, and aggressiveness are symptoms consistent with PTSD. Disorganization, interrupting, and carelessness are primarily symptoms of ADHD.

40. A) Denial
Denial is a pathological defense mechanism characterized by refusal to accept reality because it is perceived as too threatening. Suppression is a mature defense mechanism characterized by a conscious decision to delay paying attention to a thought or emotion to cope with the present reality. Undoing a neurotic defense mechanism occurs when a person tries to cancel out a threatening thought or feeling by engaging in a contrary behavior. Projection, an immature defense mechanism, occurs when ego-dystonic thoughts and desires are attributed to another person.

41. C) Resolve conflicts
The purpose of defense mechanisms is to resolve conflicts associated with Egodystonic stimuli. The fight-or-flight response alerts to danger. The Ego mediates between the Id and the Superego. The Superego operates as the moral conscience of the psyche.

42. C) Repression
Repression is a neurotic defense mechanism in which the person consciously expresses pleasurable emotions accompanied by unexplainable amnesia or lack of awareness of an ego-dystonic event. It is an unconscious mechanism employed by the ego to keep disturbing or threatening thoughts from becoming conscious. Denial is a pathological defense mechanism characterized by refusal to accept reality because it is perceived as too threatening. Suppression is a mature defense mechanism described by a conscious decision to delay paying attention to a thought or emotion to cope with the present reality. Sublimation is a mature defense mechanism in which the unhelpful emotions or tendencies are transformed into a constructive expression of emotion.

43. D) Undoing
Undoing a neurotic defense mechanism is when a person tries to cancel out a threatening thought or emotion by engaging in a contrary behavior. Repression is a neurotic defense mechanism in which the person consciously expresses pleasurable feelings accompanied by an unexplainable amnesia or lack of awareness of an ego-dystonic event. Denial is a pathological defense mechanism characterized by refusal to accept reality because it is perceived as too threatening. Suppression is a mature defense mechanism described by a conscious decision to delay paying attention to a thought or emotion to cope with the present reality.

44. C) Bulimia nervosa
Bulimia nervosa is characterized by average height and weight and involvement in sports in which a particular weight and shape are required. Binge eating disorder is observed in individuals who are typically obese. Anorexia nervosa is less common in males and is characterized by patients who are less than 85% of expected body weight. Anxiety-induced eating disorder is associated with anxiety, provoking events, and atypical depression; patients may be overweight.

45. D) Referral to supportive psychotherapy by a therapist who speaks the language

Culturally competent psychotherapy is most appropriate to build a therapeutic alliance and to understand the etiology of the problem. Medications are not preferred first-line interventions. Using a family member to interpret violates the patient's confidentiality and may not provide the best insight. Involuntary admission is for patients who have a diagnosed mental illness and pose potential harm to self or others as a result of the mental illness.

46. B) Risk of increased suicidal thoughts

Increased risk of suicidal thoughts or behaviors should be mentioned explicitly to people under 25 years of age when prescribing psychotropic medications with black box warnings. Increased impulsive behavior, sexual side effects, and dysuria are not included in black box warnings.

47. A) Not leaving the house for many days, declining social events

Not leaving home for days, declining social invitations are consistent with Cluster C (anxious and fearful) personality traits. Grandiose declarations, increased goal-directed behaviors are consistent with Cluster B personality disorders (dramatic and emotional). Guarded and reluctant information sharing with flat affect is congruent with Cluster A (odd, eccentric).

48. B) Oppositional defiant disorder

Oppositional defiant disorder is a significant risk factor for antisocial personality disorder, which cannot be diagnosed until 18 years of age. Psychotic disorders and mood disorders are not independent risk factors for antisocial personality disorder.

49. D) In the primary psychiatric disorder

The *DSM-5* no longer stratifies personality disorders according to the multi-axial system of classification, but rather it should be described in the primary psychiatric disorder. In the *DSM-IV-TR*, it had been classified under Axis II.

50. D) Blood pressure, pulse, height, weight, and 12-lead EKG

Baseline measures of blood pressure, pulse, height, weight, and 12-lead EKG are recommended before starting stimulants in children. The rating scale should be completed by the primary caregiver and other caregivers, such as teachers or coaches, to evaluate the child in multiple settings. A diagnosis of bipolar disorder does not preclude the child from being treated for ADHD. There is no specific blood work required to start the patient on stimulants for ADHD.

51. C) Avoidant personality disorder, dependent personality disorder, obsessive compulsive personality disorder

Cluster C personality disorders are considered the anxious avoidant type and include avoidant personality disorder, dependent personality disorder, and obsessive-compulsive personality disorder. Cluster A personality disorders are considered the odd, eccentric type and include paranoid personality disorder, schizoid personality disorder, and schizotypal personality disorder. Cluster B personality disorders are considered the dramatic type and include antisocial personality disorder, borderline personality disorder, histrionic personality disorder, and narcissistic personality disorder.

52. D) Validate her and inform her that the white noise sound machine muffles the sounds of the session, and it would be hard to hear the conversation outside the office

Validating the reasonable concern and stating the objective reality allows the conversation to move to something constructive. Asking her to ruminate on the paranoid ideation serves to reinforce the thought and does not challenge the cognitive distortion. Using humor can be perceived as invalidating and can harm the therapeutic alliance. Distracting her from the topic can override her legitimate concern and harm the therapeutic alliance.

53. A) Paranoid personality disorder, schizoid personality disorder, schizotypal personality disorder

Cluster A personality disorders are considered the odd, eccentric type and include paranoid personality disorder, schizoid personality disorder, and schizotypal personality disorder. Cluster B personality disorders are considered the dramatic type and include antisocial personality disorder, borderline personality disorder, histrionic personality disorder, and narcissistic personality disorder. Cluster C personality disorders are considered the anxious avoidant type and include avoidant personality disorder, dependent personality disorder, and obsessive-compulsive personality disorder.

54. A) Do not challenge his negative views or recollections of past events

Do not challenge recollections and focus on present problems through collaborative problem-solving to reduce cognitive distortions while enhancing the therapeutic alliance. Confronting his memory is unhelpful in enhancing the therapeutic alliance and will likely trigger psychological paradox. Spending time reviewing specific details and heightening emotions will erode the therapeutic alliance as the patient may perceive time-wasting. Grandiose thoughts and ideas are often manifestations of defense mechanisms, which are protective.

55. A) Enhance the client's ego strength and encourage the use of mature defense mechanisms

The primary goal of psychotherapy for someone with a personality disorder is to enhance ego strength and encourage the use of mature defense mechanisms. Reviewing the antecedents to the pathological personality profile and paying attention to trauma may be helpful but does not address the present behavior problem or restore function. Having the client form a secure attachment to the parents may not always be possible or desirable. The aim of psychotherapy is not to change someone's personality.

56. B) Antisocial personality disorder, borderline personality disorder, histrionic personality disorder, narcissistic personality disorder

Cluster B personality disorders are considered the dramatic type and include antisocial personality disorder, borderline personality disorder, histrionic personality disorder, and narcissistic personality disorder. Cluster C personality disorders are considered the anxious avoidant type and include avoidant personality disorder, dependent personality disorder, and obsessive-compulsive personality disorder. Cluster A personality disorders are considered the odd, eccentric type and include paranoid personality disorder, schizoid personality disorder, and schizotypal personality disorder.

57. A) Affirming and reflecting

Affirming and reflecting acknowledge the patient's concern and demonstrates the clinician observation. Interrupting and reassuring are not consistent with motivational interviewing. Open-ended questions, summarizing, and clarifying are consistent with motivational interviewing but are not reflected in this scenario.

58. D) "It sounds like you value luxury items. Tell me more about that"

This statement uses the elements of therapeutic communication while turning the attention back on the client and elicits more information. Simply acknowledging the statement foregoes the opportunity to build the therapeutic alliance and gather more information. Seeming defensive may alienate the therapeutic alliance and stifle further disclosure from the patient. Identifying with the client's taste and focusing the conversation on the object may encourage the patient to be overly familiar and erode professional boundaries.

59. A) Assess for hemodynamic stability and call the physician

A CIWA-A scale score >15 is consistent with severe withdrawal and hospitalization should be considered; a score of 10 to 15 is consistent with moderate withdrawal, and benzodiazepines should be utilized to reduce the risk of seizures; scores <10 can be managed with nonbenzodiazepine supportive measures unless there is a prior history of seizures or delirium tremens.

60. B) "Let me check your vital signs to see if you would be able to tolerate a clonidine patch"

Clonidine is often used to reduce symptoms of withdrawal and anxiety associated with opioid use disorder. It is important to treat anxiety symptoms in these patients as untreated anxiety symptoms are one of the biggest triggers for relapse within the first 90 days.

61. C) Heightened sensitivity to external stimuli

Heightened sensitivity, including paradoxical anxiety, is an adverse effect associated with the use of tetrahydrocannabinol (THC). Cannabis use also impairs motor skills and cognition and decreases motivation.

62. D) Isolation and intellectualization

Defense mechanisms in patients with Cluster C traits are often reinforcing isolation and include intellectualization and isolation. Cluster B trait defense mechanisms include projective identification, regression, somatization, denial, externalization, and dissociation. Cluster A fantasy-based defense mechanisms include projections, avoidance behaviors, and procrastination.

63. C) ANC less than 1,000

Clozapine should be stopped in a patient with an ANC less than 1,000. Clozapine can continue as long as the ANC is greater than 1,000; prior to starting, the ANC should be greater than 1,500.

64. A) Benzodiazepines cause memory problems and confusion in clients with a history of traumatic brain injury

Benzodiazepines cause cognitive impairment and confusion in patients with a history of traumatic brain injury and should not be used long term. Benzodiazepines do not increase the risk of subsequent traumatic brain injury, and they raise the seizure threshold.

65. A) High risk for a 1-year mortality rate

Delirium is highly correlated with a 1-year mortality rate. Aspiration, sepsis, and urinary tract infections are major risk factors for delirium.

66. D) "Help me understand what's going on so we can figure out how to proceed"

Inquiring regarding circumstances enhances the therapeutic alliance without drawing unfounded conclusions. Declaring the client's ambivalence, or assuming the client does not want treatment, and focusing on the charge for missed appointments does not enhance a therapeutic alliance and projects the psychiatric-mental health nurse counter-transference.

67. C) Antiretroviral therapy
Antiretroviral therapy is indicated for treating HIV neurocognitive deficits (HAND) and AIDS-related complex dementia. Anti-Parkinson agents and acetylcholinesterase inhibitors are ineffective in this type of dementia, and nonpharmacological supportive measures are enhanced with the use of antiretroviral therapy.

68. C) "While most brain development occurs early in life, we still form new brain cells in various areas of the brain throughout our lives. Continue with your activities because they offer the best protection of cognitive function"
Providing specific psychoeducation and promoting her current strengths is the best response. Offering further information that does not answer the question of concern and that highlights possible risks can increase anxiety. The evidence for supplements is limited and not as robust as the evidence for exercise and cognition. Telling the patient that there is nothing that can be done is disempowering and harmful to the therapeutic alliance.

69. B) Contemplation
The patient is in the contemplation stage, as he recognizes that there is a problem. In precontemplation, the patient does not believe there is a problem. In preparation to take action, the patient announces intentions and makes plans to act in the future. Action is when the patient is doing the desired behavior and lasts for 6 months, at which time the patient enters the maintenance phase.

70. B) No, the student does not meet the criteria for mental illness
No, the student does not meet the criteria for mental illness. Alcohol use disorder requires a maladaptive use pattern leading to significant impairment or distress associated with two other consequence criteria. Adjustment disorder requires clinically significant emotional or behavioral symptoms, not qualifying for a mood disorder. Social anxiety disorder is characterized by considerable fear or anxiety about social situations in which the individual fears scrutiny by others.

71. D) Duty to care, breach of a standard of care, and injury related to the breach of the standard of care
Negligence requires that the professional had a duty to care, there was a breach in the standard of care, and the injury was sustained due to the breach in the standard of care. Deceit and intent to harm are not elements of the negligence tort. Violation of ethics and patient abandonment are not sufficient elements to claim negligence. Ethical principles and breach of standards without duty and harm are not adequate to claim negligence.

72. B) Radical acceptance and change
Dialectical behavioral therapy aims to enhance distress tolerance by helping the client radically accept the reality of a situation and facilitate effective coping strategies leading to behavior change. Psychoanalysis would help the client understand experience and avoidance based on understanding unconscious elements as motivations for unconscious behavior. Experiential therapy reconciles the tension between crisis survival and radical acceptance by using specific tools and activities to allow the patient to reenact and reexperience emotional situations from the past and present. Interpersonal therapy is a time-limited manualized approach to improve the client's interpersonal relationships of knowing how and when to confront and when to avoid, improving social functioning and relieving distress.

73. D) The patient likely had a traumatic event in his childhood in which thoughts and feelings have become locked together and are inaccessible to the conscious mind
The patient is experiencing a feeling seemingly out of the blue, consistent with the core concept phenomena of TA, known as transference and countertransference, which describes how memories from past relationships can impact current relationships, more specifically how perception can impact how one conducts current relationships and life scripts. Experiencing a period of separation from parents affecting current ability to love and experience happiness, being forced into a parentified roll, and distorted thought patterns affecting interpersonal relationships are consistent with psychoanalytic theory and more commonly observed in patients with borderline or narcissistic personality traits.

74. B) Equity and efficiency
Equity and efficiency are economic concepts concerned with return on investment and serving the highest number of people. Affordability and quality are concepts concerned explicitly with accessibility and outcomes. Harm reduction is a health promotion strategy when abstinence is not feasible. Opportunities are elements in the environment that a business could use to its advantage, and risks are potential threats that can obstruct outcomes.

75. C) Serum glucose or hemoglobin A1C, lipid profile, weight, body mass index, blood pressure, waist circumference, and review of family cardiovascular disease
The prescribing guidelines do not require a physical exam before starting an antipsychotic, but they do specify the following at baseline and ongoing with continued use: serum glucose or hemoglobin A1C, lipid profile, weight, body mass index, blood pressure, waist circumference, and review of family cardiovascular disease. Antipsychotics are known to cause metabolic syndrome (hypertension, dyslipidemia, hyperglycemia, obesity, insulin resistance), in rare cases agranulocytosis, and QTc prolongation. Baseline measure should be assessed. Family history alone, CBC alone, and lipid profile with HgbA1C are not sufficient as baseline measures.

76. C) Negative symptoms
Negative symptoms are characterized by a pervasive loss of function and manifest as apathy, anhedonia, alogia (impoverished speech), and affect flattening. Positive signs are characterized by perceptual disturbances as a result of psychosis; they include hallucinations, delusions, and paranoid thoughts. Psychosis is defined as the inability to test reality and manifests as gross disorganization, including delusions and hallucinations. Self-care deficit is characterized by a failure to meet one's basic needs according to the first two levels of Maslow's hierarchy of needs (physiological needs and safety).

77. A) Tactile hallucinations
Tactile hallucinations are more common in substance induced and withdrawal delirium. Auditory hallucinations congruent with delusions are more common in psychosis. Visual hallucinations are the least common and most associated with delirium, seizure, or dementia. Combined hallucinations are most associated with substances or sleep disorders.

78. C) Tertiary prevention
Tertiary prevention focuses on improving function, chronic symptoms/disease management, and reducing morbidity and mortality after the disease has occurred. Primary prevention focuses on preventing new diseases. Secondary prevention focuses on early detection of existing illnesses. Preventive care is a comprehensive approach and includes all elements of prevention. Primary prevention focuses on preventing new diseases.

79. D) Encourage an appointment with a psychiatrist or psychiatric-mental health nurse practitioner for obstructive sleep apnea
Encourage an appointment with a psychiatrist for obstructive sleep apnea best describes these symptoms. Attention-deficit hyperactivity disorder cannot be diagnosed from the symptoms presented. He does not meet the criteria for caffeine-use disorder and does not have symptoms consistent with alcohol withdrawal syndrome.

80. A) Drugs are metabolized more slowly through the liver
Drugs are metabolized more slowly in elderly patients. Treatment duration is unaffected by age, but the dosage might be. Therapeutic doses are usually lower in the elderly than in children. Titration should be slower in the elderly.

81. C) She is hypomanic
Hypomania best describes these symptoms. Psychosis requires gross disorganization, delusions, or hallucinations. Euthymic describes a normal mood. Venlafaxine can cause elevated mood symptoms.

82. D) Call the patient's primary care provider to explain the situation, coordinate an appointment, and plan for medication refills

Collaborating with the patient's primary care provider ensures that the psychiatric-mental health nurse is not practicing outside the scope of practice. Asking the pharmacist for a refill without proper supervision and follow-up exposes the psychiatric-mental health nurse to exceed their scope of practice. Advising the patient to go to the emergency department for signs and symptoms is acceptable but does not make provision for the pressing problem. Sending the patient to urgent care contributes to the added expense and further fragments care.

83. A) Just culture

Just culture is the American Nurses Association's (ANA) statement on promoting open and fair interprofessional collaborative relationships aimed at reducing human error. Personnel policies are institution-specific operating procedures. Standardization of health information technology is a recommendation of the U.S. Department of Health and Human Services. Civil disobedience is the refusal to comply with particular laws as a peaceful form of political protest.

84. D) Autonomy

Autonomy is the right to self-determination, which includes the right to accept or refuse care. Beneficence is the ethical principle of promoting good. Justice is the moral principle of equality concerning risks and benefits. Nonmaleficence is the ethical principle of not doing harm.

85. B) Secondary prevention

Secondary prevention focuses on the early detection of existing diseases. Tertiary prevention focuses on improving function, chronic symptoms/disease management, and reducing morbidity and mortality after the illness has occurred. Preventive care is a comprehensive approach and includes all elements of prevention. Primary prevention focuses on preventing new diseases.

86. B) Primary prevention

Primary prevention focuses on preventing new diseases. Secondary prevention focuses on the early detection of existing illnesses. Tertiary prevention focuses on improving function, chronic symptoms/disease management, and reducing morbidity and mortality after the disease has occurred. Preventive care is a comprehensive approach and includes all elements of prevention.

87. A) Psychiatric interview

The psychiatric interview is the process by which the psychiatric-mental health nurse identifies signs and symptoms of mental illness. The physical exam is the process by which underlying medical conditions are excluded. Interdisciplinary treatment planning discusses the various therapy modalities for a particular condition. The neurological examination is a focused physical exam.

88. B) XI
The XI spinal accessory nerve controls the ability to shrug shoulders. The XII hypoglossal controls tongue movements. The IX glossopharyngeal nerve controls the elevation of the soft palate and uvula position. V is the trigeminal nerve, which controls facial sensations.

89. C) The Centers for Disease Control and Prevention recommends the human papillomavirus (HPV) vaccine for all children at age 10 because HPV can cause cancer in both men and women. The vaccine protects against the three most common forms of the virus. What is your concern?
Providing evidence-based information is the best answer and allows the mother to express her concerns. Advice should not be anecdotal or personal in nature but professional at all times. Encouraging the mother to skip the vaccine for anxiety may establish a pattern of avoidant behavior.

90. B) Yes, the psychiatric-mental health nurse must report
The psychiatric-mental health nurse is a mandated reporter. If the psychiatric-mental health nurse believes the child is in potential harm or danger, whether due to deliberate or inadvertent reasons, the welfare of the minor must be protected.

91. D) XII-hypoglossal nerve
Cranial nerve XII is the hypoglossal, and it is tested with tongue movements. The optic nerve is responsible for focusing the eyes. The oculomotor nerve is responsible for eye movements. The vagus nerve is responsible for the gag reflex.

92. C) Vestibulocochlear
Vestibulocochlear nerve VIII receives auditory impulses. Optic nerve II is responsible for central and peripheral vision acuity. Trigeminal nerve V controls facial sensations. Facial nerve VII controls facial muscles.

93. C) Moderate cognitive impairment
A mini-mental status exam score between 10 and 18 indicates moderate cognitive impairment; a score of 9 or less indicates severe cognitive impairment; a score between 19 and 23 indicates mild cognitive impairment; a score above 24 indicates a normal exam.

94. A) "The people on television are talking to me"
An idea of reference is a delusion in which innocuous events are considered to have significant personal meaning. "The voice in my head is telling me I should die" is an example of an auditory hallucination. "I see little people at the end of my bed" is an example of a visual hallucination. "You think people are watching us?" is an example of paranoid ideation.

95. B) Immediate safety of people involved
Crisis intervention principles focus on the immediate safety of the people involved. Once immediate safety has been established, the current living situation and coping skills must be assessed. Gathering collateral information and assessing for allergies to medications occur later in the crisis intervention process.

96. D) Hopefulness
Hopefulness is one of the therapeutic factors of the dynamic group process. Reflection on existential matters often occurs in individual therapy. Psychological relief is a mental process in the transtheoretical model of change. Peer support can happen in a variety of group settings.

97. A) Imitative behavior
This phenomenon is called "imitative behavior." Confrontational behavior occurs when group members openly discuss maladaptive coping strategies, exacerbating current problems. Avoidant behavior is characterized by group members walking on eggshells concerning other members. Mocking behavior is done to belittle another group member, usually motivated by an inferiority complex in the mocker.

98. D) Continue with the discharge as the test is negative
Continue with the discharge planning as the induration is less than 15 mm. In a non-immunocompromised patient with tuberculosis, the skin test is considered negative if it is less than 15 mm induration. If the patient is immunocompromised or under 4 years of age with induration of 10 mm or more, it is considered a positive indicator of latent tuberculosis.

99. C) Strategic therapy
Strategic therapy often uses the paradoxical directive to effect a change in behavior. Psychoanalysis seeks to clarify unconscious motivations responsible for current behaviors. Narrative therapy is a technique that helps people see themselves separate from their problems by encouraging reliance on skills to minimize distress. Psychodynamic therapy is a derivative of psychoanalysis but focuses on the patient's relationship to the external world.

100. A) Mindfulness, meditation, and emotional regulation
Mindfulness, meditation, and emotional regulation are all elements of dialectical behavioral therapy. Systematic desensitization is an element of cognitive behavioral therapy. Attachment and reintegration are elements of trauma-focused therapy. Aversion therapy is an element of a relapse prevention strategy.

101. A) Place the patient on contact isolation for possible scabies
Scabies is characterized by intractable pruritus primarily on the flexor aspect of the wrist and interdigital web spaces and causes pruritic papules and vesicles, and requires contact isolation/precautions. Impetigo is characterized by an erythematous macule that evolves into a blister, usually occurring around the mouth and appearing honey-crusted. Shingles is a vesicular rash occurring along a dermatome, often not crossing the midline, and requires contact precautions until vesicles are scabbed, and the rash should be covered. Dermatitis is an erythematous skin eruption due to irritation or infection usually requiring topical hydrocortisone.

102. D) Pica
Pica is the behavior of eating nonfood items and is a late symptom of iron deficiency anemia. Irritability, pallor, and fatigue are all symptoms of microcytic hypochromic anemia, which occurs within the first 6 months of the disease state.

103. B) Liver function and ammonia level
Liver function and ammonia level, hyperammonemia, and hepatic encephalopathy can occur at any time in some patients taking valproic acid. An MRI of the brain is not the priority screening test in this acute state. Renal function and complete blood count can help exclude other etiologies for encephalopathy but not rule in the etiology. Cardiac enzymes are not indicated in this scenario.

104. D) A 16-year-old boy with only one close friend with whom he likes to hunt
The 16-year-old boy engaging in recreational and social activities is at the lowest risk for suicide. Elderly White men with a recent major life stressor, people with substance use disorders, and people with first-degree relatives who have committed suicide are all at high risk.

105. A) Thyroid function
Thyroid function should be evaluated while on lithium as it is known to cause hypothyroidism. Liver function, cardiac enzymes are not indicated in lithium therapy. The 12-lead EKG is sometimes done at baseline and follow up, but this is not a standard of care and the evidence is of varying quality.

106. C) Anticipatory guidance regarding normal physiological changes with age
Anticipatory guidance helps normalize and validate the patient's experience with a normal physiological process and is consistent with vasomotor phenomena associated with menopause. These symptoms are not compatible with a mood disorder or anxiety.

107. A) Notify the nurse practitioner
A chest x-ray is indicated to rule out active tuberculosis in this immunocompromised patient; this order must be placed by credentialed healthcare provider (NP, DO, MD, PA). The 10-mm induration is considered positive in immunocompromised patients. If the patient is not actively coughing, there is no need for airborne precautions. Latent tuberculosis does not require hospitalization.

108. B) Renal function
Impaired renal function is a contraindication. Cardiac enzymes, liver function, and complete blood count are not explicitly indicated for lithium therapy.

109. B) Alzheimer's disease
Alzheimer's disease is a common comorbid condition in people with Down syndrome. Delirium is characterized by an acute onset of symptoms affecting the level of consciousness. A cerebrovascular accident would be associated with a focal neural deficit lasting longer than 24 hours. Attention-deficit hyperactivity disorder is not supported by the symptoms presented.

110. D) Disclosing a diagnosis to the spouse
Disclosing a patient's diagnosis without permission is a breach of confidentiality. Release of records to an insurance company, or under subpoena, or under public health mandate are all permissible disclosures without violating confidentiality law.

111. A) Convey expertise in the field of psychiatric-mental health
The psychiatric-mental health nurse conveys expertise in the field of psychiatric mental health to the public and to colleagues and reflects current knowledge of national standards of care. Certification is not intended to restrict access to care, preserve the reimbursement structure, or encourage litigation.

112. B) Comprehensive psychiatric evaluation with collateral information
Comprehensive psychiatric with collateral information is the best way to assess for dementia. An MRI of the brain and PET scan of the brain can suggest microvascular changes and hypometabolic activity consistent with dementia, but the clinical correlation is essential to make the diagnosis. An EEG is used to diagnose a seizure disorder.

113. A) State Nurse Practice Act
The State Nurse Practice Act regulates the practice of the professional registered nurse. Medicare regulations determine the necessary conditions for reimbursement. The collaborating physician does not make the regulations. The institution can determine practice only in the institution (and must not be broader in scope than state law), but the practice of the professional registered nurse is governed by the state.

114. D) Selective serotonin reuptake inhibitors
Selective serotonin reuptake inhibitors are the most commonly prescribed medication in high doses to treat obsessive compulsive disorder as monotherapy. Tricyclic antidepressants, benzodiazepines, and antipsychotics are sometimes used to augment treatment for obsessive compulsive disorder (off label).

115. A) Diphenhydramine, digoxin, oxybutynin
First-generation antihistamines, anticholinergics, and medications with a narrow therapeutic index are known to cause delirium in the elderly. All medications can theoretically predispose or cause delirium, particularly in polypharmacy states. However, it is important to treat pain, constipation, and infections because those conditions are also precipitants of delirium.

116. C) Anxiety
Anxiety is the symptom consistent with obsession. Behaviors such as handwashing, checking the gas, and ruminating are all examples of compulsions.

117. B) 1 hour before intended alcohol use
The Sinclair method involves taking naltrexone 1 hour before intended alcohol use; it is not to be used when not intending to drink alcohol. The harm reduction method requires daily naltrexone medication regardless of intended use. Another alternative is a monthly injection for harm reduction. Antabuse is considered aversive therapy.

118. D) A consistent and attentive caretaker
A consistent and attentive caretaker is not characteristic of a perpetrator of elder abuse. However, delayed medical care, new onset of sexually transmitted infection, or a patient over 80 years of age with a high care burden are all risk factors of elder abuse.

119. B) Alzheimer's disease
Alzheimer's disease is the most common type of dementia in the United States. Multi-infarct dementia and Parkinson's dementia are the next common type. Frontotemporal dementia accounts for less than 5% of cases in the United States.

120. B) Alpha blockers
Alpha blockers are commonly used to treat nightmares associated with PTSD. SSRIs are often used in PTSD to treat depression and anxiety symptoms. Beta blockers are sometimes used for performance anxiety. Benzodiazepines should not be used long term for anxiety as they are highly addictive.

121. A) Rate of onset
Rate of onset distinguishes delirium from dementia as delirium comes on much more quickly and has an intermittent waxing and waning quality. Delirium-like dementia can manifest in confusion, prolonged symptoms, and cognitive impairment. Delirium is reversible when the underlying cause is identified. Dementia is generally irreversible and is expected to decline.

122. C) Serum lipase
Serum lipase is a more sensitive indicator of pancreatitis. Renal function is not necessarily altered in pancreatitis, transient blood alcohol levels are not reflective of pancreatitis, and brain natriuretic peptide is elevated in congestive heart failure.

123. B) Panic disorder
Panic disorder can also mimic symptoms of acute myocardial infarction. Generalized anxiety disorder is characterized by consistent and persistent worry and rumination over real or imagined events. Factitious disorder is characterized by an unconscious manifestation of symptoms for secondary gain. Malingering disorder is characterized by a conscious manifestation of symptoms for secondary gain.

124. C) High premorbid and social functioning
High premorbid and social functioning is a good predictor of a better prognosis. Negative symptoms such as persistent apathy or anhedonia, delayed onset of psychotic symptoms, and persistent flat or blunted affect are a predictor of a poor prognosis (higher morbidity).

125. B) Check the client's body for signs of infestation
Check the client's body for signs of infestation before assuming tactile hallucinations. Maslow's hierarchy of needs prioritizes physiological needs over psychosocial needs. Only after ruling out a physical cause should the nurse begin reality testing. Tactile hallucinations can be caused by substance-induced psychosis, but the physical exam should be performed first as infestation may require the patient to be placed on contact isolation precautions.

126. C) "That must be frightening as it seems so real, but I don't see dead people"
Acknowledging it must be frightening, and the reality of the experience to the patient shows empathy and promotes therapeutic alliance. This should be followed by presenting reality. Making challenging statements, asking provocative questions, or unwittingly validating the hallucination limits therapeutic alliance and is counterproductive, as it does not help with reality testing or reorientation and can garner hostility and defensiveness.

127. A) Having little or no interest in work or social activities
Having little or no interest in work or social activities is one of the symptoms of schizophrenia and apathy; other symptoms include anhedonia, alogia, and blunted affect. These are considered negative symptoms and have worse prognosis than patients with positive symptoms. Echolalia, continuously repeating words and phrases; ideas of reference thinking that people on television are talking about them; and auditory hallucinations are all examples of positive symptoms.

128. C) Establish a therapeutic relationship with the client

Establishing a therapeutic relationship by building a therapeutic alliance must occur before offering other therapies. The patient is in the admission phase to an acute care facility; discharge planning with the patient is not yet appropriate. Reinforcing the need for medication adherence will not be useful if the patient does not trust the care team.

129. A) Expressly stating the rules of the group while allowing for peer pressure to govern social interactions

Establishing social rules and using peer pressure for conformity is the hallmark milieu therapy. The use of role-play is a psychoeducation technique and not characteristic of milieu therapy. Individual therapy lacks the characteristic requisite of therapeutic peer pressure to modify behavior.

130. B) Place the patient on 1:1 observation with a consistent staff member

Patients with paranoid delusions are often extremely suspicious of others and their actions. It is essential to help the client build a trusting relationship with a consistent staff member otherwise; all other interventions will be suspect. Frequently rotating staff members (A) reduces the likelihood of building a therapeutic alliance with any individual staff member. While the patient is actively paranoid, attending group activities (C) can be misinterpreted. It should be reserved for when the patient is more stable. Prior to providing any psychoeducation (D), therapeutic alliance must be established.

131. C) Psychotherapy requires a lot of patience, and his clients often relapse in the process

Psychotherapy requires patience because the client will need to learn and apply new behaviors, and relapse is common. Psychotherapy is often long-term, and lasting changes are not realized immediately. Neuroplasticity has shown the effectiveness of psychotherapy but not in short-term treatments. Psychotherapy is often successful over time.

132. A) The psychiatric-mental health nurse should establish a relationship that is respectful of the client's dignity

Establishing a therapeutic alliance requires honesty and trust with communication that is respectful of privacy and dignity. Conveying closeness or excessive warmth or friendship is likely to be met with confusion and suspicion in dealing with a client with schizophrenia. Any patient relationship should be professional and therapeutic in nature and not based on any false pretenses of friendship; professional boundaries must be maintained. Paternalism without first establishing therapeutic alliance will likely be met with resistance.

133. D) Thank the client for trusting you enough to share their delusional thought

By appreciating the client for trusting you to share their delusional thought, this enhances the therapeutic alliance which is essential before any other intervention. Therapeutic alliance builds relational equity, which must be drawn upon in psychotherapy when presenting ego dystonic information.

134. C) Attaching consequences to coping mechanisms

Attaching consequences to coping mechanisms is a behavioral approach to helping patients realize the power of their own actions. Focusing on the client's feelings is inconsistent with a behavioral approach to therapy; the client is empowered to do or not do regardless of feelings or motivation. While establishing therapeutic alliance is important, it is a characteristic of an interpersonal approach rather than a behavioral therapy approach. Performing psychoeducation regarding medications is not an example of behavioral therapy.

135. B) Some clients who developed schizophrenia have had schizoid personality traits early on

Some clients with schizoid personality disorder go on to develop schizophrenia. Not all people with schizoid personality disorder go on to develop schizophrenia, but many patients do have schizoid personality and characteristics in their premorbid state. The psychiatric-mental health nurse must make sure that the thrust of the question posed is being answered completely, confirming the client's suspicion regarding the development of schizophrenia is the most important part of the answer the nurse may go on to elaborate. Identifying the patient's feeling in a group setting when not expressly stated is an example of jumping to conclusions. Asking the patient to tell you what they know about schizophrenia does not answer their primary concern.

136. A) Apply a bed alarm

Applying a bed alarm is the priority to ensure safety overnight. Encouraging bedtime routines or dietary modifications do not address the safety risk.

137. B) Explain the effects of tolerance and how it indicates alcohol use disorder

The patient is describing tolerance which occurs when increasing amounts of substance are needed to achieve similar results. This is characteristic of a use disorder. The client is not reporting misinformation, direct confrontation is not recommended. Withdrawal is not relevant to what the client has stated. Reframing statements are helpful but incorrect as the client is not minimizing his reality.

138. D) Refocus on the client's objective accomplishments and past struggles that have been overcome

Helping the client remember past accomplishments and past success enhances self-efficacy and promotes agency. Encouraging group attendance depending on the topic may not be most helpful in this instance. Encouraging the client to focus on feelings would reinforce her negative self-worth. There is no indication that the client lacks assertiveness.

139. B) Take the medication exactly as prescribed as onset of actions can be delayed as much as 3 weeks

Many psychotropic medications take up to 3 weeks to work and require 6 to 12 weeks for full effect (patients may be inclined to skip doses if they do not feel the medication is working). Avoiding alcohol is not explicitly recommended without the specific mention of a specific class of drug. The patient's feelings may necessitate and increase or decrease augmentation in medication. Antidepressant levels are not checked for toxicity or therapeutic efficacy as the serum values do not consistently correlate.

140. D) Tremor

Alprazolam is a benzodiazepine that when abruptly stopped can show symptoms of central nervous system (CNS) arousal including tremor. Increased sedation is consistent with increased use, diarrhea, and piloerection (goosebumps) are noted in opioid withdrawal.

141. C) Ativan

Ativan is a benzodiazepine indicated for short-term use in instances of acute anxiety or predictable panic-inducing events. Clozapine is an antipsychotic, lithium is a mood stabilizer, and Lexapro can use used for generalized anxiety disorder but not for acute episodes.

142. B) Complete a focused physical exam of the cardiopulmonary system including vital signs

Physical needs must take priority over psychosocial needs, and all psychiatric disorders are applied by exclusion. A physical exam must be completed first, and hemodynamic stability ensured given the report of poor oral intake. There is no information indicating potential harm to self or others.

143. B) The patient states it may take several weeks to achieve the anti-anxiety effect of the Lexapro

Escitalopram is the generic name for Lexapro and can take serval weeks to experience desired effects. The patient should not mix alcohol with sedating medication such as gabapentin, and it should be taken as prescribed. If the patient experiences panic attack, this should be addressed with the prescribing provider.

144. D) Sit with the patient and engage them with a calm and directive approach

Sitting with the patient who is in acute distress and using a calm and directive approach to engage them to help reduce their symptoms of severe anxiety. During heightened anxiety, it is inappropriate to encourage further expression of feelings; this should be done when anxiety is low. Placing the patient in seclusion is inappropriate as it may heighten their anxiety. When a patient is heightened in anxiety, they are not in the frame of mind to concentrate on group activities.

145. B) After obtaining consent, corroborate the information with others who know the patient

Obtaining collateral information is the best way to validate the report of history present illness. Instructing regarding illicit drugs, clearly documenting their self-report, and teaching about detox will not help validate the history of present illness.

146. B) "Trazadone is an antidepressant that can stimulate your appetite"

Trazadone is an antidepressant often prescribed to help with insomnia. It is not classified as an antianxiety medication or antipsychotic medication. The primary symptom targeted in depression is the sleep quality because it may diminish other neurovegetative symptoms as well.

147. C) "I realize that recovery is a lifelong process"

It is not correct that the goal of recovery is to reduce drinking but rather to stop it altogether. Harm reduction is an example of controlled addiction rather than recovery. Detox is only the first step in the recovery process. Al-anon is not for people who are alcoholic but rather for the family members of alcoholics.

148. A) A 31-year-old male with rapid, pressured speech and poor personal boundaries

The patient who is pressured, and with poor physical boundaries may escalate into violent acting out. This client needs to be attended first. The patient with homicidal ideation is currently admitted, and the president is not in imminent danger. The patient with poor sleep is not having an acute crisis, and medication may need to be adjusted for bedtime. The patient who is isolating and not attending groups can be delayed until the milieu is made safe.

149. A) "What do flowers mean in your culture?"

It is important to assess and inquire when a patient expresses an emotion. Commenting on the friendliness of the neighbor, the hatred of flowers, or assuming she is crying because she thinks the neighbors are particularly thoughtful would not reveal that in the Vietnamese culture the sending of flowers is reserved for the rites of the dead.

150. B) Help the patient complete activities of daily living

Helping the client complete activities of daily living builds self-efficacy and reduces the feeling of helplessness. The patient has not demonstrated impulsive behaviors. While the patient is heightened in anxious symptoms expressing feelings can further exacerbate the distress. The patient needs a lower state of anxiety in order to learn and participate in reframing exercises.

Index

Abnormal Involuntary Movement Scale (AIMS), 81, 155
abstinence violation effect (AVE), 43
abuse, 107
ACT. *See* assertive community treatment (ACT)
ACTH. *See* adrenocorticotropic hormone (ACTH)
active psychosis, schizophrenia, 154
acute stress disorder, 217
adaptation, 44
addiction, 107
    medication-assisted treatment for, 115–116
adjustment disorder with disturbed conduct, 250
adrenocorticotropic hormone (ACTH), 212
    depressive disorders, 194
advanced directives, 26
Adverse Childhood Events scale, 22
afferent fibers, 75
agonist, 85
agoraphobia
    assessment and diagnosis, 218
    cluster C personality disorders, 274
    cultural implications, 219
    evaluation, 219
    incidence and prevalence, 218
    intervention, 218–219
    patient case study, 217
    planning, 218
AIMS. *See* Abnormal Involuntary Movement Scale (AIMS)
akathisia, 156
akinesia, 156
alcohol dependency, laboratory indicators of, 111, 112
Alcohol use disorder (CAGE-AID), 81
allele, 80
alpha-blockers
    attention-deficit hyperactivity disorder, 245
    generalized anxiety disorder, 216
amantadine, 157
American Nurses Association (ANA), 18

American Nurses Credentialing Center (ANCC), 18
    board certification exam map, 15
    psychiatric-mental health nurse board certification exam, 9–12
American Psychiatric Nurses Association (APNA), 18
amygdala, 74
ANA. *See* American Nurses Association (ANA)
ANCC. *See* American Nurses Credentialing Center (ANCC)
anorexia, 252–253
anorexia nervosa, 252
antagonist effects, 85
anticipatory guidance, 26–27
antidepressants, 90
    insomnia, 179
antidiuretic hormone, depressive disorders, 194
antiepileptic drugs, 92
antipsychotics
    first-generation, 86–87
    schizophrenia, 155
    second-generation, 87
antisocial behavior in psychosis, 250
antisocial personality disorder
    cluster B personality disorders, 269–271
    cluster C personality disorders, 274
anxiety disorders
    agoraphobia, 217–219
    generalized anxiety disorder, 211–217
    obsessive compulsive disorder, 219–222
    panic disorder, 222–224
    phobias, 224–225
    posttraumatic stress disorder, 225–228
anxiolytics, 90
APNA. *See* American Psychiatric Nurses Association (APNA)
Artane, 157
assertive community treatment (ACT), 156
astrocytes, 76
Ativan, 157

atomoxetine, 245
ATT. *See* Authorization to Test (ATT)
attention-deficit hyperactivity disorder (ADHD)
    assessment and diagnosis, 244
    conduct disorders, 250
    cultural implications, 245–246
    evaluation, 245
    incidence and prevalence, 243
    intervention, 244–245
    oppositional defiant disorder, 241
    patient case study, 243
    planning, 244
screening tools and early intervention, 244
atypical antipsychotics, 88
authoritarian leadership, 19
Authorization to Test (ATT), 10
autism spectrum disorder (ASD)
assessment and diagnosis, 247
    cluster A personality disorders, 266, 267
    cultural implications, 248
evaluation, 248
incidence and prevalence, 246
intervention, 247–248
patient case study, 246
planning, 247
autocracy, 19
autonomic nervous system, 75
AVE. *See* abstinence violation effect (AVE)
avoidant personality disorder
cluster A personality disorders, 267
cluster C personality disorders, 274

Barnes Akathisia Rating Scale (BARS), 81
basal ganglia, 73
basal ganglia-associated structures, dysfunction of, 74
Beck, Aaron, 52
Belsomra, 179
Benadryl, 157
benzodiazepines, 91, 92
    generalized anxiety disorder, 215–216
    obstructive sleep apnea, 178
    substance use disorder, 115
benztropine, 157
beta-blockers, 60, 157
generalized anxiety disorder, 216
binge eating disorder, 252, 253
bioamine theory, 194
biofeedback, 59
biological therapies, 59–60

biopsychosocial model, 49–50
bipolar 1 disorder, 200
bipolar 2 disorder, 200
bipolar disorders, 197
board-certified registered nurse (RN-BC), 3
borderline personality disorder
    cluster B personality disorders, 270, 271
    cluster C personality disorders, 274
brain, 72–75
brain stem, 75
brief psychotic disorder, 154
Broca's area, 73
bulimia, 253
bulimia nervosa, 252
buprenorphine, 25, 83–85
    substance use disorder, 115
bupropion, 245
buspirone, 216

carbamazepine, 89
Catapres, 245
    schizophrenia, 157
caudate nucleus, 74
central nervous system, 75
cerebellum (hindbrain), 75
cerebral cortex (gray matter), 72
cerebrospinal fluid testing, narcolepsy, 175
cerebrum, 73
certification, 16–17
child/adolescent and developmental disorders
    ages and stages, 241
    attention-deficit hyperactivity disorder, 241–246
    autism spectrum disorder, 246–248
    conduct disorders, 249–251
    eating disorders, 251–254
    milestones growth and development, 242
childhood-onset schizophrenia, 247
Children's Yale-Brown Obsessive Compulsive Scale (CY-BOCS), 83
cholinesterase inhibitors, dementia, 135
chromosomes, 79
chronic insomnia, 173
chronic obstructive pulmonary disease (COPD), 178
chronic traumatic encephalopathy (CTE), 137
cisgender, 23
Clinical Institute Withdrawal Assessment of Alcohol Scale–Revised (CIWA-Ar), 83

Clinical Opiate Withdrawal Scale (COWS), 83–84
clonazepam, 157
clonidine, 245
   schizophrenia, 157
cluster A personality disorders
   assessment and diagnosis, 268
   cultural implications, 269
   evaluation, 269
   incidence and prevalence, 267
   intervention, 268–269
   patient case study, 267
   planning, 268
   prevention and screening, 267–268
cluster B personality disorders
   antisocial personality disorder, 269–270
   assessment and diagnosis, 272
   borderline personality disorder, 270
   cultural implications, 273
   evaluation, 273
   histrionic personality disorder, 270
   incidence and prevalence, 271
   intervention, 272–273
   narcissistic personality disorder, 270–271
   patient case study, 271
   planning, 272
cluster C personality disorders
   assessment and diagnosis, 275–276
   avoidant personality disorder, 274
   cultural implications, 277
   dependent personality disorder, 274
   evaluation, 277
   incidence and prevalence, 275
   intervention, 276
   obsessive compulsive personality disorder, 274
   patient case study, 275
   planning, 276
   prevention and screening, 275
codependence, 107
Cogentin, 157
cognitive behavioral therapy, 52
   generalized anxiety disorder, 213, 216
   hypersomnolence, 171
   insomnia, 175
   obstructive sleep apnea, 178
cognitive distortions, 8–9
cognitive theory, 44
   depressive disorders, 195
complementary and alternative therapies
   biological therapies, 59–60
   manipulative physical interventions, 59
   mind–body interventions, 59
conduct disorders
   assessment and diagnosis, 249–250
   attention-deficit hyperactivity disorder, 243
   cluster B personality disorders, 269
   cultural implications, 251
   demographics, 249
   evaluation, 251
   patient case study, 249
   planning, 250
   treatment, 251
Connors Rating Scales-Revised (CRS-R), 81
COPD. *See* chronic obstructive pulmonary disease (COPD)
coping strategy, 43
corpus callosum, 73
correctional nursing, 24
COWS. *See* Clinical Opiate Withdrawal Scale (COWS)
cranial nerves, 76
Creutzfeldt–Jakob disease, 132
cross-tolerance, 107
CRS-R. *See* Connors Rating Scales-Revised (CRS-R)
CTE. *See* chronic traumatic encephalopathy (CTE)
cues to action, 38
cultural care, 49
cultural competence, 21–22
curative factors, of group psychotherapy
   altruism, 55
   catharsis, 56
   corrective refocusing, 56
   existential factors, 56
   group cohesiveness, 55
   imitative behaviors, 55
   increased development of social skills, 56
   installation of hope, 56
   interpersonal learning, 55
   universality, 55
CY-BOCS. *See* Children's Yale-Brown Obsessive Compulsive Scale (CY-BOCS)
cyclothymic disorder, 200

Dantrolene, 157
defense mechanisms, 48
delirium
   vs. dementia, 135
   diagnostic reasoning, 131
   incidence and prevalence, 130

delirium (*cont.*)
  patient case study, 130
  screening, 130
  subtypes, 129–130
delusional disorders
  agoraphobia, 217
  cluster A personality disorders, 266
  schizophrenia, 153
delusions, 153
dementia
  cultural implications, 136
  vs. delirium, 135
  diagnostic tests, 133
  differentials, 133
  etiologies for, 133
  evaluation, 136
  incidence and prevalence, 131–132
  mental state exam, 133–134
  patient case study, 131
  pharmacological management, 135–136
  planning, 135
democratic leadership, 19
Depakene, 87, 89
dependence, 107
dependent personality disorder
  cluster B personality disorders, 270
  cluster C personality disorders, 274
depolarization, 86
depression, 136
depressive disorders
  assessment and diagnosis, 197
  bipolar disorders, 197
  cultural implications, 200
  dysthymia, 193–195
  evaluation, 200
  incidence and prevalence, 196
  intervention, 198–200
  mood symptoms for, 197
  pathological characteristics of, 193
  patient case study, 195
  planning, 197–198
detoxification process, substance use disorder, 114–115
dialectical behavioral therapy, 52–53
diphenhydramine, 157
disruptive mood dysregulation disorder (DMDD)
  attention-deficit hyperactivity disorder, 243
  depressive disorders, 200
DNA, 79
dopamine reuptake inhibitor, ADHD, 245

dopaminergic pathways, 73
dual diagnosis, 107
dysthymia, 199
dystonia, 156

eating disorders
  assessment and diagnosis, 252–253
  cultural implications, 254
  epidemiology, 252
  evaluation, 254
  patient case study, 251
  planning, 253
  screening tools and early intervention, 252
  treatment, 254
eclectic psychotherapy, 38
ECT. *See* electroconvulsive therapy (ECT)
EDS. *See* excessive daytime sleepiness (EDS)
EEG. *See* electroencephalogram (EEG)
efferent fibers, 75
ego, 47
electroconvulsive therapy (ECT), 199
electroencephalogram (EEG), 79
  obstructive sleep apnea, 178
endocrine dysfunction, depressive disorders, 194
enzyme inhibitors, 86
ependyma, 76
epigenetics, 80
EPS. *See* extrapyramidal symptoms (EPS)
EPSE. *See* extrapyramidal side effects (EPSE)
Erikson's stages of development, 44, 45
erotomaniac delusions, 153
Eskalith, 89
eszopiclone, 179
ethics, 20–21
etiological theories
  depressive disorders, 194
  schizophrenia, 152
evidence-based studying techniques, for PMH-BC™ ANCC exam
  cognitive behavioral strategies, 6
  distraction free environment, 5
  justification, 6
  note-taking, 6
  practice answering questions, 6
  rehearsing technique, 6
  rereading, 6
  self-verbalizing strategy, 6
  synthesizing, 6
  timeline creation, 5
  visualization process, 6

excessive daytime sleepiness (EDS), 173
exercise, 26
existential therapy, 53
extrapyramidal side effects (EPSE), 155
extrapyramidal symptoms (EPS), 155
eye movement desensitization and
   reprocessing, 55

FGAs. *See* first-generation antipsychotics
   (FGAs)
first-degree relatives, 80
first-generation antipsychotics (FGAs),
   86–87
fish oils, 60
fluorodeoxyglucose (FDG)-PET, 79
follicle stimulating hormone, depressive
   disorders, 194
forensic nursing, 24
Frankl, Viktor, 53
Freud, Sigmund, 47, 52, 213
frontal lobe, 73
frontotemporal dementia, 132

gabapentin, 216
gamete cell, 79
gamma-aminobutyric acid (GABA), 212
ganglia, 75
GDS. *See* Geriatric Depression Scale (GDS)
gender identity disorder, 23–24
generalized anxiety disorder (GAD)
   assessment and diagnosis, 214–215
   cultural implications, 216–217
   evaluation, 216
   history, 213–214
   incidence and prevalence, 212–213
   intervention, 215–216
   patient case study, 212
   signs and symptoms, 211
genetic counseling, 80
genetic predisposition, schizophrenia, 152
genetics, 79–81
genogram pedigree, 80
genomics, 80
Geriatric Depression Scale (GDS), 82
glial cells, 76
grandiose delusions, 153
group dynamics, phases of, 56
group therapy, 55–56
   schizophrenia, 155–156
growth hormone, depressive disorders, 194
guanfacine, 245

hallucinations, 153
HAM-D. *See* Hamilton Rating Scale for
   Depression (HAM-D)
Hamilton Anxiety Rating Scale, 220
Hamilton Rating Scale for Depression
   (HAM-D), 82
HAND. *See* HIV-associated neurocognitive
   deficits (HAND)
HBM. *See* health belief model (HBM)
health behavior guidelines, 26
health belief model (HBM), 38
healthcare power of attorney, 26
Health Insurance Portability and
   Accountability Act of 1996 (HIPAA), 16
health promotion and maintenance, 20
health-specific anticipatory guidance, 27
health status management, 20
high-risk situations, 42–43
HIPAA. *See* Health Insurance Portability and
   Accountability Act of 1996 (HIPAA)
histrionic personality disorder
   cluster B personality disorders, 270, 271
   cluster C personality disorders, 274
HIV-associated neurocognitive deficits
   (HAND), 132
hoarding disorder, 274
HPA. *See* hypothalamic-pituitary axis (HPA)
humanistic therapy, 54–55
Huntington's disease, dementia, 132
hyperactive delirium, 130
hypersomnolence
   assessment and diagnosis, 170–171
   cultural implications, 173
   evaluation, 173
   incidence and prevalence, 170
   nonpharmacological interventions, 171–172
   patient case study, 170
   planning, 171
   screening tools and early intervention, 170
hypoactive delirium, 130
hypomanic criteria, depressive
   disorders, 200
hypothalamic-pituitary axis (HPA)
   depressive disorders, 194
   generalized anxiety disorder, 212–213
hypothalamus, 74

id, 47
Inderal, 157
individual therapy, schizophrenia, 155
informed consent, 17

insomnia
  assessment and diagnosis, 174
  chronic, 173
  cultural implications, 175
  evaluation, 175
  incidence and prevalence, 173
  intervention, 174
  patient case study, 173
  planning, 174
  screening tools and early intervention, 174
  short-term, 173
intellectual disability, 247
intermittent explosive disorder
  attention-deficit hyperactivity disorder, 243
  conduct disorders, 250
interpersonal development, Sullivan's stages of, 46–47
interpersonal therapy, 55
interpersonal theory, generalized anxiety disorder, 213
Intuniv, 245
inverse agonist, 85
involuntary commitment criteria, 17
ion channel blockers, 85–86
ischemic heart disease, 214

jealous, delusional disorder, 153

Klerman, Gerald, 55
Klonopin, 157
Klüver–Bucy syndrome, 132
Kraepelin, E., 212

laissez-faire leadership, 19
Lamictal, 89
Lamotrigine, 89
language disorders, 267
Lazarus, Arnold, 52
leadership styles, 19–20
left and right hemisphere, 73
Leininger, Madeleine, 49
Lewy body dementia, 132
licensure, 16
lifestyle factors and substance use disorder, 117
light control
  hypersomnolence, 171
  insomnia, 175
  obstructive sleep apnea, 178
Linehan, Marsha, 52–53
lithium, 89

living will, 26
lorazepam, 157
Lunesta, 179

major depressive disorder (MDD), 194
  agoraphobia, 217
  depressive disorders, 198
mania, 271
manipulative physical interventions, 59
MAOIs. *See* monoamine oxidase inhibitors (MAOIs)
Maslow's hierarchy of needs, 41–42
MATA. *See* medication-assisted treatment for addiction (MATA)
MDD. *See* major depressive disorder (MDD)
medical foods, dementia, 136
medication-assisted treatment for addiction (MATA), 115–116, 215
medulla oblongata, 75
melatonin, 60
mental illness grid, etiology of, 50
mental status exam
  conduct disorders, 250
  dementia, 133–134
  eating disorders, 253
  schizophrenia, 154
  substance use disorder, 111
mesocorticolimbic pathways, 73
methylphenidate, 244
MI. *See* motivational interviewing (MI)
microglial-phagocytes, 76
midbrain, 75
mind–body interventions, 59
mixed delirium, 130
MOCA. *See* Montreal Cognitive Assessment (MOCA)
monoamine oxidase inhibitors (MAOIs), 90
  depressive disorders, 199
Montreal Cognitive Assessment (MOCA), 82
mood disorders
  cluster A personality disorders, 266
  conduct disorders, 250
  depressive disorders, 193–200
mood stabilizers, 87, 89
motivational interviewing (MI)
  principles of, 41
  vs. traditional counseling, 40
motor type Ranvier node, 76
movement disorders, 179
  schizophrenia, 156

MSLT. *See* multiple sleep latency testing (MSLT)
multiple sleep latency testing (MSLT), 175

narcissistic personality disorder
    cluster B personality disorders, 270–271
    cluster C personality disorders, 274
narcolepsy
    assessment and diagnosis, 176
    cultural implications, 177
    evaluation, 177
    incidence and prevalence, 176
    intervention, 177
    patient case study, 175
    planning, 177
    screening tools and early intervention, 176
nervous system, 72–78
neuroadaptation, 107, 108
neurobiological theories, 212
neurodevelopmental disorders, 152
neuroimaging, 79
neuroleptic malignant syndrome, 156
neurons, 76
neuropsychiatric assessment, substance use disorder, 111
neuropsychological tests, 81–84
neurotransmitters, 77–78, 86–87
neurotransmitter theory, depressive disorders, 194
nigrostriatal pathways, 73
N-methyl d-aspartate glutamate receptor antagonists, dementia, 135
nonpharmaceutical intervention, traumatic brain injury, 137
nonpharmacological management, 178
    agoraphobia, 218–219
    attention-deficit hyperactivity disorder, 245
    dementia, 136
    generalized anxiety disorder, 216
    insomnia, 171–172
    obsessive compulsive disorder, 221
    panic disorder, 223
    phobias, 225
    posttraumatic stress disorder, 227
    of psychosis, 155–156
nonpharmacological treatments
    complementary and alternative therapies, 59–60
    family therapies, 57–59
    individual therapy, 51–55
    substance use disorder, 116

    therapeutic alliance, 50–51
nurse–patient relationship, maintenance of, 20
Nurse Practice Act, 16
nursing theorists, 49

obsessive compulsive disorder (OCD)
    agoraphobia, 217
    assessment and diagnosis, 221
    cultural implications, 222
    evaluation, 221
    generalized anxiety disorder, 212
    incidence and prevalence, 220
    nonpharmacological management, 221
    patient case study, 220
    planning, 221
obsessive compulsive personality disorder
    cluster B personality disorders, 271
    cluster C personality disorders, 274
obstructive sleep apnea (OSA), 175
    assessment and diagnosis, 178
    cultural implications, 179
    evaluation, 179
    incidence and prevalence, 178
    nonpharmacological interventions, 178
    patient case study, 177
    pharmacological interventions, 178–179
    planning, 178
    screening tools and early intervention, 178
occipital lobe, 74
OCD. *See* obsessive compulsive disorder (OCD)
ODD. *See* oppositional defiant disorder (ODD)
oligodendrocytes, 76
omega-3 fatty acids, 60
oppositional defiant disorder (ODD)
    attention-deficit hyperactivity disorder, 241
    conduct disorders, 250
orexin receptor antagonist, 179
OSA. *See* obstructive sleep apnea (OSA)
Overall Anxiety Severity and Impairment Scale, 220
oxcarbazepine, 89
oxytocin, 194

PANDAS. *See* pediatric autoimmune neuropsychiatric disorders associated with streptococcal infections (PANDAS)
panic disorder
    assessment and diagnosis, 223
    cultural implications, 224

panic disorder (*cont.*)
  evaluation, 223–224
  incidence and prevalence, 222
  nonpharmacological management, 223
  patient case study, 222
  planning, 223
  signs and symptoms, 222
paranoid personality disorders
  cluster A personality disorders, 266, 267
  cluster B personality disorders, 270, 271
  cluster C personality disorders, 274
parasympathetic nervous system, 75
parietal lobe, 74
Parkinson's symptoms, 155
partial agonist, 85
Patient Health Questionnaire (PHQ-2/9), 82
pediatric autoimmune neuropsychiatric disorders associated with streptococcal infections (PANDAS), 220
Peplau, Hildegard, 49
perceived benefits, 38
perceived severity, 38
perceived susceptibility, 38
peripheral nervous system, 75
persecutory delusions, 153
persistent depressive disorder, 199
personality disorders
  cluster A personality disorders, 266–269
  cluster B personality disorders, 269–273
  cluster C personality disorders, 273–277
  diagnosis of, 265
PET. *See* positron emission tomography (PET)
pharmacological management
  attention-deficit hyperactivity disorder, 244–245
  dementia, 135–136
  generalized anxiety disorder, 215
  obstructive sleep apnea, 178–179
phenotype, 79
phobias, 224–225
PHQ-2/9. *See* Patient Health Questionnaire (PHQ-2/9)
Piaget, Jean, 44
Pick's disease, 132
pituitary gland, 74
PMH-BC™ exam. *See* Psychiatric Mental Health Nurse board certification (PMH-BC™) exam
PMHN. *See* psychiatric-mental health nurse (PMHN)
polysomnography (PSG), 175
pons, 75
positron emission tomography (PET), 79
posttraumatic stress disorder (PTSD)
  agoraphobia, 217
  assessment and diagnosis, 227
  avoidance symptoms, 226
  cultural implications, 228
  evaluation, 227
  incidence and prevalence, 226
  nonpharmacological management, 227
  patient case study, 226
  persistent hyperarousal symptoms, 226
  planning, 227
  reexperiencing symptoms, 226
power of attorney, 26
premenstrual dysphoric disorder, 199–200
primary prevention, 25
prodrome, 154
professional organizations, 18
prolactin, 194
propranolol, 157
pseudo-Parkinson's, 156
PSG. *See* polysomnography (PSG)
psychiatric-mental health nurse (PMHN), 3
  objective of, 15
  scope of practice, 16–17
Psychiatric Mental Health Nurse board certification (PMH-BC™) exam, 3
  cognitive behavioral strategies, 6
  cognitive distortions, 8–9
  evidence-based studying techniques, 5
  exam eligibility requirements, 4
  exam prep exercise, 9
  multiple-choice questions, 12–13
  post examination requirements, 13–14
  self-care, 7–8
  test content map, 11–12
psychoanalytic therapy, 52
psychodynamic theories
  depressive disorders, 194
  generalized anxiety disorder, 213
psychoeducation, restless legs syndrome, 181
psychological stages of human development, 44
psychopharmacology, 50, 72
  depressive disorders, 198–200
  pharmacodynamics, 85
  pharmacokinetics, 84
  in pregnancy, 92
  treatment, 37
psychosexual stages of development, 47–48
psychosis, 136. *See also* psychotic disorders

psychosocial theories, 37
psychotherapy, 37–38
psychotic disorders
   cluster A personality disorders, 266
   negative symptoms, 151
   positive symptoms, 151
   psychosis, 151
   schizophrenia (*See* schizophrenia)
psychotropic classifications, 86–92
pulmonary embolism, 215
Punnet square, 80
putamen, 73–74

quality of care, 25
Quick Inventory of Depressive
   Symptomatology (QIDS), 82

Ramelteon, 179
Ranvier node, 76
relapse prevention
   abstinence violation effect (AVE), 43
   coping strategy, 43
   high-risk situations, 42–43
   self-efficacy, 43
   substance use disorder, 117
repolarization, 86
residual phase, schizophrenia, 154
restless legs syndrome
   assessment and diagnosis, 180–181
   cultural implications, 182
   evaluation, 182
   incidence and prevalence, 180
   intervention, 181
   patient case study, 180
   planning, 181
   screening tools and early intervention, 180
Rett syndrome, 247
reuptake inhibitors, 86
risk management, 25
Rogers, Carl, 54
root cause analysis (RCA), 25
Rozerem, 179

Saint Louis University Mental Status
   (SLUMS), 81–82
Sam-e (S-adenosyl-l-methionine), 60
schemas, 44
schizoaffective disorder, 154
schizoid personality disorders
   cluster A personality disorders, 266, 267
   cluster C personality disorders, 274, 275

schizophrenia
   assessment and diagnosis, 154
   cluster A personality disorders, 266
   cultural implications, 158
   evaluation, 157–158
   incidence and prevalence, 152
   intervention, 155–157
   patient case study, 152
   planning, 155
   treatment, 157
schizophreniform disorder, 154
schizotypal personality disorder
   cluster A personality disorders, 266
   cluster B personality disorders, 270, 271
   cluster C personality disorders, 274
secondary prevention, 25
second-degree relatives, 80
second-generation antipsychotics (SGAs), 87
sedative hypnotics, 179
selective mutism, 247
selective (serotonin) norepinephrine reuptake
   inhibitors (sSNRIs), 91
selective serotonin reuptake inhibitors
   (SSRIs), 90, 198
   generalized anxiety disorder, 215
self-care, during exam preparation
   avoid marathon study sessions, 7
   eating consistent meals, 7
   enhancing self-efficacy, 7
   exercise, 8
   personal hygiene, 8
   radical acceptance, 7
   relationships and social interactions, 8
   sleep hygiene, 7
self-disclosure, 24
self-efficacy, 38, 43
sensory type Ranvier node, 76
sentinel event reporting, 25
separation anxiety disorder, 217, 274
serotonin, generalized anxiety
   disorder, 212
serotonin-norepinephrine reuptake inhibitors
   (SNRIs), 199
   attention-deficit hyperactivity disorder, 245
servant leadership, 19
sexual identity, 23
SGAs. *See* second-generation antipsychotics
   (SGAs)
Shapiro, Francine, 55
short-term insomnia, 173
situational leadership, 19

sleep disorders
  hypersomnolence, 169–173
  insomnia, 173–175
  narcolepsy, 175–177
  obstructive sleep apnea, 177–179
  restless legs syndrome, 179–182
SLUMS. *See* Saint Louis University Mental Status (SLUMS)
SNRIs. *See* serotonin-norepinephrine reuptake inhibitors (SNRIs)
social anxiety disorder, 217
social learning theory, 43
Socratic questioning method, 53–54
somatic delusions, 153
somatic nervous system, 75
special populations
  homeless people, 22
  sexual minorities and classification, 22–24
sSNRIs. *See* selective (serotonin) norepinephrine reuptake inhibitors (sSNRIs)
SSRIs. *See* selective serotonin reuptake inhibitors (SSRIs)
stages of cognitive development, 44, 46
Strattera, 245
structural brain abnormalities, 194
substance use disorder
  abstinence violation effect, 117
  adolescence, 117
  connecting to support groups, 117
  coping skills, 117
  cultural implications, 118
  current level and history, 110
  detoxification, 114–115
  diagnostic tests, 111
  evaluation, 117
  family system care, 116
  high-risk situations, 117
  incidence and prevalence, 109–110
  intervention, 114–116
  lifestyle factors, 117
  management and plan, 114
  medication-assisted treatment for addiction, 115–116
  mental status exam, 111
  nonpharmacological treatment, 116
  older adults, 117
  outcome expectancies, 117
  patient case history, 109
  pattern of use, 110
  physical exam, 111

  physical/psychological consequences, 111
  positive and negative reinforcement, 109–110
  relational aspects, 110
  risk factors, 109
  screening tools and early intervention, 110–111
  social consequences, 110
  symptoms, 108
  treatment plan, 114
  urges/cravings, 117
Sullivan, Herbert Stack, 46, 213
Sullivan's stages of interpersonal development, 46–47
superego, 48
suvorexant, 179
Symmetrel, 157
sympathetic nervous system, 75

talk therapy, 50
tardive dyskinesia, schizophrenia, 156
TCAs. *See* tricyclic antidepressants (TCAs)
Tegretol, 89
telehealth, 3
temporal lobe, 74
tertiary prevention, 25
thalamus, 74
theory of interpersonal relationships, 49
therapeutic index (TI), 85
thyroid stimulating hormone, depressive disorders, 194
tobacco use disorder, 156
tolerance, 107
traditional counseling vs. motivational interviewing, 40
transcranial magnetic stimulation, depressive disorders, 199
transformational leadership, 19
transgender, 23–24
transient schizotypal traits in adolescents, 267
transtheoretical model (TTM), 38
  decisional balance, 39
  process of change, 39–40
  self-efficacy, 39
  stages of change, 39
traumatic brain injury
  assessment and diagnosis, 137–138
  evaluation, 139
  incidence and prevalence, 137
  intervention, 138–139
  patient case study, 137
  planning, 138

tricyclic antidepressants (TCAs), 89–90
    depressive disorders, 199
    generalized anxiety disorder, 216
    insomnia, 179
trihexyphenidyl, 157
Trileptal, 89
tryptophan, 60
TTM. *See* transtheoretical model (TTM)
tuberoinfundibular pathways, 73

urine screen toxicology drug of abuse, 112–113

vagal nerve stimulation (VNS), depressive disorders, 199
valproic acid, 87, 89
vascular dementia, 132
ventral tegmental area, 75

Watson, Jean, 49
Weissman, Myrna, 55
Wellbutrin, 245
white matter, 73
withdrawal, 107, 108

Yale-Brown Obsessive Compulsive Scale (YBOCS), 83
Yalom, Irvin, 55
Young Mania Rating Scale (YMRS), 83